Freedom *from* Anxiety

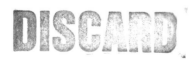

Freedom *from* Anxiety

A Holistic Approach to Emotional Well-Being

MARCEY SHAPIRO, MD

Foreword by Barbara L. Vivino, PhD

North Atlantic Books
Berkeley, California

Published by
North Atlantic Books
P.O. Box 12327
Berkeley, California 94712

Cover photo by Star Woodward
Cover and book design by Susan Quasha
Printed in the United States of America

Freedom from Anxiety: A Holistic Approach to Emotional Well-Being is sponsored by the Society for the Study of Native Arts and Sciences, a nonprofit educational corporation whose goals are to develop an educational and cross-cultural perspective linking various scientific, social, and artistic fields; to nurture a holistic view of arts, sciences, humanities, and healing; and to publish and distribute literature on the relationship of mind, body, and nature.

North Atlantic Books' publications are available through most bookstores. For further information, visit our website at www.northatlanticbooks.com or call 800–733–3000.

MEDICAL DISCLAIMER: The following information is intended for general information purposes only. Individuals should always see their health care provider before administering any suggestions made in this book. Any application of the material set forth in the following pages is at the reader's discretion and is his or her sole responsibility.

Library of Congress Cataloging-in-Publication Data

Shapiro, Marcey, 1957–
    Freedom from anxiety : a holistic approach to emotional well-being / Marcey Shapiro, MD ; foreword by Barbara L. Vivino, PhD.
        pages cm
    Includes bibliographical references and index.
    Summary: "Based on Dr. Marcey Shapiro's decades of clinical experience and research, this book presents hundreds of safe, practical, and effective tools and techniques to alleviate anxiety, an epidemic that affects nearly 20 percent of Americans."—Provided by publisher.
    ISBN 978–1–58394–675–6
    1. Anxiety—Alternative treatment—Popular works. 2. Holistic medicine. I. Title.
RC531.S45 2013
    616.85'22—dc23 2013012833

1 2 3 4 5 6 7 8 9 SHERIDAN 19 18 17 16 15 14
Printed on recycled paper

*For Star Woodward, my partner in life,
with great love and appreciation!*

Acknowledgments

Ideeply appreciate the many supportive people who have helped this book come to fruition.

First and foremost is my amazing spouse and partner in life's journeys, Star Woodward, for her unwavering support, encouragement, good cheer, and love. She took the beautiful cover photo and supported me with multiple rereads, edits, moments of inspiration, provocative discussions, laughter, fun, and helpful suggestions. Plus, I gratefully acknowledge her support in pulling me away from writing at those moments when I was joylessly pushing myself to "get it done," by gently reminding me to stay in my own alignment as I write. All that, in addition to so many little things: cups of tea, mountains of clothes cleaned and dishes washed, extra dog walks, and bowls of soup…. You are simply the best!

Also thanks to many others:

Julie Klenn, my dear friend, whose editorial comments are detailed, cogent, and extremely useful. As in my prior book, I incorporated many of the changes you suggested. I love how your mind organizes things!

Susan Gorell for reading and commenting on the manuscript, and helping me to shape and clarify the phrasing. Also thanks for the appreciation you expressed at several points in the editing round.

Ruth Segal for reading the manuscript and offering pithy advice for honing it.

Barbara Vivino, PhD, for writing an awe-inspiring foreword, for her friendship, laughter, and general good advice, and for reviewing the acupuncture chapter.

Terry Trotter, MSW, for advice about somatic therapies and for many good conversations about therapeutically supporting patients in overcoming anxiety.

Liz Olivas for her contribution about manual lymph drainage for support of persons with anxiety, and for being a loving, supportive friend.

My patients and others who have lent me their trust, sharing their secret fears and worries with me in order to let go of them, bravely finding new ways to wholeness and greater peace.

I also thank the wonderful staff at North Atlantic Books including:

Richard Grossinger for vision, advice, encouragement, philosophical musings, and his own insightful books.

Doug Reil for his passion for a better, kinder world, and for his visionary thinking and deep conversations.

Emily Boyd, my project editor, thank you for your flexibility, insight, and support.

Kathy Glass, my fantastic copyeditor, for understanding me and for your detailed notes, thoughtful suggestions and tips, and clear communication. This is the second project we have done together, and I cannot imagine a better editor for my works.

There are many others, some of whom I know personally and others I have not yet met, who influence my work and life with their teachings. While some have books that are mentioned in the bibliography, others have had a broader, less specific influence on my thought. A few of these others I would love to mention here—these include several inspirational and spiritual teachers from a broad sampling of perspectives who have helped shape my thought and teaching, including:

Esther and Jerry Hicks for presenting the teachings of Abraham, Law of Attraction, and for their humor and good-heartedness. Their work and ongoing contribution are deeply appreciated and respected.

Wayne Dyer for his pioneering works in self-help psychology and the deeply personal spiritual vein he shares.

Eckhart Tolle for his teaching and insight on the power of the present moment.

Marianne Williamson for making the *Course In Miracles* material more accessible, and for sharing so much of herself.

Darryl Anka for sharing the timely teachings of Bashar.

Sanaya Roman and Duane Packer for sharing the teachings of Orin and Daben, and for their many lovely meditation CDs.

Thich Nhat Hanh, the Dalai Lama, Pema Chödrön, Tenzin Palmo, and others, each for sharing their unique interpretation of Buddhist traditions and teachings.

John Kabat-Zinn for his pioneering work on mindfulness.

Deepak Chopra for his spiritual understanding of health and copious writings and self-help materials.

Ted Kaptchuk for his wisdom and teaching in the field of Chinese Medicine.

Candace Pert and Bruce Lipton for their pioneering work on the science of the mind/body connection.

Rudolf Steiner for his enormous contributions, including Anthroposophic medicine.

Finally and especially for the many osteopaths who listen within, sharing and teaching the wise beauty of the osteopathic understanding of health and disease: the breath of life, primary respiration, and the wholeness of the body, mind, and spirit. Special deep gratitude to my teacher, James Jealous, DO, and to the earlier osteopaths who shared their writings: A. T. Still, MD, William Garner Sutherland, DO, Rollin Becker, DO, and Tom Schooley, DO.

Thanks to anyone I may have forgotten to thank. I stand on many shoulders, and I want to acknowledge each one, in my heart if not on paper.

Contents

Foreword

Iam impressed and moved by the contents of this book and even more so by my personal relationship with Marcey Shapiro. Marcey's open-minded pursuit of healing methods to assist her patients is courageous and has resulted in a compendium of healing approaches that is remarkable in its breadth, depth, practicality, and inspiration. Marcey's unusually candid discussion of her personal journey toward relief from anxiety serves as a template for the book and allows the reader to normalize their own experiences while staying open to her suggestions, even if they are unfamiliar.

Through a series of synchronistic events I connected with Marcey at conferences that we both attended over the span of a couple years. We had a lot in common and would engage in animated conversation over lunch or during breaks. I was aware that she had a certain wisdom, but it was a while before I realized that she was a physician. More ironically, we eventually discovered that our respective practices were on the same street within one mile of each other! Upon learning this, we began to meet more often and share thoughts about clinical practice. I then recognized that she was an open-minded doctor indeed. Rather than simply treating the psychological symptoms like anxiety in the traditional way with prescription drugs, Marcey asked the important questions. Not only did she ponder the physical imbalances that might be at play for her patients, she also questioned and explored the emotional under-pinnings and spiritual roots of the imbalance. As Wayne Dyer says, "An open mind allows you to explore and create and grow. ... Progress would be impossible if we always did things the way we always have." Marcey's cutting-edge, heart-centered approach shows great progress in the treatment of anxiety.

Every day as a psychologist in private practice I see anxious people. Anxiety is an issue that impacts every human being. It seems to affect everyone from professional academics to students, to couples, to parents and children.

When I was the Director of Clinical Training at a Clinical Psychology Doctoral Program, I supervised a lot of anxious clinicians and patients and worked with anxious professors. In my current clinical practice, anxiety is the number-one reason that patients seek psychotherapy. Over the years I learned that compassion and acceptance are essential steps in the process of change. Marcey makes a beautiful point in this book by suggesting that it is through our hearts that we connect with our deepest wisdom and our well-being. She urges us to compassionately listen to our own symptoms for guidance. In my training and licensure both as an acupuncturist and as a psychologist, I know how important it is to incorporate the wisdom from alternative medicine and traditional approaches. Marcey has done an exceptional job of identifying a variety of approaches to anxiety that incorporate the body, mind, and spirit.

Marcey's soul-searching approach leads the reader through a journey of treatments for anxiety from herbs and gems to breathing and meditation. Anxiety has often been considered to be an inevitable part of life. Freud said that "the act of birth is the first experience of anxiety." Yet Marcey offers hope in overcoming anxiety's distress and urges the reader to consider looking within for answers to their anxiety. According to Marcey, an "inner divinity" is present within each of us and we already possess what we are looking for. She suggests that we can tap into the self-healing love that is always within.

I'm honored to play a small role in bringing this hopeful message to those seeking freedom from anxiety. Marcey observes that many people today are no longer aware of the "still small voice" that resides within us. Clearly, Marcey is listening to her "still small voice" which allows us to be the fortunate recipients of her wisdom and inspiration. Marcey offers guidance not only in freeing ourselves from anxiety but in connecting with our "inner divinity," which has unlimited potential for healing.

—Dr. Barbara L. Vivino, Psychologist, Acupuncturist
Berkeley, California, May 2013

Introduction

"Healing" literally means "to make whole." *Freedom from Anxiety* is written to help people overcome anxiety by learning ways to find the sense of wholeness that is always available inside each of us. The process is a journey of self-discovery. *Freedom from Anxiety* acknowledges that we exist simultaneously as body, mind, and spirit. We are unified beings in every moment of our lives. Each of us is a cohesive whole, always expressing a blend of both our physical and non-physical selves. Body, mind, and spirit are not separate parts. Instead they are more like lenses, or ways of focusing. The awareness of oneness, and the peace it brings, can be nurtured by anyone who is interested.

I like to refer to this book as an "insider's guide" since I personally grappled with various forms of anxiety for many years of my life. On my personal journey I found anxiety to be an excellent spiritual teacher. It provided a powerful platform for growth through self-awareness and self-acceptance. Most people who meet me now are not aware of my past struggles and their legacy of positive growth, because I am now (usually) a calm and serene person. That I am now fairly "mellow" is living proof that our emotional set points and patterns of reactivity can be shifted over time. If I can truly feel better, I am confident that you or your loved one can, too!

I have cultivated inner peace throughout my life through study, practice, research, and commitment to well-being. Along my path I discovered hundreds of effective tools to find a way to help find more ease in stressful times, when emotional balance is off-kilter. The tools I collected over the years have helped me as well as many others with whom I have connected. In *Freedom from Anxiety* I share some of my own experiences, along with insights and stories from others.

All real healing is self-healing. True healing, though, may look different than a medical cure. Conventional medicine offers many simple and elaborate "band-aids," but these heroic efforts are almost exclusively aimed at managing symptoms rather than examining or shifting underlying causes. Healing, on the other hand, requires a transformation of consciousness, an "ah-ha moment" where we understand ourselves anew. Healing is entirely an "inside job," providing a fresh comprehension that shifts our experience of reality.

All healing is inevitably heart-centered. It is through our heart that we connect with our inner divinity, sense of knowing, and deepest wisdom. As we nourish our heart space, we come to an increased sense of unity with our inner being. We allow the wisdom of the heart to guide us in the direction of wholeness. Together, throughout this book, we will explore the practicalities of cultivating a heart-centered, peace-enhancing life.

While emotional well-being is its own reward, it also provides a wellspring for physical health. Feelings of inner peace, joy, and well-being may result in profound physiological benefits. These can become apparent even on a cellular level, as I discuss in the first two chapters.

Chapters 2 through 4 delve into various psychological and emotional tools for shifting thoughts and feelings. We are often more empowered than we think or believe. When considering various emotional or physical health problems, including anxiety, we always have a choice regarding how to focus. We can continue ruminating about the problem as we now see it, or we can pivot, nurturing a willingness and ability to observe and focus upon health and wholeness despite current circumstances. At times, redirecting one's focus may seem difficult or even impossible. In those moments our best choice may consist of finding greater peace within the moment, by letting go and by developing greater kindness and compassion for current circumstances and oneself. Chapter 3 offers many tools for letting go and for being with ourselves, with compassion.

We always have a choice to release old emotions and to create peace within. Chapters 3 and 4 look more deeply at how focus can affect daily life experience, recommending practical tools to facilitate release of old dysfunctional patterns. As we develop an ability to remain focused upon health—in our culture, our environment, our physical well-being, and in our lives—we are able to be more compassionate with ourselves. We can then experience a freer flow of emotions and improved emotional health.

Emotional flow or well-being is a part of the energy of our life force. Health, emotional health, and vitality are like water: continually in motion, constantly changing, and essential to life. They will flow naturally toward areas where there is no restriction of movement, toward the direction of ease. The human body, spirit, and emotions are adaptive and constantly renewed. We are naturally drawn toward well-being. We are naturally self-corrective. When emotionally unencumbered, we always move toward freedom, joy, and love. We can celebrate the emotional flow while gently dissolving any obstruction, just like water erodes even the greatest rock over time. Several chapters examine emotional flow in more detail, and practical tools for clearing our internal obstructions are explored, especially in chapters 3 through 8.

In each of us there is internal knowledge, a gentle voice, beckoning us toward well-being. It tells us to let go, to stay in the river of present experience, not to dam up our lives by worrying about potential futures or bemoaning past mistakes. Many people in our civilization have learned to ignore that inner voice. They no longer have any awareness that this "still small voice" resides within us.[1] When we ignore it or are no longer aware of it because of habits, beliefs, and conditioning, we dam our emotional flow, and our energy and vitality may suffer. Many of the techniques throughout this book are intended to help us wake up and remember how to find, and hear, the voice calling each of us to inner peace.

There is a powerful but gentle current of self-correcting love within each of us. This love is intertwined with compassion, self-esteem, and self-acceptance. Each person can discover his or her own personal stream of self-worth. The techniques in *Freedom from Anxiety* can help individuals notice where their emotional flow is dammed, even if that blockage is longstanding, causing chronic discomfort, fatigue, fearfulness, or anxiety. A key element of healing is developing tools for focusing on and allowing emotional health. Thus many exercises teach readers how to get in touch with their own sense of positive, supportive inner guidance. Such tools and exercises are explored in greater detail throughout the book, especially in chapters 5 through 9.

This material is presented to empower you to improve your life and health by improving your emotional state. There are dozens of techniques throughout this book that can help you do so, including laughter, meditation, letting go, time in nature, deep breathing, distraction, homeopathy, flower essences, and many more.

The tools and exercises in this book are best utilized on an ongoing basis. The more you do them, the easier the practices will become. I liken the choice and use of various tools to a program of strength training at a gym. If you decide, for example, that you want to have firm and toned biceps, you would not go to the gym just once and expect a buff body after lifting a few weights. You would understand that improvement takes time. You would expect to be rewarded by evidence of your progress as you continue to visit the gym and use the facilities. You would undoubtedly also learn that a balanced strength-training program is not limited to the biceps, even if improving them was your original goal. Muscles work in tandem with one another, so in order to strengthen one group you must strengthen the whole. Still, if there were some machines or weights or classes you preferred over others, at a well-stocked gym you could select among those you most enjoyed, thereby devising an excellent program to ultimately achieve your overall fitness goals.

Like the choices at the gym, these tools to relieve anxiety can be utilized in many ways. You have "emotional fitness" goals for yourself, or you want to support someone you love. These goals might include greater ease, greater peace of mind, more calmness, more joy, more comfortable harmonious thoughts, more of a sense of well-being, and a greater ability to feel and think things that support well-being. When working with any guidebook, it is good to remember that there is no one right way for everyone to proceed. At a gym you might choose a type of equipment or class with which you are familiar and comfortable, or ask an employee to walk you through and describe all the available options. Or you might select equipment or a class because it is intriguing and you are curious.

Similarly, not every exercise and tool in this book is meant for each reader. There is no "right" perspective. That is okay. Each of us walks our own unique path.

The unity of mind, body, and spirit, for example, is a premise shared by many but not everyone. An understanding that we are more than our physical bodies—that we are also, at all times, our inner being expressing itself in the wholeness of existence—can help many people to cultivate deep peace and happiness. It can be soothing to know, or to believe, that our soul is interwoven through our entire life experience, and to understand that we can consciously connect with its guidance. Those who choose to engage in cultivating awareness of communication with their soul often notice that their conscious participation increases the strength and ease of the connection. You will find exercises and advice to nurture this connection throughout the book.

Some readers, however, may be skeptical of what they might term "spiritual stuff" and simply want herbal and natural remedies that support feeling calmer and more at peace. This, too, is fine. If you don't resonate with the spiritual aspects of *Freedom from Anxiety,* I trust you will decide for yourself what works for you. You might prefer the nutritional supplements, aromatherapy, or herbs suggested for anxiety in chapters 10, 11, and 14, or perhaps homeopathy, flower essences, or color and light (chapters 15, 17, and 18). There are as many paths as there are individuals; thus many different types of resources are addressed in these pages.

Self-awareness and self-acceptance include learning and acting upon what is most harmonious in the present moment. There are many ways to be true to yourself and to trust your inner guidance. Alignment with the whole self is deeply calming to the nervous system. It is a profound antidote to anxiety.

So use this information however you see fit. Go where you are drawn in the book. Many tools are free, such as breathing techniques and meditations. Others, such as herbal remedies and flower essences, are inexpensive. Some tools, like self-massage, calming herbal baths, and self-acupressure, can be utilized without assistance, while bodywork, acupuncture, and psychotherapy require the skills of a trained practitioner. *Freedom from Anxiety* includes many low-cost methods, since many people are anxious about money. It can be comforting to rely upon resources that are free or inexpensive. Fortunately, some of the most effective and self-empowering techniques cost very little. Emotional well-being is available to everyone, regardless of his or her life path or financial resources.

I establish a framework of the medical and psychological understanding and treatment of "anxiety disorders" late in the book, in chapters 20 and 21. Anxiety disorders are among the most prevalent health problems in the U.S. today, where diagnosable anxiety problems currently affect about 18 percent of the population,[2] or almost a fifth of people you meet. Biomedically, there are many varieties of anxiety. The six most common forms of anxiety disorder are addressed in this book: 1. Generalized anxiety; 2. Panic attacks and panic disorder; 3. Post-traumatic stress disorder (PTSD); 4. Obsessive-Compulsive disorder (OCD); 5. Social anxiety; and 6. Phobias. Specific approaches to these are discussed throughout the book.

The medical examination of anxiety disorders is placed late in the book because, while it may be useful to some, I do not like to pigeonhole people. I observed early in my medical education that a pinch of diagnosis is often accompanied by a large dose of self-fulfilling prophecy on the part of the patient. Each of us is constantly evolving, expanding, and shifting. We are always new, never the same from moment to moment. This book builds from that perspective, rather than merely a biomedical approach.

Freedom from Anxiety evolved as a compendium of useful implements I have compiled and utilized for many years. It is my hope that you will choose what is most appealing to you from amongst the potpourri of tools offered for feeling better. As a result, I hope that you will learn how to soothe yourself in difficult moments, and strengthen your connection with your deepest wisdom. I sincerely hope this book will be of benefit to you and those you love, and that in it you will find the perfect tools for you, right now, on your unique path to wholeness in body, mind, and spirit.

CHAPTER 1

Emotional Well-Being and Physical Health

Emotional well-being and physical health are intricately linked. There is quite a lot of contemporary science that leads us to the eye-opening conclusion that there is no action more important for improving your health than cultivating your sense of happiness. This chapter is offered as further encouragement toward stretching one's self to feel greater ease. It provides a playful romp through some highlights of important current findings in various fields of science that demonstrate a link between emotional and physical health.

Optimism and Pessimism

In the past ten years, the study of optimism, a topic that was once shunned in psychological research, perhaps because it was thought to be too "new age," has achieved great popularity and credibility. A large body of evidence compares various parameters, including health outcomes, prosperity, and general well-being, in optimists and pessimists. The conclusion of a majority of these studies is that true optimism is good for health.

Optimism is generally defined as "a tendency to expect the best possible outcome, or to dwell upon the most hopeful aspects of a situation."[1] It is a habit of positive anticipation. Optimists view life as an exciting, interesting adventure, full of opportunities, and generally expect things to work out well. When encountering a challenge, optimists are likely to look for the "silver lining," extracting meaning and pearls of wisdom, even from difficult situations.

They focus on what they have gleaned from mistakes in order to prevent repeating them in the future.

One reason optimists may seem to have a greater ability to succeed is that they do not give up. They are tenacious, mainly because they believe in the likelihood of a positive outcome. The adage "if at first you don't succeed, try, try again" is an optimistic credo. Optimists assume that eventually, with perseverance, success will arrive. The experiences in their life support this belief, perhaps because of their persistence as well as their expectations.

Pessimism is generally defined as "a tendency to stress the negative or unfavorable or to take the gloomiest possible view."[2] In contrast to optimists, pessimists have no confidence that persistence will eventually lead to success, so they give up more readily, especially in the face of challenges. Pessimists are more cynical than optimists and are likely to focus on the futility of effort. When confronted with a challenge, pessimists are more likely to focus on their personal frustration, complain to themselves or others about negative aspects of the event, and believe things will turn out badly. They can become preoccupied with negative expectations, seeing challenges as experiences that are likely to lead to disappointment.

People can develop habits of optimism in certain areas and pessimism in others. This is especially true if the person's underlying beliefs have not been examined, or the individual has picked up associations from family, culture, or personal exposure that he or she has not reexamined. For example, a person born into a wealthy family might be very optimistic financially, but the same person might be quite pessimistic about love, especially if heartbreak has occurred in their past.

A person's overall level of optimism can be assessed with various psychological tools. When I refer to health associations of optimism and pessimism, I am referring to people who are generally optimistic or pessimistic in most areas of their life. In psychology, the level of overall optimism or pessimism can be measured in standardized assessments. Studies of optimism versus pessimism usually focus upon the differences between people who have ingrained habits of thought that place them decidedly in one camp or the other, rather than people who tend to be in the middle, with a blend of both.

Optimism and pessimism are fluid, changeable states. Pessimists can learn to become optimists, or at least be more optimistic. There are many methods to retrain thought patterns and assist individuals in examining their underlying beliefs and assumptions, in order to discard those that no longer serve them. Many people who suffer from anxiety have habits of thinking pessimistically that can exacerbate the anxiety. Choosing to shift to more optimistic perspectives feels better, alleviates anxiety, and may improve physical health outcomes as well.

Optimists Have Stronger Immune Systems

Studies suggest that immune function improves as optimism improves. While many studies look at the differences in overall immune health between optimists and pessimists, a few, like one done by Dr. Suzanne Segerstrom, studied the immune health of individuals whose optimism levels varied over time. In 2010, she examined the effects of stress on cell-mediated immunity, an important parameter of immune health, in 124 first-year law student volunteers. In her study, Segerstrom administered a questionnaire that measured participants' level of optimism or pessimism about the upcoming year. Her researchers then injected them with two harmless substances, in order to provoke a normal immune response, and they measured the level of each student's responses. Both the questionnaire and the injections were repeated five times, over the course of a year of law school. The results showed that immune function, as measured by cell-mediated immune response, actually improved in optimistic individuals who remained optimistic but fell in those who had experienced setbacks that decreased their optimism.[3]

Optimism and Longevity

In Holland there was an intriguing nine-year study of 941 elderly men and women, aged 65 to 85. Participants were assessed for their level of optimism using a questionnaire that evaluated a number of parameters, including optimistic viewpoint, health, self-respect, morale, and relationships. Over the course of the study, almost four hundred of the participants died of various causes. But the findings revealed that those who rated high in optimism had a 55 percent lower mortality from all causes, as well as an almost 25 percent reduced risk of heart disease compared to those who ranked low. Participants were divided into quartiles based upon their response to statements like: "I still have positive expectations regarding my future" and "I often feel that life is full of promise."[4] Thirty percent of those in the most optimistic quartile died during the nine-year study, while 56 percent of the participants in the most pessimistic quartile died.

The study was carefully controlled to rule out excess mortality in either group due to confounding factors like high blood pressure and smoking. In their analysis the authors noted:

"Our results, combined with the finding that hopelessness was associated with an increased incidence or progression of disease, suggest that dispositional optimism affects the progression of cardiovascular disease." The researchers further state. "Although optimism reduces the risk of cardiovascular death through mechanisms largely unaffected by baseline values of physical activity, obesity, smoking, hypertension, and lipid profile, pessimistic subjects may be more prone to changes across time in risk factors that affect the progression of cardiovascular disease (e.g., the development of smoking habits, obesity, or hypertension) than optimistic subjects. Dispositional optimism may also be associated with better coping strategies that are adhered to throughout life."[5] The same researcher studied optimism in 545 men ages 64–84 over a fifteen-year period, and again found that increasing levels of optimism were correlated well with a decreased risk of cardiovascular mortality, with the most optimistic overall having the lowest mortality.[6]

Happy Little Immune Cells

Our bodies naturally produce many biochemicals that induce good feelings. One large grouping of these is the endorphins, neuro-hormones that give us a "natural high." Runners, for example, are well known to get persistent feelings of joy and decreased perception of pain after a long run. Any sort of sustained vigorous exercise releases one's endorphins into the circulatory system.

Our bodies produce about twenty different endorphins, and some of these are identical to molecules produced by poppy plants, the source of many narcotic drugs. In fact, the reason opiates and narcotics work to reduce pain and induce euphoria in humans and animals is because we have built-in receptors for them to utilize the benefits of naturally occurring biochemicals that our bodies already make. (This includes our own internal cannabinoid system—our bodies naturally create cannabinoids, the "active" factor in marijuana, and our cells have receptors for them.) Since we synthesize cannabinoids and opiates in nature's laboratory, our brain and body, both the ones we make ourselves and those we take as medications work psycho-actively in people, as nature intended.

What is the relevance of opiates and cannabinoids to anxiety relief and the immune system? Although I am not encouraging experimentation with illegal substances, these naturally produced compounds induce feelings of well-being, euphoria, happiness, and exhilaration. They also are extensively connected with proper immune function. Optimal functioning of the immune system, it turns out, is dependent upon feeling good. This was discovered through study of the drug receptors on various types of cells. So let's examine those in greater detail.

Understanding Cell Receptors

Every cell of our body functions cooperatively in the community of cells that comprise our organs and tissues. Each cell can communicate with other cells, tissues, and organs. When cells need to give each other messages, or when we have thoughts, which also give information to our cells, how are the messages transmitted? Cells communicate via various physiologic messaging systems, including chemical messages transmitted through the blood and lymph.

Just as you can choose to ignore your phone when it is ringing, cells decide which messages and types of messages they will accept from other cells and tissues. Cells "answer the phone" by placing biochemical receptors on their surface, signaling their receptivity for specific types of information.

Internal Cannabinoids, Endorphins, and Immune Health

It was pointed out to me by caring reviewers that this section is a little technical, and all readers may not be interested in such details. The take-home point is that our cells' immune system is strengthened by internal biochemicals of happiness. The immune system creates many of these biochemicals in response to our emotional state. So to have a healthy immune system, it helps to be happy. Now, if you want more scientific information to back this up—read on, otherwise, skip to the next section.

An interesting fact is that everyone's immune cells have receptors for opiates and for cannabinoids—lots of them! Researchers have found that more than 90 percent of receptors on our immune cells, like T cells and B cells, are for endogenous (made by our bodies) opiates (endorphins) and cannabinoids. Ninety percent of these immune-system receptors are seeking information to notify the cells about our state of well-being, or lack thereof.

If we dig a bit deeper, we discover that our internal endorphins and cannabinoids come from several unexpected areas. One major site of production is the immune system. In 1984, J. Edwin Blalock, a prominent researcher in the field of psychoneuroimmunology, described the immune system as "our sixth sense."[7]

The endocrine glands that respond to stress, particularly the adrenal glands, produce these "feel good" chemicals. There are many short proteins, normally called "brain peptides" in medical science, that are actually predominantly produced in, and frequently received by, cells of the immune system. They then cross-communicate with other systems of the body, especially the endocrine (hormonal) system and the brain/central nervous system. For example, interferons, a type of immune cell, synthesize both endorphins and adrenocorticotrophic hormone (ACTH). ACTH modulates our physiologic response to stress. It was previously believed to be a hormone produced exclusively in the pituitary gland of the brain. But ACTH can be produced as well as interpreted by cells of the immune system. There are also receptors on immune cells for additional neuropeptides normally made by the brain.[8] It is clear that our immune system actually can, and does, produce and respond to much of what researchers normally think of as products of our hormonal system.

The immune system is essential for health. It protects us against all sorts of diseases and infections from bacteria, fungi, viruses, and parasites, and it monitors the body for abnormal cellular processes like cancers and inflammatory conditions. So it would seem extremely important to understand the vital connection between our natural happiness neurochemicals (the endorphins and cannabinoids) and optimal immune function. A great deal of the research on endorphins has demonstrated that they are key to immune function, and more study is underway. Research into the cannabinoid system is still in its infancy, because of the unfortunate legal status of cannabis. Some of the early research indicates that various cannabinoids are especially powerful balancers of mood and immune function, and others are beneficial mediators of inflammation. Regarding mood, one notable study of a drug that blocked some of the cannabinoid receptors responsible for appetite was discontinued when an alarming number of participants became depressed and suicidal in just a few days.

An out-of-balance immune system can cause severe disease, as is seen in autoimmune ailments. The immune system goes haywire, confusing self and other, and attacking the self. Autoimmune disease may one day be proven to be caused to a large degree by a deficiency of endorphins and cannabinoids. This would certainly be suggested by the strong predominance of receptors for these compounds on immune cells. Science has begun to verify the connection. A 2003 study reported in the *New England Journal of Medicine* noted, "Preclinical evidence indicates overwhelmingly that opioids alter the development, differentiation and function of immune cells, and that both innate and adaptive systems are affected." So our own little bliss hormones seem to affect, at a fundamental level, the development and growth of our entire immune system.

A great deal of the cross-talk between our emotions, our endocrine system, and our immune system serves to inform the immune system about our state of well-being. If we are generally happy, embracing life and its possibilities, then the immune system is more able to work at its optimal capacity. But if we are chronically glum, feel ambivalent about life, or are perpetually discouraged, this may be expressed in a weakening of our immune system that can lead to various diseases, including cancers. Both situations are normal, physiologic responses to predominant states of mind. Disease and health are both organized processes. If you are enjoying life, your body will do its best to keep you thriving, so you can feel great while making the most of it. But if you are unhappy, your body may reflect this with lack of vitality and illness. If your malaise is protracted, your immune system may ultimately help you move on (die). If we want to thrive physically, we owe it to ourselves to learn to be happy.

Stress and Health

In my early days as a physician in North Carolina, I had a patient who was a devoted minister. He was a truly inspiring man who loved his work and his congregation, and he worked long hours to help his community. But he tended to worry about his flock. We would track his blood pressure during office visits, and when he worked too long and hard, or did not get enough sleep, especially over time, it would rise.

Arteries are blood vessels that lead away from the heart, bringing nourishing blood to the tissues of the body. They are surrounded by smooth muscle. Through complex biochemical and electromagnetic feedback loops, this muscle constricts when we are tense, and it can remain tight if we are chronically stressed. Our blood pressure is literally the pressure that the blood has to exert to move through the arteries to reach the tissues, where it can deliver its nourishment. When the muscles that wrap the arteries constrict, it takes more pressure to send the blood through them. I liken this to water pressure in a garden hose. If there is a kink in the hose, which tightens it, more water pressure is required to deliver water to the garden.

Whenever this patient's blood pressure became too high and difficult to manage, I would prescribe he go on a meditation retreat. During these ten-day retreats, he became very relaxed. After just two or three days of quiet contemplation in nature, he did not need to take any medications at all, as his blood pressure returned to normal. Once he returned to work, he would continue meditation and contemplation, but over time, he would return to his ingrained habits of worry about his congregation. His blood pressure would rise, and he would once again resume medications to stabilize his condition.

These findings are similar to those observed in two studies of stress reduction and hypertension, discussed in an article published in the *American Journal of Cardiology*. Health outcomes were followed for 202 hypertensive men and women. They were taught a technique called Transcendental Meditation (TM), and instructed in other behavioral stress-reduction techniques. The individuals were followed for up to eighteen years. Statistically significant improvement was recorded for those who meditated regularly, as compared with the control group. Compared with average people, those who meditated experienced a 30 percent reduction in cardiovascular mortality, and a 49 percent decrease in mortality from cancer.[9]

Dozens of studies demonstrate the profound benefits of stress reduction for overall health. Large insurers like Kaiser Permanente Foundation have paid attention to these reports and now offer classes in yoga, stress reduction, and meditation in order to improve health outcomes in their clients.

Don't Worry about Worrying

There is a potential pitfall once people understand that feelings and emotions impact health. There can be a tendency to then shift the focus of worrying about other concerns to anxiety about feeling bad and how this may affect your health. People learn that it is physiologically better for their health if they think positively, and then they "worry themselves sick" because they are not thinking positively all the time or haven't thought positively in the past. They essentially add stressing about all the stress to their stress.

This can be a normal, temporary response to changing thought patterns. The key to continuing to shift is to recognize that this is one potential response, and to keep the emotions moving, not getting locked in this new story. Humor can help, as can the recognition that this type of worry is an extension of the same negative mental tapes that the individual has already been running. It is just another access point into the mental file of "things that feel bad."

If this happens to you, be gentle with yourself. If you notice that you have shifted from worrying about the economy or your children to worrying about the potential health effects of too much worry, observe that while the names and topics have changed, the game is still the same. None of that is worthwhile. So let yourself off the hook. Your improved awareness is a first step to greater wholeness and ease.

To feel better, individuals can strive to turn off the negative self-talk about the negative self-talk. Fortunately, there are many ways to get out of this vicious cycle. Before we can shift a pattern, we have to notice it is there. Noticing all of this can be seen as a positive improvement, as it begins to show the anxious person some of the persistent mental traps that may have been previously hidden. Relax in knowing that your awareness of the problem is the first step toward its resolution.

"Don't worry, be happy."

This quote, often attributed to singer Bobby McFerrin, is actually a quote from the teachings of Meher Baba, a twentieth-century Hindu spiritual master. I remember frequently seeing photos of his joyous, smiling face during the seventies, with this simple, lovely quote. Really, "don't worry, be happy" is the pure essence of well-being.

Scientists have demonstrated that it is possible to change one's brain chemistry by changing attitudes and thoughts.[10] Even pessimists and worriers, over time, can change their predominant habits of thought. Once you shift your thoughts for the better, your world begins to shift with them.

CHAPTER 2

Neurobiology:
Anxiety and Calm

Why, when we are down or anxious, is it so easy to globalize? "Globalizing" in this context can be understood as the way we seem to be easily able to recollect and ruminate on many more negative experiences, worrisome ideas, and self-deprecating thoughts once we are already feeling bad. In popular culture, the term "globalizing" usually refers to negative emotions only, as people don't mind globalizing positively. We do not worry about having excessive numbers of happy thoughts, one after another, or recalling too many good experiences, or anticipating more upcoming joy. But, in fact, we usually globalize, either positively or negatively, when we think without intentionally choosing what we focus upon. Our brains are hard-wired to amplify and give us more evidence of our current emotional state—positive, negative, or neutral.

There is a simple, neurobiological basis for why we globalize. The mind stores and categorizes memories and thoughts by their emotional content. Items that feel emotionally similar are stored in the same group. That is one reason our trains of thought seem to skip around. For example, when we are thinking of one thing that happened when we were eight years old, we do not next begin to recall the catalogue of experiences of our eight-year-old self. Instead we next recall something equally emotionally memorable and intense.

One friend reported a typical happy, amusing thought train that occurred in less than a minute. When she learned that her son had adopted a new calico cat, she skipped in her mind from that event to her love of cats in general, and then recalled her pleasure on the day she got her first grey kitten at age seven. She loved how the kitty would purr, play, and frolic, and would then conk out exhausted and sleep on a pillow in her bed. Next she thought of the time she fell in love at age sixteen and how sweet, funny, and gentle her beau had been. She next recalled nursing her son, just after he was born, and the feelings of love she felt for him. How tiny and how perfect he was. These thoughts are not unrelated, though they may seem so. They are linked by emotional content, and not chronology. All felt great, all included love, so my friend's mind grouped them together.

This is how images and thoughts associated with joy or deep peace are collected together and "color-coded" by their emotional content. Likewise, thoughts, beliefs, and memories that prompt a feeling of overwhelm are collected with others of the same emotional "flavor." The coding is biochemical, communicated from cell to cell by tiny short-lived protein molecules called peptides.[1] Researcher Candace Pert, PhD, discusses this connection in more detail in her outstanding book *Molecules of Emotion*. We make neuropeptides in response to our thoughts, observations, and experiences.

The mix of peptides present in the brain at any moment signals which areas of the brain are "on" or lighting up, and which are off. I liken this to strolling in various rooms in a house and looking at the objects in it. Imagine that you had many storerooms in your house, where you collected and grouped things emotionally instead of by function. You have a room where you have gathered only objects that are funny and light-hearted, another room where everything is sad, a room where everything is peaceful, and another room where everything is frightening. Neurochemicals are like the keys that open the doors to the rooms of our minds. The mix of neuropeptides in one's system will determine whether the lights are on or off in any particular mental room.

When we are anxious, the lights in the worry/stress/frightening room are "on" and we can easily view the distressing collection of anxiety-producing thoughts, memories, and upsetting projections that we have accumulated within that space, just like we could see the furnishings of a brightly lit living room. If we have been anxious frequently in our life, this mental nervousness "room" is now more like a vast cluttered storeroom of horrors. It becomes easy to globalize about how bad it is, because there are so many readily apparent thoughts, similar in emotional tone, to the one that first triggered the feeling of anxiety. As we focus upon details of each of these, we walk deeper and deeper into the room, brightly lighting more lights and making more reinforcing neurochemicals, and so we find more and more unpleasant confirmatory details. This is like some modern supermarkets, where the freezer case "lights up" as we walk down the aisle. Details of how worthless we are, details of how we have done things wrong, details of what we fear might happen to ourselves and our loved ones, details about our insignificance, details of how no one likes us, and awful details of terrible things that can and have happened to ourselves and others we care about—all demand attention. Anxiety is truly a horrible room, and it can seem terribly overwhelming.

But if we were in a house, we could just close that door and walk away, right? We could get rid of all that dreadful stuff—let someone come and haul it away who might have a better use for it—and never look at it again. We can do this in our mind too, but it takes some practice. Consider that we can really only focus on one thought at a time, just like we can only be in one room in our house at a time. So when the light is on in the room of anxiety, then the light is off in other, more pleasing rooms, rooms like joy, silliness, ease, and peace. The other rooms do exist even if we haven't been spending enough time in them. For a much more pleasant experience, we can learn to switch off the lights in the anxiety room, close the door, and to illumine other, more peaceful mental spaces instead.

It has been very empowering for many of my patients to learn that the mix of peptides that "color-codes" our emotional state can be quite transient. These important neurochemicals that amplify, group, and light up the emotional content of our thoughts are not permanent. Nor are cell receptors for neurochemicals permanent. Some individual peptide molecules persist less than one minute. The cell receptors are more long-lived, but even they can be dramatically shifted over a period of a few days or weeks.

If this is true, why then do we seem to feel some emotional states for hours, days, or months? The answer is: simply because new neurochemicals are constantly created from our current emotional state, in response to it. These biochemicals reflect and perpetuate our current state of mind. When we are anxious, we create anxiety peptides, so then we remember more things that are "color-coded" to the "anxiety room" of our mind. Our anxiety increases, and we create still more peptides that reflect this. This disagreeable loop effect can go on and on. Similarly, when we are calm or feel joy, our bodies create more peptides of happiness, and then our thoughts and memories reflect our well-being, and additional good-feeling peptides are created.

This one simple fact has revolutionary implications. Without an understanding that we are empowered, many of us remain for a long time within the anxiety room, believing it is our only option. We continue picking up assorted stressful thoughts and mulling them over, so we continue to make stress peptides that functionally keep the lights on in that room. As we do so, we collect and recall more confirmatory memories and experiences, since the filter of our emotional state colors our experience of life. If we do not flip the switch, we might eventually work ourselves up more and more, illuminating the dark gnarly corners of the room that show us our most despairing and defeated thoughts, memories, and beliefs. In this way we can inadvertently blind ourselves to the things that are going well. We do not see them because we are not looking in that direction, because the lights are off in the well-being rooms.

But we are in charge. We can emotionally walk away from the thoughts that fill us with fear. We can let go. We can turn off the lights, close the door of the unpleasant room, and go somewhere else nicer, just about as quickly as we can walk from our bathroom to our bedroom. It takes less than a minute to consciously change our feelings by intentionally changing our focus. This starts to shift the balance of our neuropeptides in a more positive direction. As we consistently insist on feeling better now, the neurochemicals of fear and anxiety dissipate within minutes.

A truly wonderful thing to understand is that we do not need to deliberately feel better about any of the topics in the stressful room. We can ignore them completely for the time being and focus on something entirely different. It is the feelings and emotions that determine the mix of peptides, thereby coding which types of thoughts are "on" and which are "off." It is our emotional state, not the specific content of our thoughts, that triggers peptide synthesis. This means, for example, that you can be worrying about your finances, relationship, or health and shift how you are feeling for the better by appreciating your warm feelings about puppies, sunsets, flowers, or hummingbirds. By shifting emotional state we can easily change the mix of peptides, and thus turn on the light and open the doors to more pleasant rooms, letting the fresh breeze of calm and ease blow through.

As someone who has grappled with anxiety, I learned it is essential to let ourselves depart the rooms where we find unhappy, anxiety-filled thoughts, however compelling they might seem in the moment. This is not denial. Re-examining painful memories merely restimulates them, bringing past distress into the present. It results in creation of more short-acting anxiety peptides that illuminate more unpleasant memories and thoughts. It also suppresses production of more durable good-feeling neurotransmitters, like GABA, serotonin, and empowering amines like dopamine and phenylethylamine, that help us with motivation, focus, and feelings of bliss.

Anxious thoughts can feel very intense. This is simply neurochemistry. Those thoughts can feel consuming only because we are flooded with anxiety-producing biochemicals as we continue to think them. It is empowering to let go, allowing the balance to change. Continuing negative patterns of thought will not help you let go. The point at which you notice your thoughts are creating misery for you is the point where you have a choice. You must do your best to let go and think about something else, something that feels better to you. One way to let go is to intentionally think about something else. Persist in doing this whenever you realize you are feeling bad, and the next time you will notice it sooner. It will get easier. This is an exercise that feels good and is good for you.

You always live now, only now, in the present moment. Your life is an accumulation of *now* moments. There is no reason to worry about potentially undesirable futures, or to replay past pains. You are the only one who is bringing the past difficulties or speculative undesirable futures into the present moment. You are the only one who can make a new choice for yourself. You can make it at any moment. Like now. Because there is "no time like the present." The only effort needed is consciously choosing thoughts that feel better. Feeling better is its own reward. Feeling better gives you tremendous relief and liberates a lot of energy.

Tools for Transformation: Emotional Fluidity

One path to feeling better involves understanding and practicing emotional fluidity. We can examine our thoughts and notice both the emotions and physical energy associated with them. We may observe that our thoughts can make us feel any number of ways: tired, ill at ease, and fearful, or energized, comfortable, free, peaceful, and easy. When we focus upon what we do not prefer, placing our awareness upon the issues causing obstruction of the emotional flow, we inadvertently add bricks to our energetic dams, making them higher. We close ourselves off. We may experience discomfort, anxiety, and even fatigue. If we notice any discomfort with a train of thought, it is possible to make a different choice. We never need to continue to be spectators of negativity in our own mind.

Emotional fluidity has a few steps that build upon the understanding that we affect our biochemistry with our thoughts. Each step will be expanded upon here, and discussed in more detail in later chapters, so don't worry about immediately "getting it right." This is just a framework that should naturally fill in for you as you read, practice, and experience.

One: Notice How You Feel

Acknowledge where you are emotionally right now. Don't judge it, just notice. If you are not sure how you feel, notice that. There are some tools in upcoming chapters to help you identify your emotional state.

Two: Acknowledge That You Want to Feel Better, Right Now

This is an important step, so claim it. "I want to feel better!" That is what you really want, right? The spiritual teacher Abraham points out that "whatever we think we want, we only want it because we believe we will be happier having it." You may think you want various things—a relationship, lots of money, vibrant health, a new red car—but what you really want, why you want those things, is because you want to feel happier, calmer, and more joyful in life. Many believe that having certain things will provide the good feelings. But those feelings are transient. There is always another shiny thing, a next object of desire. What you really want is what is enduring. That is peace of mind, joy, health, and wholeness.

To illustrate: Think about when you got something that you had wanted for a long time. It can be an item or an experience. How long did that make you happy before you were looking toward the next desire? For many of us, it is a few moments or a few days. Happiness is not about getting stuff, unless you are deprived of fundamental needs like food, shelter, or warmth. This has been demonstrated over and over again, worldwide, in diverse cultures and lands.[2]

By continually shifting your point of focus toward well-being, your perspective on the experiences of your life changes. The more you do this, the more you create a durable sense of well-being. Nothing is more important than feeling better, right now. There is really no reason to knock around in any more bad-feeling emotional spaces. There is a tendency to think, incorrectly, when you are stressed or anxious, that you must first "figure things out" before you can feel better. You cannot. Abraham once said: "You can't get to the bottom of it. There is no bottom." Thoughts and solutions generated during an anxious state of mind are seldom productive. Choices made from fear rarely get you what you really want, and actions taken from anxious states of mind rarely turn out well. The anxious state of mind is a dead-end, leading to more anxiety-ridden experience.

So simply acknowledge, "What I really want now is to feel better. I want to feel happier—to feel as good as it is possible for me to feel right now." Just acknowledging that gives relief. Feeling a little better is doable right now. You are unlikely to have a new financial situation, a different body, or items that you have been craving in this very moment. But you can feel slightly happier, exactly as things are right now. The door cracks open when you notice and claim that it is the feelings of happiness, peace, or wholeness that you really want. Let yourself acknowledge that you are open to allowing well-being in, and to knowing how to create it, in any of life's circumstances.

Three: Think of Better-Feeling Stuff

Think of some things that help you feel better. Get into the sensing place of this. If you are really in turmoil, then just feeling a little better will give a lot of relief. You are not, at this moment, striving for the best feeling you have ever had. You are merely trying to find something that feels a little better than what you were currently thinking about when you noticed feeling bad. Even slightly better is an improvement to be applauded.

Make a list of things that feel good or neutral to you. Write them down, perhaps in a journal. You may want to keep this around, periodically adding more notes to your list. Items can be memories, fantasies, experiences, or connections. They can be things from the natural world, or pleasant things you anticipate.

Here are some personal examples, gleaned from my own list and the lists of some of my patients. Each provides a good-feeling vignette to contemplate.

> Walking in the woods.
>
> Sitting on the beach and watching the waves and seagulls, while smelling the fresh sea air.
>
> Falling in love.
>
> A good first date.
>
> The birth of children.
>
> Playing fetch with my dog.
>
> Playing with a grandchild.
>
> Driving my new car.
>
> My five-year-old birthday party, when my uncle came as a clown.
>
> Christmas morning when I was little.
>
> Chanukah when I was little.
>
> Singing in a choir.
>
> Dancing.
>
> Thanksgiving Day.

Talking to my best friend.

My nephew or niece.

My upcoming vacation.

Skiing.

As you write your own list, include some things that feel great and others that feel okay, serene, or peaceful. As you practice, you will find that depending on how you are feeling, some of these items are easier to recall and remember. If you are very anxious, it may be easier to remember the feelings of a calm day, where nothing much of consequence happened, rather than the emotions of one of the high points of your life.

Four: Remember

Remember the feelings. Remember the emotions. "Remember" is an interesting and quite literal word. You are re-making it physical for yourself, re-experiencing the good or peaceful feelings, and re-letting them course through your mind and body. You are consciously and deliberately choosing to change how you feel, by changing what you are thinking about, and then letting the new, more enjoyable emotions suffuse you.

Pick three things from your list and let yourself remember or imagine them. Feel the feelings. Feel how delicious they are. Recall or invent details. If there is a place involved, what are the colors, the scents, and the sounds? The more you can fill this in, the more real it is for you. It is most important to really experience the improved emotions. Spend at least one minute enjoying each of your scenarios. Longer is fine. Try doing this now.

Here is an example that works well for me:

A walk in the woods

I am in a forest, hiking on a lovely trail in springtime. It is a pleasantly warm day, and there is a light breeze. As I walk, I hear my footfalls crunch on dried leaves and pine needles. The pine needles release a fresh light aroma, and I enjoy catching whiffs of it as I stroll. Birds are singing, with a call and response. As I walk, I spy various woodland animals: chipmunks, frogs, and a rare red fox. A woodpecker flies by, and as my gaze follows it, I notice a glade with a shaft of sunlight pouring down. It illuminates a grassy patch lively with California spring wildflowers; tidy tips, goldfields, poppies, and lupines bloom luxuriously amidst wild grasses. Seeing the sunbeams gleaming on wildflowers always give me a feeling of peace and the knowledge that all is well. I rest in this feeling.

Five: Practice, Practice, and Practice

You will get better at this over time. The more you practice, the easier it becomes to shift your emotions. The more you play with this, the more you show yourself that you are able to do it.

When people say that this is hard for them, I am understanding and encouraging. Each new skill we take on is difficult until it becomes easy. When I learned to play guitar as a teenager, there was a lot of pluck, pluck, pluck, then pause, rearrange my fingers on the frets, then pluck, pluck, pluck, and repeat. I wasn't fluid right away. I was clunky! But I kept practicing, because I really liked the guitar and wanted to be good at it, and eventually my fingers knew what to do. In a relatively short time, I no longer needed to think about it every time I changed the chord, or to look at where my fingers were placed when I was strumming.

A good bodyworker knows the same thing. Many years ago, my partner Star completed training at The Florida School of Massage, then spent many more years studying Ortho-Bionomy. While learning, she had to focus and practice—this amount of pressure here, these are trigger points, etc. Now, after many years of experience, she often just "follows her hands." Anyone who learns anything knows this. What at first is difficult eventually becomes easier, then with even more practice, it becomes second nature.

Shifting emotionally is essentially the same thing. At first it may seem choppy or even difficult. You will probably not be great at it right away. Effort and focus are involved. Do not get discouraged. You can practice, just as if you were learning to play an instrument or give a good massage. Really, you are learning to play the most important instrument, the harp of your mind and emotions. It is a vibrational tuning and receiving device that is unparalleled in its potential for creating feelings of joy and well-being.

And just like learning to play an instrument, you do not start to practice on the day of your big performance. No one expects to wait until a really important moment to try and learn how to play an instrument. This is also true of shifting our emotions. I counsel patients to practice many times a day, in many settings, and not just begin trying when they are feeling most miserable and most in need of a shift. Certainly you can learn to shift your emotional state when things feel bleak, just like you can eventually perform your musical piece in front of a big audience, or even on television. But that is not where you start. You start by showing yourself you can do this. By practicing over time, you make it easy.

Be kind to yourself as you practice. No self-criticism is allowed. Self-criticism dumps you back into an anxiety loop. Most people would never dream of saying to another person the damaging things they say to themselves. If you notice you are being self-critical, try to be compassionate, just as you would be to another person. Try humor or patience. Of course you are wobbly when you are first learning. Think of a colt standing for the first time. This baby horse will someday be a smooth and elegant stallion. He will someday run swiftly and surely. And you will too, but maybe not at first. Let yourself be amused, just like you would be observing a clumsy, shy colt taking his first steps. Allow yourself to learn and grow. Let yourself be kind to yourself.

Six: Mix It Up

Part of being fluid is practicing a variety of different good-feeling emotional states. Try calm, peace, happy, silly, playful, and serene. You will want a repertoire of many pleasant-feeling emotions. Sometimes peace and ease will work, sometimes playful and light is perfect, and other times joy is just the ticket. Write down scenarios that elicit various good feelings and practice a wide range of them.

Seven: Relax and Enjoy

When you have achieved a good-feeling state, let yourself relax and enjoy the emotions. There is no need to quickly move on to other tasks. Deliberately and consciously nurture the good feelings. Pleasantly examine why they feel good, what you like about them. Think of more things that feel good in a similar way, then muse pleasantly about what is good about them as well. What, for example, is similar about loving your pet, your spouse, and your grandchild? What is similar about fishing on a quiet stream, listening to your favorite jazz music, and conversing deeply with your trusted friend? This type of associating starts to create new, more desirable mental and emotional pathways. As your brain chemistry changes with your improved feelings, it will become easier to allow good thoughts to run rampant. Let the feelings of well-being, love, ease, and peace course through your entire body. Good feelings will nourish your cells, organs, and bones. Tell your body you love it, tell your mind you love it, tell your heart that you love you, and bathe it in the goodness you are feeling.

In summary, here are steps for emotional fluidity:

1. Acknowledge how you feel right now.
2. Acknowledge that you want to feel better right now.
3. Think of things that give you good feelings. Make a list of them and add to it frequently. Keep it in an accessible spot.
4. Remember the feelings of well-being using your list. Feel ease in your body and emotions, not just your thoughts.
5. Practice often. Your skills improve with time and practice.
6. Mix it up, practicing lots of more pleasant-feeling emotions each day. Try experiencing a variety of positive states, some playful and some more profound. Show yourself all the ways you can feel good.
7. Relish the positive feeling for a while. Let yourself relax and enjoy the good vibes.

CHAPTER 3

༼ ༽

The Wellsprings of Inner Peace
and Letting Go:
A Spiritual Look at Emotional Health

Within you there is a stillness and a sanctuary to which
you can retreat any time and be yourself.

—HERMANN HESSE

A lake of inner peace exists within each of us. This pool is deep, wide, restful, and soothing. It is a patient, ever-present refuge, a private internal oasis of renewal that is always available, for free. We simply need to know how to find it. The inner lake of peace is accessible to those who have cultivated their own paths to it. These people can dive into its refreshing waters at any time, even after stressful events, to restore themselves in serenity and calm. You may have met some of those people and wondered how they manage to remain so unflappably peaceful and happy, despite life's challenges.

For many folks in contemporary society, the road to our inner lake of peace can be murky and unclear. Many of us have no confidence that we will find peace when we want it. It can seem the most elusive when our need seems most profound. When anxious, depressed, or discouraged, it may seem that the path has disappeared completely.

And yet there are those times, when we seem to stumble upon feelings of peace, as if by accident, unsure how we arrived there. Almost everyone has times when they feel tranquil and untroubled, times when things "came together." But often we think these interludes "just happened" and fail to give ourselves credit for creating the feeling of well-being. If we do not understand that we are empowered, we do not understand that we can do it again.

The goal of this chapter is to help you find your own reliable internal road map to inner peace. There are many paths and we each have a number of emotional trails that lead to well-being. We can all learn which tools work best in each situation. By applying them, our confidence and understanding that we have a variety of resources will grow. Following are several key principles that are frequently helpful in developing inner peace.

The First Principle: Feelings Matter

One key to finding peace is to accept our emotions, whatever they are. We do not need to run from them. It is alright to have feelings and emotions. Once we can identify how we are feeling, we can begin to understand what our emotions are telling us.

Years ago I had a disagreement with a dear friend. I cried and poured my heart out, explaining how a situation between us was affecting me. I talked specifically about each emotion. Throughout my explanation, she was very quiet. When I was through and had said all I could say, the silence continued. I wondered if she was angry but then thought that I could be projecting my worry onto her. I had no real knowledge of her emotional state. So I asked her, "What are you feeling about this situation?" She thought for a long while then answered simply, "I do not know." I then asked her how she was feeling about what I had expressed, and again, after a long pause, she answered, "I don't know."

A light bulb lit up for me. She really did not know how she felt! This insight deepened my understanding about what was going on. My initial frustration dissolved into compassion. The reason that she could not respond to my outpouring of emotion was she had not yet located herself. She could not communicate her feelings because she was simply unaware of them.

Over the years I have met many good people, like my dear friend, who are unaware of how they feel much of the time. Some actively run away from feeling emotion, overfilling their lives with distracting activities. Some periodically get caught up in gusts and eddies of emotion, not understanding where they came from. When this happens, they may claim "something came over me" or "it hit me like a ton of bricks."

This is not surprising. In contemporary society, many of us have been trained to ignore our feelings. We may believe we should be rational, thinking things through dispassionately, rather than paying attention to our emotions. Some believe that emotions actually get in the way of "rational" thought. As a result, we may need a "ton of bricks" to break through the barriers to our feelings. Unfortunately, many of the things that "hit us hard," thereby demanding our attention, are not pleasant. This can reinforce the belief that emotions are troublesome. The question remains, how can a person feel better if they are unaware of how they are feeling, unless the emotions are so extreme that they feel overwhelmed by them?

Just as a sailor has to measure longitude and latitude to know his or her position on the ocean and determine the best course to their destination, we need to know where we are emotionally in order to orient ourselves toward feeling better. A first step, then, in finding ways to feel good is to understand how we are feeling throughout our day. A ship's navigator has instruments to calibrate the precise position of the vessel. We too have the ability to notice and precisely locate our emotions. This involves repeatedly checking in with one's self. It is a practice, and like any practice it improves with repetition.

One method to learn how we feel is to merely inquire. Ask yourself, throughout your day: "How do I feel now?" "How do I feel in response to this comment?" "To that belief?" "To this scene?" As you practice checking in, your emotional self-awareness will increase and expand. Be sure, as you check in, that you describe your feelings to yourself.

Some people find it difficult to remember to check in with themselves periodically about their emotions. Setting an alarm that chimes every hour or so is one way to remind yourself to observe what you are feeling in relation to what is happening at the time. Journaling these observations and reflecting on them later can help bring you closer to your emotional self-awareness goal.

Here is a short example from one woman's emotional journal: "8:15 eating breakfast, pretty calm. 9:15 late to work because there was lots of traffic, my anxiety is high. 10:15 boss is cranky, and taking it out on us. I feel frustrated with her. 11:15 doing work, I'm bored, but not upset, pretty calm. 12:15 eating lunch with a co-worker, the choices in the cafeteria were tasty, and we are having fun poking fun at some of our boss's more outrageous comments. Feel amused."

When we check in frequently, using whatever method works, we encourage greater self-awareness. We begin to notice that we have a wide range of emotions throughout a day. Let yourself enjoy and celebrate the richness of your emotional experience.

You do not need to judge your emotions. They are neither good nor bad. Emotions can be described in any number of ways: comfortable, uncomfortable, neutral, pleasant, stressful, serene, or joyous. But feelings, however we describe them, are really only information about our current state of mind. Emotions inform us about how we feel about our thoughts, observations, intentions, and focus. Emotions are a response. They tell us how we feel about our current life experiences. We generate emotions as we consider various thoughts, topics of focus, beliefs, stimuli, and actions.

Where we focus our thoughts is the key to our emotional state. Emotions occur in response to our thoughts, as well as our interpretation of them. This is true no matter what we are responding to, even physical stimuli. Another way to learn to discern our emotions is to deliberately pay attention to our thoughts about various stimuli, and then observe the emotions that arise. If we smell something we deem unpleasant, there is a thought that goes with that judgment—something like "Yuck!" or "Get me out of here!" There is a corresponding emotion, in this case of dislike, which will match the thought. Or if we pet a soft, cuddly kitten, we might think something like "Mmmm" or "This is nice." A matching, soothing emotion will simultaneously present itself. Exploring emotional responses to physical stimuli such as these can sometimes be an easy way for people who are unsure of how they feel to begin to check in with themselves.

Example of Checking In: Inner Peace

Checking in about our emotional responses to life experiences as they are occurring is essential for improving one's state of mind. We saw that we can find our emotional location by various periods of checking in with ourselves throughout the day. Knowing where we are, we can then chart a course to better-feeling states. It is also useful to understand our feelings and beliefs about a variety of topics and ideas. This is another form of checking in.

Since one major theme of this chapter is developing inner peace, we can use a "check-in" about this topic as an example of how to proceed. Our feelings around inner peace provide an ideal opportunity for self-examination, and exploration of underlying beliefs and emotions surrounding them.

Take a few moments and ask yourself the following questions. You may want to journal your responses to look at later.

What does inner peace mean to you?

Do you want inner peace?

Why? (Whether the answer is yes, no, or maybe)

Do you believe inner peace is possible for you?

When is the last time you remember having even a brief feeling of peace or well-being?

Can you describe what peace felt like to you?

What was happening in your life at that time?

Was there any period of your life when you recall experiencing protracted feelings of well-being, for days, weeks, or months?

If so, what were the circumstances of your life then?

How are you feeling right now?

How would you like to feel right now?

Principle Two: Emotions Provide Guidance

Emotions, as we noted previously, are a response to our focus. Our emotions can give us accurate guidance on how to navigate and direct our thoughts and focus. I was first introduced to this life-changing concept via the teachings of Abraham,[1] and it has been very useful to me and to others. Understanding that emotions are a response, we can use them as an internal compass. Emotions can show us whether our thoughts are pointing us toward feel better or hindering our progress.

Our inner store of well-being is like a radio antenna. It broadcasts a constant message to our personality self, saying: "All is well, you are loved, and you are love." This inner being dwells fully and completely in harmony, unconditional love, and joy.[2] Our true spirit can never become diseased or distressed.

Emotions can tell us whether we are tuning in to the harmonious frequencies of the perpetual broadcast of our divine inner self, or whether we are dialing in to static. A surge of good-feeling emotions like peace, calm, joy, and love indicates that we are setting our internal tuner to receive our inner well-being bandwidth, whereas feelings of increasing anxiety, worry, and fear let us know that we are tuning into static and disharmony. It may be that anxiety is merely a message from the spirit, a call to balance, encouraging us to "tune inward" in order to find the broadcast of joy, inner peace, and love.

Certain emotions are always associated with peace and feelings of internal connectedness. As you progress, identify what emotions sustain you the most. In my own journey toward peace, I have found the "love feeling," a feeling of well-being that is profoundly beautiful and serene, to be the most reliable indicator of connectedness to my deeper self. When I feel the "love feeling" I am always calm, knowing wholeness and trusting my inner wisdom. The "love feeling," and other emotions like it, let me know I am on the right "bandwidth."

Emotions are our guidance. If thinking about a topic in a particular way feels emotionally satisfying, continue. If it feels worse, change the channel. You might look at a sunset, listen to some soothing music, or play tug with your dog.

Some people worry that it is selfish or frivolous to pursue happiness. Nothing could be further from the truth. It is good to be happy and to feel at peace. Peace Pilgrim, a spiritual teacher during the Cold War era who walked across the United States many times, taught that peace in the world begins with inner peace. True peace in the individual marks the road to greater peace in the whole.

When we experience anxiety, we are simply out of touch with the ease that is at our core. Illness or disease, whether emotional or physical, is never a punishment for a past thought or action. Anxiety is a result of dialing into static, an indication that we are dwelling upon thoughts and behaviors that feel bad rather than tuning in to the broadcast of our truest inner self. This is the case even if the impetus for our thoughts began with the words or actions of others.

With practice, each of us can manage and direct our own thoughts. We can choose different ones. We own our thoughts. No one else controls our thoughts; no one else forces us to continue to think about stressful topics. We generate our own thoughts and they persist because we keep on thinking them. The founder of the Biodynamics of Osteopathy, James Jealous, DO, observed in a class I attended that "most everyone is living in a movie that they are projecting, but that is not actually happening."

It may seem like our thoughts are out of our control, when we simply have ingrained habits. It is good to remember that there is a continuous broadcast from our inner being, guiding us gently toward harmony and balance. It provides a much nicer movie to live than our unpleasant projections, because it is real and healthy. In truth, we are constantly, inexorably moving toward health. Healing is a process of transmutation that results in a greater expression of wholeness. Anxiety simply lets us know there is an imbalance, a misunderstanding between the vibration of our true nature and what we are expressing in the present moment.

Well-being does not just happen. We are not passive participants. We are active creators of our experience. You are ultimately responsible for the spiritual journey toward your emotional health. Anyone or anything else along the way—health practitioners, books, seminars, movies, energy healers, shamans, or friends—is just a vehicle for you to get in touch with you. I discuss some more ways to utilize emotions as guidance in the next chapter, "Moving Up the Scale."

Principle Three: Making Peace in the Present Moment

Many believe that the circumstances of their lives are the cause of their unhappiness. People say things to themselves such as "If I only had more money, I would be happier" or "I am miserable because my boss is so horrid" or "If I had a relationship, my life would be much more fulfilling" or "To feel good I must lose at least fifty pounds." How we are feeling at any moment is just a jumping-off point for where we are headed. We are always headed somewhere. The current experiences of our lives are just where we are at now. There is always a juxtaposition of where we are now and where we are going. There is always something more that we will want, because that is part of being alive. Understanding this, and making peace with it, is a central task in finding emotional balance and freedom from anxiety.

The wealthy are statistically no happier than the poor. In my medical practice, I see patients from a wide range of income brackets. Some have meager resources and others are extremely well off. Some of my happiest patients have very little in the way of material wealth, while a few of the wealthiest are among the most troubled. Wealth or lack of it, beyond basic necessities, does not engender happiness.

Happiness is an inside job. It is how we see our experience, how we think about it that provides happiness. Wanting more, and different, experiences is the nature of physical existence. But if we wait until we "get there," ironically, we may never arrive to collect the pot of gold we think lies at the destination. Instead we may miss the true gold that is contained in the beauty of the journey.[3]

Find some good in your current situation. For example, I worked with a patient I'll call Steve, who became ill and lost his job. He had to move back in with his ex-wife and kids, and he felt very bad about this. He had been living in Hawaii but was now back in Oakland (California). Steve was initially quite focused on the noisiness of the children (ages four, seven, and nine) and felt certain their ruckus impeded his healing, as he believed he required a quiet, contemplative environment to recuperate. He was also bickering with his ex-wife in ways that were all too familiar. When we spoke initially, Steve could not come up with any positives of this situation. He felt trapped, because he believed it was impossible for him to heal in this environment. He felt he was stuck, as he also believed there were "no other options" for him financially. But Steve was genuinely interested in feeling better and was willing to examine and possibly change his beliefs.

Principle Four: I Can Be Happier Now

We do not have to change external conditions in order to feel happier in any moment. Steve's situation is a perfect example. He was interested in seeing things differently, partly because he was so miserable, and he understood that feeling stuck gave him no relief. I explained that there are always other options of thought that have to do only with our perspective, and do not require changing circumstances that are seemingly out of our control. Painstakingly, we looked at all the limiting beliefs he had trucked in with him during his move back to Oakland. Not surprisingly, he soon discovered that this type of limiting thought was present in the circumstances that resulted in his illness and job loss in the first place.

Steve started to notice that he had many stuck beliefs layered on top of one another, and began to unpack them. He worked with me, as well as with an excellent psychotherapist, to shift his negative thoughts and make peace with his current situation, finding the good in it. Steve considered himself a spiritual person and was able to see the effort he was taking to make peace and feel better in the present as part of his inner journey. He used lots of the tools in this book, and eventually he began to think about how to look at his life differently.

He was able to acknowledge the sweetness of his children and could reframe their boisterousness as exuberance for life. He acknowledged that he wanted more exuberance about his own life, and some of his frustration about their noisiness fell away. He noticed that it was nice for him to see them grow, and he enjoyed participating more in their daily lives rather than just having brief visits. And he began to feel his appreciation for his ex-wife for letting him move back in when he was down and out. He stopped bickering so much with her, practicing breathing techniques, yoga, and taking walks when his irritation increased. He realized that how he interpreted their inter-actions was up to him. Although they did not reconcile their marriage, he and his ex-wife embarked upon a friendship. As all these changes happened, Steve slowly began to realize that he could heal in this environment, and in fact he was healing because of the changes in his character. His focus on his symptoms became less consuming, and he grew more optimistic about recov-ering his health.

Even in extreme circumstances, we can be happier. Psychologist Jill Leb-eau explains in her book *Feng Shui Your Mind* that painful life experiences are inevitable, but suffering is an option. Great saints have lived, and flourished, in tiny cells. Nelson Mandela used his long incarceration at Robben's Island as an opportunity for spiritual growth that ultimately benefited all humankind.

Principle Five: Being Kind and Compassionate to Myself

Most of us have compassion for others. We can also be compassionate to ourselves. "Always be kind to yourself" is a sentence I have written on patient instruction sheets for as long as I have had a medical practice. Throughout the years, I have noticed that many people are distinctly unkind to them-selves. They judge themselves harshly and even ridicule or belittle themselves when they do not live up to impossible standards. They are their own worst critics. Many good, kind people have told me horrible things about them-selves, such as that they are "total failures" or they "have no self-discipline." Ironically, these same people are also good-hearted, and they would never treat others the way they treat themselves. They would never say to others the unkind things they say to themselves.

Anxious persons can be particularly self-critical, self-limiting, and harsh. When we are cruel to ourselves, we dig ourselves further into a hole. As a result, anxiety increases. This may ring true for you. If it does, notice that the more the self-taunting voice belittles, the more your anxiety level rises. Eventu-ally, as we step back and don the perspective of our inner observer, we realize that negative self-judgment is a learned, damaging, and totally useless habit.

Negative self-judgment never comes from one's inner being. Our soul, spirit, or inner divinity never finds us unworthy. It knows our wholeness and our health. It knows we reside in love. It beams a constant ray of love, encouragement, and support to guide us toward a deeper inner connection and feelings of unity, health, and wholeness.

Some conventional streams of psychotherapy encourage people to delve into the roots of these self-critical messages. This may involve a lengthy examination of various influences, extending back to early childhood. I rarely encourage this sort of exploration, especially in the earlier stages of freeing oneself from anxiety. Exploring the roots of a problem may keep people hooked in to the problem rather than the solutions. Generally, if one needs to understand a reason for a thought pattern to find relief, insight about it will come up in the present, without having to dig around in past unpleasantness.

To shift, try dedicating to self-acceptance and inner peace. This may not be easy at first. If an individual has been self-critical for a long time, he or she may find a need to return to kindness, patience, and humor over and over again. That is okay! Once again, practice, practice, practice. Interrupt negative self-talk whenever you notice it, and you will begin to hear less of it.

Remember that you are doing the best you can. I know this. Through years of my own anxiety and working with patients who struggle, I saw that no one wants to feel anxious. So when your mind chatter begins to gnaw at you, you can respond to yourself, "I am doing the best I can. I am trying to feel better." There may be a voice inside you that will argue with that, telling you that you are bad, wrong, unworthy. You do not need to argue or reason with that unkind voice. It is not rational. It is not your inner being, or your soul. You can acknowledge that the self-critical voice is there, but you are now letting yourself focus elsewhere.

Dialogue of Kindness

It can be helpful to regard the self-deprecating inner voice as one would a small child who does not know better. There is an art to learning gentleness with ourselves. Think about how you would treat a baby, a kitten, a puppy, or a tiny bird. Most of us would treat them gently, indulgently, and patiently.

We deserve this for ourselves too. You are that baby, that small child, that little bird. A self-critical inner voice is often formed early in childhood as a protective response to uncontrollable life stressors. Many of us are unaware that we have a choice whether to identify with that fearful self-deprecating voice or with the quiet, peaceful, loving, inner wisdom. One way to unhook from our self-critical thoughts is by a dialogue of kindness with them. Instead of mentally arguing with them, we can appreciate and thank them for their past contributions to our well-being. Let yourself understand that you developed these habits of thought by trying to protect a younger, more vulnerable part of yourself. Explain to the thoughts that you no longer need or want this type of protection.

We can feel our emotions compassionately. We can be kind to ourselves no matter what we are feeling. Even difficult emotions are never a justification for beating ourselves up. Compassion also means letting go of negative self-talk about negative self-talk. Saying things like "Why is this taking so long?" "I am just not getting this," or "I am no good at this" are all more ways to dig the emotional hole deeper.

Look at your beliefs about yourself. Allow yourself to shift those that no longer serve you. Another way you can let them drop is by deliberately telling new, kinder stories. For example, you might replace self-defeating thoughts with milder ones. Here are some examples: "I will get better at this eventually," "I really want to feel better, and I know that my feelings will improve," "It is okay if it takes a while," "It is okay for me to develop my skills at self-soothing and shifting my feelings," "Improvement will take as long as it takes, and I know it will be helpful if I can be as nice as possible to myself along my journey."

More Tools for Letting Go

Letting go gives us freedom, and freedom is the only
condition for happiness.

–Thich Nhat Hanh[4]

1. Developing Our Inner Observer

Another important group of tools for finding our inner lake of peace involves
letting go. When we participate in our seemingly incessant internal dialogue,
we may eventually wonder who, exactly, is listening? Inside our heart is a
quiet, peaceful, nonjudgmental observer. Our observer is not affected by
emotional ups and downs, our personal life dramas, or by the events of the
external world. It is our observer, at the core of our being, that teaches us
to let go as we begin identify with it rather than with all the hubbub of
our moment-to-moment experience and our mental chatter about it. We can
learn to come into alignment with the observer, to find the freedom and
peace that is always present. Merely asking the question "who is listening to
all this?" starts to bring the observer into awareness. There are many effective tools to let go and *be* the observer who is always at the heart of you, free,
serene, and peaceful. Here are some that I have found particularly useful.

2. Movie on a Screen

Early in my process of spiritual development, I learned the idea of visualizing
all of our experience, including our internal banter, as a movie on a screen.
This was during the early 1970s. At the time a process called "Sensurround"
that supposedly enhanced the audio experience of movies was widely adver-
tised. The 1974 movie *Earthquake* was the most famous example of this audio
technology. While I never saw that movie, I did think a lot about how the
external world surrounds our senses. As a science fiction buff, I speculated
about movies and performances that might have not only enhanced audio
but also 3-D visuals as well as tactile and olfactory inputs. Clearly I was not

the only one to think this way; the idea is the basic concept of the dystopian movie *The Matrix.*

Metaphorically, it was very easy to see "the world stage" as part of a holographic, very compelling movie. I realized that we are living in that "movie," and that it is quite persuasive. In *As You Like It,* Shakespeare said something similar, in one of his most famous passages:

> All the world's a stage,
> And all the men and women merely players:
> They have their exits and their entrances;
> And one man in his time plays many parts.

But with a movie or a play, there is always someone watching. I speculated about that too, asking myself, "Who is watching the movie of my life?" I perceived the events of my life passing by on my personal screen. I recognized that my opinions, beliefs, observations, and judgments were all part of the movie. All my interactions, my conversations, and my activities were there, and I noticed too that there was someone who was also me, who was gently, uncritically, and peacefully observing, without categorizing or assigning meaning. This inner me knew it was all a movie. I found the inner observer quite intriguing. The observer seemed to uniformly enjoy and appreciate every show, without judgment, and with compassion. Over time, I noticed that my inner observer was not limited in location to my physical body—it could be "bigger" than me—and I began to play with that concept too.

Remembering that this inner observer exists is deeply comforting to me. There is a coming-home feeling in noticing the presence of the inner peace that listens non-critically. I believe this observer is our spirit, our divinity, and our deepest inner sense of knowing. It forms a space in and around each of us, in which we are always invited to reside in wholeness and love.

During the same time period of my life that I was thinking about "Sensurround," when I was eighteen years old, I had a powerful experience where I briefly, but fully, donned the perspective of the observer. It was as if I completely switched channels to the broadcast of eternal divine love, and knew the wholeness and perfection of all. I knew that everything was okay and always would be. I was aware of myself as "Marcey" the whole time, but I had a feeling of utter peace and wholeness. Ironically, this actually happened in a movie theatre, during a movie I cannot even recall. The experience seemed timeless, but probably lasted about ten minutes. I wrote about this in more detail in my first book, *Transforming the Nature of Health*.

So try this for yourself. See if you can imagine that your life is a play, a holographic movie, or a vivid illusion. Step back, throughout your day, and "watch the movie" of your life. Notice your roles. Observe your responses. See if you this helps you locate your inner observer.

3. Just Ask

Another way to be the observer is simply to ask it of yourself in any moment. Say to yourself that you would like to see things as your soul sees them, or as your inner being sees them. It is like changing lenses or looking at the world from a different perspective. Then relax. It is difficult to receive an answer while you are still focused on asking the question. I find it helpful to ask and then focus on my breathing, or the ringing of some lovely wind chimes I have positioned outside my bedroom, and then let the shift happen. Sometimes this is just for a flash or a moment, and then I am back into my "monkey mind." But even that flash is enough to notice that the whole world opens up, and things that I thought were worrisome are, in fact, no big deal.

4. Being with What Is

Another way to let go and experience our inner observer is simply being with what is, without trying to change it, or push it away. All our feelings, even those that seem painful, are deeply empowering. We can sit with our feelings, noticing them, without digging in, judging, or justification, just as our inner observer does. Without saying to ourselves "this is good or this is bad." Without commenting internally or externally. Merely acknowledging a feeling and sitting with it, experiencing it, breathing into it, or feeling it in our body is very empowering and soothing. To flow, emotions need to be allowed and experienced. They have information for us. When we try to escape them, they can feel more insistent. This is certainly the case with anxiety.

One way to be with a painful feeling like fear is merely to gently acknowledge it. You can notice and feel the feelings without digging in deeper. Even through unpleasant feelings we can simply be with our self, with kindness. You might say to yourself something like "This anxiety feels terrible right now; I am in an uncomfortable place," or "I do not like this feeling." As you just sit with your emotions and breath, often there is naturally a shifting. Emotions can shift to a place of greater ease, even peace, rather quickly when we let ourselves simply experience them rather than trying to force them away.

5. Dropping the Thoughts

Another way to let go is to focus on the feelings alone and not the thoughts that trigger them. It does not usually matter why you feel anxious right now. In this moment, there is little you can do to change the current circumstances in your life. There is nothing you can do about the past, and very little you can do about the future. Right now there is only Now. You cannot affect the presentation you will give tomorrow, whether your loved one will recover from his illness, whether what you said to a friend made her angry with you, whether the bank will repossess your house, how the U.S. political situation will affect the global economy, or the global climate. Worrying about those thoughts, and others like them, just digs your emotional hole deeper. But you can say to yourself, "Right now I feel anxious" or "Right now I feel sad," without having to mentally add some reason or justification about why you feel how you do. You can feel the emotion and at the same time drop the story line. This provides a great deal of relief and allows the emotions to flow.

At happier moments, we can allow pleasant emotions to flow without a story line. While it is seemingly easy to experience pleasant emotions, in actuality, often we skip over them. We can be hurrying on to the next experience, or be busy comparing the present to a past moment. *Be Here Now* was the delightful title of a book by spiritual teacher Ram Dass, and is a fun contemporary song by Ray Lamontagne. It is worthwhile for our emotional flow to practice "being here now" by relaxing and noticing delightful feelings when they occur.

6. Finding Emotions in One's Body

Another tool for letting go is to note where you feel your emotions in your body. Different ones might show up in different places. Often people who are distressed are not aware of their body, yet their body is giving them valuable information about the situation. Personally, my tension generally goes into my shoulders. If I am very tense I can also get heartburn or feel like my stomach is in a knot. I have worked with patients who had various physical symptoms of anxiety.

Asthma, for example, is widely acknowledged, even among conventionally minded physicians, to have a significant emotional component. Chinese medicine explains that breathing is about the present moment, and often shortness of breath reflects a discomfort with being in the here and now.

When we notice our emotions in our body we can consciously begin to release the tension in those areas. Again we can drop the story line, as we work out the physical kinks. We can apply body-centered breathing techniques. We can stretch with yoga or movement. We can get some bodywork or do some self-acupressure or self-massage. There are many ways we can consciously encourage a tense body area to relax.

In his book *Waking the Tiger,* Peter Levine observed that after a stressful event, animals in the wild instinctively tremble, shake, stretch, yawn, or do any number of other physical releases to allow their nervous systems to rebalance. I have found deliberate shaking, trembling, howling, and yawning to be very helpful for myself and many of my patients.

7. Notice That You Have a Range of Emotions Every Day

This is a letting-go technique that expands upon the tools for awareness of emotions. I have heard some people say that they "always" feel terrible, anxious, or worried. It gives us substantial relief to acknowledge to ourself that this is an exaggeration that we do not want to claim as our identity. In twenty-five years of medical practice, I have never met anyone who "always feels anxious" in every moment of every day. Just observe, for example, that if you read the sentence above and felt amused, irritated, or annoyed, you were not feeling anxious at that moment. Statements such as "I always" can indicate a self-limiting belief. Notice the things you say to yourself that might be self-limiting beliefs, and let them drop. You do not need to claim an identity that feels uncomfortable to you. There is a big difference between the statements "I frequently feel anxious" and "I always feel anxious."

The feeling of anxiety is certainly compelling and unpleasant. When it is persistent, it seems consuming. But we each have a range of emotions every day. If we are in a difficult period of our lives, our daily emotions may predominantly shift through fear, anxiety, anger, frustration, irritation, and boredom. None of those feel too good. I have felt this way myself. But I realized that even at my worst, I did not always feel horrible. Sometimes I felt neutral; sometimes I was even distracted by something pleasant. Even in very anxious periods of time, I might be momentarily amused by a mockingbird's song, appreciate a lovely cloud formation, or be moved by the beauty of the Milky Way. I might enjoy the scent of fresh pine needles, be mesmerized by a flickering flame, or appreciate the flavor of a delicious food.

Mark or note the emotions you feel in a day. Anxious persons may tend to notice over and over again when they are anxious, while ignoring or discounting the other feelings they have. Prove to yourself that you have a range of emotions by checking in with yourself as often as possible. When you repeatedly ask yourself, "How do I feel now?" the answers will vary.

8. I Will Not Always Feel This Way

Noticing the fluidity of our emotions helps us to feel less stuck, while noticing an unpleasant emotion repeatedly and perseverating on it makes us feel more stuck. Feeling stuck increases anxiety. Arguing for limitations, as in "No, I really *do* feel anxious all the time," increases the tension. Even if you are feeling anxious in a moment, it will pass. Try saying this to yourself when you are noticing worried thoughts. "This feeling will pass. I will not always feel this way." This sentence was one important nugget from my personal journey. Sometimes when I felt horribly tense I would just say to myself: "Well, I will not always feel like this." This was a breath of fresh air and always took the tension down a notch, nudging me toward my quiet, contented observer.

9. Looking at the Bigger Picture

This is another letting-go tool I learned from Abraham. When in distress, try backing out and focusing on the bigger picture. What does this mean? Abraham explains that when we are anxious or fearful, we are usually focusing specifically on something unwanted. Our specific focus on negative details is what triggers escalating stress. The more we do it, the worse it gets. Abraham advises "backing out" by finding more general things along the same lines to think about. Eventually, as we back out, consciously choosing to be less negative, we usually find that our emotions are more calm and neutral.

For example, I used to worry that a loved one's plane might crash. I knew this was unreasonable, but at times I would get anxious about it. Continuing to worry and mentally paint undesired scenarios certainly would increase my anxiety. But I found that I could back out, go more general, and find relief. Thoughts such as "I and my loved ones have traveled safely often," "Even our bumpy flights in inclement weather landed safely," and "Airplane accidents are big news precisely because they are so rare," and "Air travel is safer than auto travel" were often quite soothing and would take me somewhat in the direction of a more general, bigger picture. Remembering the words to Rheinhold Neiber's Serenity Prayer can also comfort me a great deal:

> God grant me the serenity
> to accept the things I cannot change;
> courage to change the things I can;
> and wisdom to know the difference.
> Living one day at a time.

I recognized that just acknowledging that my loved one's aircraft was not something I had control over could allow me to relax and enjoy the present moment. I found relief with bigger-picture thoughts such as "This is not something I have control over, and my worrying will not make it better or worse for them, it will only make my experience more unpleasant right now," or "If it is their time to go, then it is their time," and "We are all eternal beings, and love persists from lifetime to lifetime."

Personally, by the time I get to "we are all eternal beings," I am always in a much better space. There is no need to argue with negative thoughts. I just notice them, back out, go general, and allow them to fade.

10. Once Again, Practice Many Times Per Day

If some of these tools feel helpful to you, practice them throughout your day. I said this earlier in the book and it bears repeating. It is great to have tools that we can apply when we are at our most stressed, but we get fluidity and ease if we show ourselves that we can improve emotionally while in a variety of situations. Try not to wait until you are in distress to practice these exercises.

CHAPTER 4

❧

Moving Up the Scale

As we have learned thus far, we can calmly get in touch with ourselves by observing our emotional responses to life's circumstances. Our feelings are information, letting us know what works, or doesn't work so well, in our lives. Physically, emotions are a response of the body and brain, mediated by various neurochemicals. Psychologically, emotions are the response (at a number of levels) of conscious awareness to subconscious and unconscious thoughts, beliefs, motivations, and actions. Our emotional responses may teach us about parts of ourselves that are not in our conscious awareness. Spiritually, how our emotions feel to us is a key to the communication and guidance that our soul/spirit is offering our physical self, to guide us toward greater well-being.

Since emotions are merely information, there are no good or bad, right or wrong emotions. But there are emotions that feel quite wonderful, and ones that feel horrible, as well as everything in between, including placidity, nonchalance, and other essentially neutral emotions. We may feel bad or good about an emotion, but it is still simply information. As we step back from feeling and observe what is being offered, we can gain tremendous insight. From a detached but curious perspective, each emotional response we generate can give us new questions and new subsequent answers to ponder, extending our self-awareness.

For example, several years ago I went for an extended weekend retreat to Wilbur Hot Springs, a serene sanctuary about two hours north of the San Francisco Bay Area. Each visitor at Wilbur brings his or her own food to prepare as they wish, with each assigned storage in a part of a refrigerator, including a corresponding shelf on the door. At this particular visit, I loaded up my shelves, putting my special raw milk and raw cream, along with some other dairy items, on the appropriate door shelf, which happened to be an upper one. When I came back that evening to prepare dinner, my milk and other door items had been moved to the bottom shelf. They were not used, discarded, or opened—just moved to the bottom shelf. Still, I had an extreme emotional reaction; I felt violated and upset. I practically started crying right there in the group kitchen, and my heart began to pound. But I could also see that the situation was absurd, and obviously inconsequential, so I was immediately able to acknowledge that my distraught emotional response could not possibly be solely due to someone moving my groceries to a different shelf. This proved to be a great opportunity for me to step back and look at many deeper interwoven issues about trust, security, and personal space. Since I had three days at Wilbur to contemplate, I was able to heal many old hurts that I found knotted up in that initial blast of emotion. I now bless whomever it was that moved my milk, because it resulted in rewarding self-exploration, self-awareness, and much greater inner harmony. By the end of the weekend, my thoughts about the incident had only positive emotional charge.

Emotions Shift as We Shift Focus

Our emotions are not static; they change as we change our thoughts and focus. My Wilbur vignette is just one simple, now playful, example of the power for personal growth that is available in any situation, even an upsetting or disturbing one. We can always step back from an emotional response to look more deeply at ourselves with eyes of love. Stepping back allows us to see that we always have more than one perspective. We are simultaneously both the person who experiences our lives and the person who observes our experience of our lives. As we step back, we can don the perspective of the observer. This is what I did at Wilbur. I had my experience and then saw it anew in its complexity, with the eyes of a loving, amused observer. From this new vantage point we may acknowledge that what we really want is to feel better. The best time to improve how we feel is always in the present moment.

The contemporary spiritual teacher Abraham offers numerous helpful and uplifting exercises. As readers probably have noticed, I have utilized and suggested several of these over the years, generally with overwhelmingly positive results both personally and professionally. To help facilitate shifting emotions, try a tool that has been profoundly useful to me and many of my patients called "the emotional scale," the essence of which is simply too good to leave out of this book. Abraham's emotional scale is best outlined in their bestselling work *Ask and It Is Given*. One chapter of the book outlines a scale of twenty-two emotions from a low point of despair to a high point of bliss. With patients, I often work with a ladder inspired by and overlapping with the Abraham-Hicks scale that utilizes many of the "letting-go" tools.

The midpoint of the emotional scale is somewhere around placidity or nonchalance. These are essentially neutral emotions. Above, in more or less ascending order, are contentment, serenity, hopefulness, satisfaction, gratitude, harmony, peacefulness, optimism, pleasure, invigoration, delight, enthusiasm, exuberance, inspiration, exhilaration, joy, radiance, euphoria, and bliss. I have observed that there is more physical and emotional energy available to individuals as the scale ascends. For example, in my medical practice, my overall happiest patients are often brimming with vitality as well. This makes some sense as we consider it. Think about four-year-old children. An exuberant child is more energized than one who is merely enthusiastic, and an enthusiastic child has more energy than a hopeful one. Still, in adults, all of these are pleasant states, and most people who are doing well much of the time will move back and forth between contentment and serenity, and enthusiasm, joy, and even bliss. The more peaceful states of well-being are nourishing resting states, allowing integration and respite, while the more dynamic states are creative and expansive. Abraham also points out that with each move up the scale, there is more personal empowerment and more alignment with our inner being and our true purpose.

Below neutral, in more or less descending order, are indifference, boredom, listlessness, annoyance, overwhelm, crankiness, disgruntlement, irritability, pessimism, confusion, frustration, apprehension, alarm, contempt, anger, rage, anguish, anxiety, powerlessness, despair, desolation, hopelessness. As the scale descends, each emotion has less energy, and I have observed that many patients who frequently experience these lower-register emotions also complain of fatigue. This is not to say that everyone who is fatigued is unhappy, and everyone who is energetic is happy. These are general trends that, like statistics, do not necessarily apply to each individual. But people who often focus in the lower range of the emotional register generally experience fewer feelings of personal empowerment. I find that an emotional lack of personal power can often translate to less physical vitality.

We can be at different set points on different topics. For example, I recently saw a patient who struggles with her chronic health problems, but who has a very happy forty-year marriage to a wonderfully supportive partner. She is in the highest part of the emotional scale when she thinks of her husband and marriage, but dips near the bottom when she worries about her health and the toll it may take on their lives.

Abraham teaches that while individuals can theoretically move all the way up the scale from despair to bliss in a half hour or so, it usually takes more time. Most of us do not leap from emotional states at the lowest end of the scale, like fear, powerlessness, or rage, to ones at the highest end of the scale, like bliss, serenity, and joy, without traveling through the intermediate territory. They teach that every improvement up the scale is worthwhile, if it is embraced with self-awareness. With each gradation of improvement, there is more personal power and greater ease. Thus anger, though it still feels awful, is a much better feeling than powerlessness, and so it is an important step on the road away from despair. Irritation, though it still feels crummy, is a much better feeling than anger, and a further step up the ladder.

The improvement that individuals feel as they shift up the scale results from a lowering of "resistance" with each incremental step. I find the concept of resistance easier to understand in physical science. In physics, resistance is friction. Friction inevitably slows things down. Perpetual motion exists only in a frictionless environment. Bliss would be the emotional equivalent of a frictionless experience. Emotional resistance is similar to a physical force, like having one's legs mired in mud. If the mud is very thick, it is like cement and very hard to get out of. But if the mud is diluted, it becomes easier to move through. I liken lowering resistance to diluting the thick mud. So, for example, if you are angry and look instead for feelings of irritation and annoyance about the same subject, you will notice a slight improvement in your emotions, and more feelings of freedom and personal power. You have watered down the difficult emotion and now have greater ease.

While occasionally some people are able to make a great shift in a brief amount of time, many will hang out in an intermediate state for a while (hours, days, or weeks) as they acknowledge and incorporate the relief that comes from the lowered resistance. As you use this tool, let yourself experience the improvement achieved through moving up the scale. Consciously feel the relief generated from moving feelings of despair into feelings of anger, or feelings of anger to feelings of irritation and mild annoyance, or feelings of irritation into boredom or placidity. Sense them in your body, heart, and mind. Notice the improvement and congratulate yourself. This affirms that although things are not yet rosy, they are moving in a better direction and you have noticed.

It is best not to take action or make decisions from a place that feels less than good. Often when we are distressed we cannot make an informed choice, because anxiety prevents us from tuning in to the full range of possibilities available. Without a clear picture, one that includes much of the good stuff, we may take actions that are not in our best interest. Whenever possible, postpone taking action or making important decisions until you have reached a state where you feel happy, relaxed, and joyful, or at least more joyful. It is when we are in the upper register of emotions that we make the best choices and have the most rewarding life experiences, since in those states we have more information available to us.

Following Emotional Guidance

Tracking how emotions feel can inform us as to whether or not thoughts and actions resonate with improved well-being. Instead of looking at emotions as pesky troublemakers, or constantly trying to override them with reason, we might instead consider relying on them as indicators of the direction of our focus. We can use this guidance as information to direct subsequent thoughts. Emotions can let you know if you are moving toward well-being or away from it. They let you know if you are moving up or down the scale.

How does this work? Simply put, "if it truly feels good, it is good for you right now," while conversely "bad feels bad."

Steps for Moving Up the Scale

These steps build upon the tools presented in the last few chapters. You can do them while in any emotional state, even if you are feeling pretty good. It can be delightful fun to move up the scale from happiness to even better emotions. Try to "move up the scale" in a variety of contexts.

1. Begin with an emotional temperature check. Notice how you feel right now. Acknowledge how you feel. Let yourself experience your emotions for a little while. Try not to judge yourself. Just feel, without taking any other action. If you are able to, you may notice where you experience particular emotions in your body. Don't worry if it is not clear to you.

2. Perhaps consider what you were doing or thinking that generated the unpleasant emotion (or current emotion if you are feeling pretty good). This step may be useful, especially if it is a frequently experienced emotion, but it is not essential. If clarity does not come quickly, move on.

3. Now let go of your story about WHY you feel the way you do, and simply feel your feelings.

4. Acknowledge that you want to feel better, right now.

5. Find a thought that emotionally feels slightly better. Abraham says here: "You are not looking for the best-feeling thought you've ever had, just something that is an improvement." This is important! When we try to reach too far too fast, it can be difficult to make the jump. The better-feeling thought may be more general, since distressing thoughts are more often quite specific.

6. Feel the emotions you have in response to the new, improved thought. You should feel freer, as if the thick mud you were stuck in has been diluted. Congratulate yourself, and notice your relief.

7. You can then rest a bit in this improved place, go on to another task, or try to move up a little more by repeating the process.

Here is an example of moving up the scale from one of my patients, a middle-aged activist we will call "Estelle." She had been noticing increased anxiety and fatigue over the previous two years and was intrigued by this technique.

1. Estelle noticed that she was feeling powerless, like things were out of control in many areas of her life. She felt scared, small, and fearful. She acknowledged how she felt and sensed the emotions in her mind and body, noticing that she experienced them mostly in her shoulders and stomach.

2. She saw had been worrying, once again, about world problems: poverty, injustice, environmental destruction, global warming, starvation, and global fascism. This was a frequent train of thought that always left her feeling disempowered, anxious, and hopeless. She would end up with very dark thoughts that compounded upon one another, thoughts like "the Earth is just going to wipe us all out" or "we are already in a fascism-controlled society and the people are asleep."

3. Next, she dropped the story line and allowed herself to feel the physical and emotional feelings without any mental focus on the "reasons."

4. She acknowledged that she wanted to feel better. This was easy to do, because the emotions she had been experiencing were painful and clearly leading her nowhere pleasant. Nor were they changing the world.

5. She looked for thoughts that felt a little better. Since she was in an emotional space of feeling despair and powerlessness, she practiced purposefully becoming angry. It was easy for her to find targets for her anger: large corporations, greedy individuals, corrupt politicians, and an uncaring, self-absorbed populace. She was used to feeling angry when focusing on these thoughts, but now she was

also noticing how the feelings of anger were an emotional improvement over powerlessness. This time she took this step consciously and noticed that the anger feelings gave her a great deal of relief from the hopeless and disempowered feelings.

6. She again dropped the story line and let herself just feel her anger, appreciating the whoosh of feelings of personal power that came with letting go of hopelessness. Anger, while still not great, did feel a lot better! How had she never noticed before all the improvement in her emotions from this shift?

7. She decided to move up a little more. Now, from a place of feeling angry, she decided to move up to irritation. She thought about one particular pet peeve, littering, and those who leave their trash strewn in public parks. Then she considered some Facebook friends who had different political beliefs from her, whom she considered misguided and misinformed, and how irritating she found their political posts to be. Whenever she noted a thought that felt better than her angry state, she gave it a boost by thinking about it a little longer, at the same time moving away from thoughts that felt like they were going back toward anger. She noticed that she could navigate by how her thoughts felt. She noticed her relief, observing greater calm in the feeling of irritation than in the feeling of anger.

8. She let herself let go of the stories again, simply feeling her emotions. This clearly felt better than how she felt ten minutes earlier, and Estelle congratulated herself. "This really works," she thought.

9. Then she noticed that she was feeling a little bored with the whole thing and felt like doing something else. Boredom, she knew from our discussions, was a further improvement up from irritation, one with little emotional charge. She let herself drop the topic and the exercise for a while, resting in the feelings of boredom that were "miles away" from where she had started out a little while earlier. Feeling and acknowledging a great deal of relief, Estelle went for a walk, with a much improved emotional state.

CHAPTER 5

Meditation

Meditation is a process that teaches us to transcend the chatter of the thinking mind. It assists with greater clarity and joy of being. Scientifically, meditation has been shown to have as much benefit for relaxation as light sleep. Meditation can be fun and easy, even for those who have not had "success" with it in the past. There are multitudes of ways to meditate, and this chapter explains several of them. By exploring a variety of techniques you can find those that appeal to you right now. The ideal choice of meditation styles is highly personal. There is not one right way.

Meditation is found in most if not all religious traditions, but there is nothing inherently religious about it. Some ways to meditate involve chanting phrases or utilizing tools of a particular faith such as a rosary or mala. But most meditation techniques are non-denominational, completely unrelated to religious beliefs. Atheists and agnostics can and do successfully meditate. Meditation is a natural condition of mind for human beings, and for animals as well. In a meditative state, our brainwave patterns become slower and more coherent.

Some people say, "I can't meditate." This is not true! Meditation is a skill that anyone can learn. All babies and most small children have the brainwave patterns of adept meditators. If you could do it at three months, you can do it now. The ability is hard-wired into our systems. If you are someone who has had a negative experience of meditation in the past, try some different techniques. For example, a movement meditation is often better for people who are squirmy. Only attempt techniques that feel good to you. The purpose of meditation is to relax, feel better, gain perspective, and calm the mind. If a technique makes you jittery or anxious, move on and try another one. Many people with anxiety find it difficult to do "traditional" sitting meditation with the eyes closed. That is fine! There are many other options including walking meditation, eyes-open meditation in a natural setting, or work with bowls or chanting. One might begin with simple breathing exercises like those in chapter 8.

The keys for successfully learning meditation can be summed up with "Practice, practice, and practice," and have fun. Remember, you are fine just as you are. A big part of the benefit of meditation comes merely from assuming a beginner's mind and making time in your day for an inward journey. My friend, writer Susan Gorell, a long-time meditator, explains: "I've heard it said that the benefit of meditation is in taking the posture of meditation, which to me means forming and carrying out the intention to do a good thing for one's self."

So don't judge your progress by anyone else's. You will actually progress faster and farther when you do not compare yourself. Most of all, enjoy your experience! Eventually you will find a form of meditation that is perfect for you and will anticipate those treasured moments of peace.

Meditation Basics

The object of meditation is quieting the thinking mind in order to allow the wholeness of being to emerge. This leads to a deep sense of inner peace. Meditation helps the inner observer move from the background into the foreground. When you meditate, you usually provide the mind something to lightly focus upon, because it keeps it occupied while you are relaxing. It is much easier, especially at first, to have something relatively mindless or repetitive to focus upon than it is to completely let go of thought. You can take your pick of objects of focus: try your breath, or the sound of the rain, or your footsteps if you are walking, or the hum of your air conditioner, or the sound of the ocean, or a mantra, or phrase that you repeat to yourself either silently or out loud. The focus could also be a visualization, such as a strong oak tree or a rainbow crystal inside your core, or a special place in nature that makes you calm.

You are likely to notice that thoughts arise. Thinking is inevitable. As these thoughts arise, release them. You might imagine them floating away in a bubble, like the one the good witch Glenda floated in on in *The Wizard of Oz*. Or see the thoughts dissolve, like sugar in water, or erase them like writing on a chalkboard, or let an imaginary vacuum cleaner suck them away, or blink, or simply turn away from them and refocus on whatever you are choosing to focus on—your steps, your breath, the sound of the wind in the trees, or the reverberations of a singing bowl. Put an overly active mind to work on two things at once, like following the breath as well as one's steps, or the breath plus a word or mantra.

Always be kind to yourself when you notice there is a thought, even if you happen to observe that you were traveling on a particular thought train for quite a while before you even noticed. An extended period of time may have passed since you last thought of your meditative object of focus. That is alright. Whenever you notice that you have a thought, just release it then. If it is something that you really want to think about, remind yourself that you can think about it later, when you are done meditating. Your perspective after meditation will usually be more fresh and relaxed.

Should your eyes be open or closed? Again, it's up to you. Many people when first studying meditation find it less distracting to have the eyes closed. Visual stimuli can be like a flood of thoughts. But there are powerful meditation techniques that employ simply being present with the visual world, eyes open, and not cataloging or mentally commenting upon it. Gazing at a candle flame, a landscape, a piece of art, or a crystal can work as a focal point, not a distraction.

While the eventual goal of meditating is having no thought, this takes some practice, and there is no hurry. This will happen eventually of its own accord in a way that is natural for you. At first "no thought" occurs in brief snippets. Sooner or later these episodes become protracted. Eventually in meditating you may get to a place where you are actually "not thinking" much of the time. Sometimes there are insights that come after these episodes; sometimes you feel that your inner being or higher consciousness is "thinking you"; and sometimes there is just a peaceful stillness, like a serene lake on a calm sunny day. At these times, people feel well-being, ease, and a sensation of knowing that all is well. Often, when meditation is deep or prolonged, a flash of insight can be experienced regarding a persistent problem, or a blast of creative inspiration arrives. These come from the deepest part of you, your essence, and your wisest inner self.

Techniques for Seated Meditation

Here are a few of the most popular and time-tested techniques for seated meditation. Many of them can also be used in walking and movement mediations.

Following the Breath

This common technique involves little more than mentally watching and following the breath as it flows in and out, in and out. There is no force or changing of the breathing pattern, except when it occurs naturally. When there are thoughts, gently let go of them and return to focus on the breath.

A subtype of following breath is to focus only on the out breath. Let the inhalation be neutral, but observe the exhalation. This out-breath meditation focus is common in certain schools of Vipassana meditation and in Continuum movement. Some people find this variation useful in letting go of attachments.

Listening to Your Heartbeat

In a silent room or space, tune in to the gentle rhythm of your heart. Place your awareness in the center of your chest. Listen inside, connecting with the rhythm of your heart. This type of meditation is simple where it is quiet but can be impossible in a noisy environment.

A subtype of this meditation is to feel the rhythm of the heart rather than listening for it. This can be performed by feeling the pulse at thumb side of the inner wrist, or by placing one's hand on one's chest. Connecting with the heart via either of these methods can be quite calming.

Breathing Words

With this technique the practitioner matches breathing with thoughts of a word or simple phrase. *Love, peace, freedom,* and *ease* are commonly used words for breathing, as are short phrases like *ease and flow, well-being abounds, all is well,* and *it's all okay.* So, for example, one might breathe in love, and breathe out love, thinking the word "love" on both the in-breath and the out-breath. Again, breaths do not have to be deep or shallow; the normal rhythm of your breath is perfect. As for choosing words or phrases, the ones above are just a few suggestions. Find words that suit you at the time of meditation.

Mantra Meditation

This is the mental or verbal repetition of a simple sound or phrase. The word *mantra* is from Sanskrit and connotes a sound, syllable, word, or group of words or phrase that can produce spiritual transformation. Repetition of the mantra can be linked with breath, or it may be purely a repeated thought, without attention to breath. Many mantra meditations are associated with various religious and spiritual groups, but there is nothing inherent in the use of these tools that requires a religious affiliation. Beginning meditators may find it useful to repeat the mantra out loud, with the outbreath.

Here are some examples of mantras I learned in my own journey. My first experience of meditation practice was at age sixteen, when I learned Transcendental Meditation (TM) and was assigned the mantra *Hay-Ying.* I did not know what it meant, or even if it had a meaning, but did I find it soothing to repeat it in my mind. I did this without focus on breath. Years later, I took a class from the Ananda Marga organization and was given another mantra, *Ham-So.* Now and then I still use either of these mantras.

Common mantras not associated with a particular faith or organization include *OM* (or *AUM*), said by some to be the original sound of creation, and *So-ham,* from the Sanskrit, meaning "I am that." A common Sanskrit phrase mantra is *Om Mane Padme Hum.* This is the six-syllable mantra of Avalokiteshvara, the Buddhist Bodhisattva of Compassion. Many languages have a common mantra such as *Shalom* in Hebrew and *Salaam* in Arabic, both words meaning "peace."

Chanting is a subclass of mantra meditation whereby a syllable, word, phrase, intention, or sound is repeated aloud for a few minutes or an extended period. This is sometimes done in groups, particularly religious groups, but (again) it can be used as desired. Chanting *OM* can be a good place to start if one is attracted to chanting but has no experience with this form of meditation. It can help tame a monkey mind to say something out loud and focus on that.

Auditory Meditations

This involves listening to something external, usually a repetitive sound, and focusing upon that. The basic tenets of meditation apply. Many different sounds can be selected for meditative listening.

One of my favorite ways to meditate is to listen to the sound of the rain. I find this quite peaceful and relaxing during the winter rainy season here in Northern California. Gentle repetitive music is also a good choice, as is the sound of waves by an ocean, or a recording of waves, or listening to waters in a fountain or the babbling sounds of a river rushing. But one could just as easily listen to the hum from an air conditioner or the sound of the dishwasher running, if you find those soothing. I have known patients with tinnitus who have embraced that, and they now listen to the high-pitched whistle in their ears to good effect. But ideally, any sound that you find soothing is best for an auditory meditation focus.

Bowl Meditations

There are a number of wonderful types of singing bowls available. Traditional Asian singing bowls, made from hammered metals (usually brass or copper), are available in various sizes. They make a prolonged, resonant ringing sound when struck by a mallet. Crystal bowls are a more modern invention, operating on the same principle. When gently struck or rubbed with a mallet, they resonate a particular note. I have three hand-hammered Tibetan singing bowls that produce beautiful harmonious sounds, and often enjoy using this meditation technique, as it involves meditatively striking the bowl, hearing sound, and feeling physical vibration. I love to feel the subtle sensation of vibration in my body as the bowls are sounded. I find the whole experience very soothing and centering.

I have a friend who loves crystal singing bowls. These are tuned to specific notes, and he has become adept at creating 30- to 60-minute healing voyages with a variety of bowls, since all types of bowls can help with attaining a deep meditative state.

Guided Meditations and Visualizations

Guided visualizations can be a segue to other forms of meditation or a preferred stand-alone method. Some people simply relax better when there is verbal guidance, either a little or a lot. There is a vast array of products for meditation support on the market. Many that I have experienced are quite lovely. I have recorded a few guided meditations myself, and they are available on my website, including one from my last book.[1]

Some of my favorites are Hemi-Sync Meditations. For more information on these, see "Binaural Beats" below. Channeled meditations are a subclass of guided meditations, offered by various channels of non-physical energy. Two that I have personally enjoyed a lot are the many meditations by Orin and Daben, and The Vortex meditations by Abraham-Hicks. You can make your own guided meditations, writing a script of something you would like to hear, with your own phrasing and pacing, then recording and listening to it.

Meditation Immersions

Many religious and non-denominational groups offer meditation and contemplation retreats. Some of these are specifically geared to a particular tradition, while others, even some in centers belonging to particular faiths, welcome anyone in a quiet, supportive environment. Some meditation immersion retreats are facilitated, with a specific program of activities and meals through the day. Others, at various convents, monasteries, and other institutions, provide support such as meals and lodging, and facilities for personal, unstructured meditation retreats. It is not necessary to go to an official institution for a meditation immersion. One can simply choose a place that is tranquil and set up one's own program.

Group Meditations

Meditation with a group may enhance each person's experience. Resonance and other field effects enhance the individual's abilities to achieve deeper meditative states. There are religious and non-denominational group meditations. Many senior centers and community centers offer meditation instruction and group meditations, and more are willing to do so when there are enough interested students.

Binaural Beats

Although binaural beats were discovered in the 1850s, they were not widely utilized until the advent of recording technology.

Robert Monroe, founder of The Monroe Institute, was an originator and pioneer of the field. A "techno-shaman," he and his researchers spent thirty years exploring and mapping the beat frequencies and combinations that easily induce desired states of consciousness, like those of deep meditation. Today Monroe Products offers many titles with embedded binaural beats, sold under the name Hemi-Sync. Listening to these can assist people in achieving deeper states of consciousness and greater calm.

A number of companies have utilized the technology that Monroe developed. Holosync is probably the most well known of these. Today several binaural beat programs are available for free—via open source on the web—and others are sold.

Visual Meditations

There are many subtypes of visual meditation. One is the contemplation of sacred geometry images such as a yantra,[2] focusing upon the image and letting thoughts go. There are several good video programs on the market that flow a variety of sacred geometry images. Light-Source is one I like quite a lot that is done with Hemi-Sync.

As mentioned above, a basic form of visual meditation is simply to sit, stand, or walk with eyes open and let the images of the world flow. Practitioners often focus on the breath as they hold their gaze neutral. This is done without reaction or mental commentary, without naming or internal description of what is seen. It is a form of meditation where one practices being with the whole of what is, without judgment or labeling. Or a specific image, object, or scene can be selected for gazing, to offer the mind a tool for peaceful visual focus. Examples of this sort of tool include gazing at a yantra, a light, a moving body of water, a stone, or any natural setting.

Walking and Movement Meditations

Walking meditations are time-honored in many traditions. They include meditative movement and movement sequences, as well as walking in particular places such as labyrinths. Walking and movement meditations are great for squirmy people, children, and others who find that they are too distracted during siting mediations.

Movement meditations do not always require walking. Patterns can be traced with the finger, or a pen, or even the eyes. Movement can be in a scooter or a wheelchair. Or there can be a meditative program of movements, as in tai qi or bagua. These are discussed in more detail in the next chapter.

Labyrinths

Labyrinths can be found throughout the world. Each has a starting point and a center. Although the two words are sometimes used interchangeably, labyrinths are different from mazes. Mazes are puzzles that allow the participant to choose between several routes. In order to complete a maze, a solution is required. On the other hand, the object of walking a labyrinth is spiritual contemplation. There is only one path into and out of a labyrinth; no choices or decisions are required. Many floor labyrinths are designed in tile or mosaic, though others are laid out with stones or etched in rock.

Labyrinths were well known in antiquity. The word is from the ancient Minoans and was translated to *labyrinthos* by the Greeks. Labyrinths figured prominently in the spiritual practices of earlier eras, among the Minoans, Greeks, Romans, and Egyptians, to name a few cultures that used them. Ancient labyrinths have been found in diverse lands including North America, India (Goa), China, and the Solovetsy Islands in Russia's White Sea. Later they were widely adopted as spiritual contemplative tools in Christianity, incorporated into cathedrals and sacred sites throughout the world. The most famous is the great labyrinth of the Chartres Cathedral in France. Its design provides the template for many others, including the two labyrinths at Grace Cathedral in San Francisco, California.

Most people who walk a labyrinth for spiritual contemplation will ask a question or set an intention at the outset. Upon entering the labyrinth, the participant walks slowly and deliberately, pacing the breathing and footfalls in a meditative manner. In the center of the labyrinth, a few meditative breaths are taken. Sometimes a participant will sit in the center of the labyrinth and meditate or pause there quite a while. That is fine too—there are no rules. When ready, the individual reverses course and walks the path, slowly and contemplatively, out of the labyrinth. Often people meditate just outside of it as well. At Chartres, for example, there are benches nearby for further contemplation. Many people consider a series of three passes into the center and out again a perfect number for an inward journey. Pay attention to any insights you notice during or after your labyrinth experience.

It is easy to make a small outdoor labyrinth. We built a Minoan-style one in our backyard, with homemade stepping stones. There are a number of labyrinth-locating websites that can assist in finding a labyrinth in your area. There are lots of them all over the world, and it is likely there is already one near you. Labyrinths can be drawn with a stick on a sandy beach, mowed in tall grass, drawn with chalk on a tennis court, or laid out on a flat patch of earth. They do not need to be permanent structures.

One simple, free way to explore labyrinths is to trace a path with a finger or with the eyes. When doing so, try the same slow, deliberate meditative pace that you might use if walking a labyrinth. A sample finger labyrinth, tracing the path of the Chartres Cathedral labyrinth, is included on the next page.

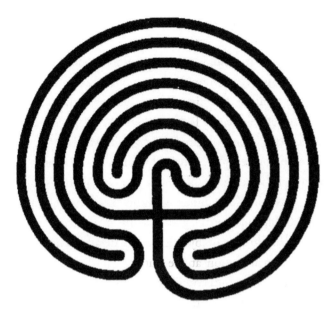

Labyrinth

Meditation during Regular Exercise

It is simple to combine many forms of exercise such as running, walking, and swimming with meditation. To do this, one might add in a mantra, a calming phrase, or a focus on a soothing word like *love, ease,* or *peace.* With each swim stroke or running footfall, mentally repeat the phrase, mantra, or soothing word. This has double benefits: it supports inner peace as well as cardiovascular fitness, and is quite popular with many of my patients.

Several of them prefer a prayer meditation with exercise. I have one friend and patient who swims daily for about an hour. She has a prayer list that she mentally recites during her swims. During her exercise she thinks of various people and situations with thoughts of loving-kindness, compassion, and well-being, holding each person in a mental embrace. This is uplifting to her, and is very likely of benefit to those about whom she prays.

Yoga, tai qi, qi gong, aikido, and bagua are movement and martial arts that can be performed as meditations. Each of these will be discussed in greater detail in the next chapter.

Locations for Meditation

Meditation can be done almost anywhere, indoor or outdoor, in a quiet spot or a busy airport. However, when first learning to meditate, it can be helpful to choose a quiet location. Many people meditate in bed, upon waking in the morning or just before sleep at night. Others have a special space, room, or altar for meditation. There is, again, no one right way.

Meditation in nature can be especially fulfilling and calming. If possible, stand barefoot on the earth, or sit in some grass, soft moss, or hay, or lean against a tree. Have physical contact with the earth to allow any electromagnetic charge that has built up in your system to dissipate into the ground. (The practice of Earthing is discussed in more detail in chapter 7.) This will further assist in your ability to relax.

There are so many settings and times of day that are wonderful for natural meditation. Find a place that inspires you. Water areas are quite popular—choose the ocean, a river, a pond, a creek, or a lake, whatever appeals to you. As to time of day, while any time is fine, some people find extra boost for their meditations just before sunrise and at twilight. In Sufism, the light that shines at dawn before the sun rises and at dusk after it sets is called the *nur*, or *noor*. It is considered to be a special spiritual time of day. Although I am not a Sufi, per se, I have noticed qualities at these times of day that greatly enhance well-being. The dawn bird chorus sings most sweetly before the sun rises and crescendos as the first rays glow on the horizon. Crickets hum, fireflies sparkle, and the air is charged as twilight deepens. Poets and artists have also noticed the special, invigorating characteristics of this time of day, and there are several poems, songs, and even a movie with the words "In the Gloaming" in their titles. *Gloaming* is the old-fashioned English/Scottish word for twilight. Early morning and twilight light are favorites of photographers and painters as well. Try meditation outdoors "in the gloaming" and see what you notice!

Tools for Transformation: "Rest and Recharge"

Here is a guided meditation that I wrote and may someday record as a free download. Feel free to record it yourself to listen to in your own voice. You are also free to share it, as long as you credit me in any re-publication.

The focus of this exercise is to help you recharge and renew at any point in your day. You can use it when there is a specific concern or just for a revitalizing break. While there are many verbal suggestions for easy focus during the journey, it is also okay if you find yourself dozing or not paying attention to the words. Allow your body and mind to recharge in the way that is best for you right now.

Begin by taking some refreshing breaths. The simple act of breathing consciously is a powerful tool for support of calm energy and inner peace. Continue gentle breathing consciously throughout this exercise.

Place your hands on your lower abdomen, below your navel. Now inhale and exhale in a natural rhythm. Feel the breath moving the abdominal muscles, expanding with inhalation and contracting with exhalation. There is no need to hold your breath or forcibly expel it. If is easy for you to do so, let the breath flow in and out through your nostrils.

As you continue this relaxed natural breathing, feeling the gentle rising and falling of your abdomen, imagine that your are breathing light or love. Love in, love out. Light in, light out. Now imagine that your breath rises from your abdomen to your heart with each in-breath. As you exhale, let the breath flow out from your heart as you open to the new.

How we feel is important to our well-being. Positive feelings contribute to mental equilibrium, immune health, and vitality. While it is fun to accomplish our goals and to do various activities, often in our busy lives we can benefit by taking more times to simply rest in quiet mindfulness, to allow a state of well-being to emerge. Resting calmly in love, serenity, or appreciation allows our vital force to replenish at a deep level.

As you continue peaceful, natural breaths, softly notice your emotions. How are you feeling right now?

Emotions may feel pleasant or unpleasant, but the emotions themselves are neither good nor bad. Our emotions are a response, giving us information about our thoughts and focus. Notice your gut, especially the solar plexus area, as you softly observe your emotional state without judgment. Let yourself be in wholeness with whatever you are feeling. Continue to focus upon your breath, letting go of thoughts. Do not try to push emotions away, but do not cling to them either. Let them be fluid as you hold awareness of your breath, letting go of thoughts. When we let go of thoughts, including thoughts about our emotions, they can gently shift and ease, of their own accord.

Continue your gentle, natural breathing—light in, light out, love in, love out—as you listen to the following narrative.

Breathing is just one of the many natural rhythms of the body. There is also a delicious slow rhythm of expansion and contraction that attunes us to the Breath of Life itself. This rhythm supports our body's natural ability to heal and regenerate, whether or not we are ever aware of it. This flow enlivens all of us, bathing each of our cells in the essence of love. It can be peaceful and soothing to learn to experience it directly. Experiencing it is not required for this meditation; it is just one possibility of what might occur. So just relax, enjoy your breaths, and let them lead you into your wholeness and ease.

Some people begin to notice this rhythm (the Breath of Life) most easily by placing the focus of attention to their breath either at the solar plexus (the area at the top of the abdomen, just below the breastbone) or at the heart center (around the center of the breastbone, in the middle of the chest). Attuning to this rhythm may feel like we are part of a slow and peaceful tide that gently expands and contracts us, cycling about twice a minute. There is an even slower rhythm that a few people tune into that feels like it comes from the horizon, which cycles every two minutes or so. Gently now, without striving or straining, and in a peaceful, playful manner, see if you can relax into a sense of either of these slow and calming rhythms of expansion and contraction, while you softly focus upon your breath.

Just let go, and let them come to you, if they do. You may notice a sensation of floating, of freedom, of peace, or nothing in particular other than your breath. It is alright if you do not feel these rhythms. They are subtle yet nourish you at all times, even if you are never consciously aware of them. Continue to gently breath naturally, and whether you perceive them now or not, know that the gentle tides of the Breath of Life are renewing and revivifying every cell, every tissue, and every organ of your body.

Continue to breathe, peaceful and easy. Light in, light out, love in, love out. Rest in your feelings of well-being.

CHAPTER 6

✥

Movement and Exercise

Physical movement is an essential part of emotional well-being and is outstanding for decreasing anxiety and improving calm and optimism. Movement is simply one of the easiest and fastest ways to improve mood. There has been lots of research showing the emotional benefits of regular exercise. In some studies exercise outperformed medication for improving mood and stabilizing emotions. Even a brief ten-minute walk has been shown to improve mood for two hours.[1]

Exercise is a natural stress reliever. When you see images in the media of people participating in social sports and exercise, they usually appear happy. This is not an accident. Vigorous exercise releases endorphins, a natural opiate. Those natural biochemicals are the basis of the oft-mentioned "runner's high." Any active exercise, such as vigorous biking, swimming, or Bikram (hot) yoga, will release endorphins. As we learned in chapter 2, endorphins are key to excellent immune function. Releasing these natural biochemicals, though, is not the only reason to move our bodies. Physical movement stimulates our reflexes and moves fluids of the body, circulating lymph and helping eliminate wastes and toxins.

Too often, people who are depressed or anxious are "in their head." This is used as a metaphor, but there is also a literal truth to this understanding. Worry, fear, despair, or any stressor may move people energetically out of awareness of the lower portion of their bodies. With exercise or conscious movement, we feel more grounded and more embodied.

Any type of exercise can help us ground, embody, and connect emotions and body. Often people find that exercise in nature has added emotional benefits. The best exercise, though, is something you enjoy since it is easy, over time, to continue to do activities that are pleasurable.

The exception to exercise helping to decrease stress is participation in competitive sports. Participation in sports that pit one person against another, according to one article in *Johns Hopkins School of Medicine Health Alerts,* can increase anxiety. So pay attention to how you feel. If you can be mellow during a quick pick-up basketball game, enjoy! But if you notice that the competition makes you more tense, then choose another activity to unwind.

I often advise patients interested in more exercise to mix it up—a combination of types of exercise can be of greater cardiovascular and emotional benefit than one practice day after day. A great program, for example, might be yoga twice a week in a class, daily brief walks in the home or work neighborhood with one or two longer hikes in nature weekly, and perhaps one afternoon of dancing, swimming, or biking.

If you are not used to exercise, start slow and gentle. Try a short walk, perhaps around the block, or do some simple stretches. Let your body guide you on how much and how fast to increase your workouts. Any sort of exercise oxygenates tissues and will likely help alleviate stress and anxiety.

Types of Recommended Exercise

Walking, especially walking or hiking in nature when possible.

Jogging can be a great stress reliever, but go gently with this one if you are not used to it.

Bicycling, stationary or outdoors. Biking in a natural area can be of dual benefit.

Swimming, indoors or outdoors. Swimming in lakes and rivers can be especially soothing.

Dancing is fun and may add a welcome social component. There are lots of types of dance: free style, belly dancing, country and western line dancing, two step, ballroom dance, hip hop, ballet, jazz, modern. Pick the style or styles that you enjoy.

Yoga can be a powerful tool in overcoming anxiety and depression. There are many reasons for its benefits. First, yoga includes exercises that support balance, focus, and concentration, helping bring practitioners into the present moment. Yoga also incorporates breath-work, or *pranayama,* which can further decrease stress and stress hormones. Yoga increases levels of the calming neurotransmitter GABA.[2] I explain several yogic breathing tools in chapter 8.

Tai Qi, Qi Gong, and Bagua (Baguazhang): These are meditative martial arts from the Chinese Taoist tradition. All involve a series of prescribed movements designed to help the body and spirit increase vitality and life force. There are many types of tai qi, bagua, and qi gong, and any of them can be helpful for people with anxiety. All are ideally done meditatively, with a relaxed internal focus. Bagua, with its profound spiritual internal practice, emphasizes walking meditation and connection with breath. There are several good videos demonstrating this soothing technique available on YouTube.

Aikido: This Japanese martial art teaches self-defense from a perspective of balance and internal harmony. Morihei Ueshiba developed aikido, and the name means "Way of Harmonious Spirit." Like tai qi, qi gong, and bagua, there are many styles of aikido available today.

Classes: In addition to aikido, qi gong, etc., many recreation centers offer a wide selection of exercise classes. Step, Kickboxing, Zumba, Pilates, and Hula Hoop are currently popular offerings. There are many types and levels available at gyms, recreation centers, and other facilities. Exercise classes are a great way to connect with others, relieve stress and tension, and improve your fitness.

The Feldenkrais Method: Feldenkrais is a method of somatic education, also called Awareness Through Movement. It was developed by Moshe Feldenkrais, a Russian-born physicist, judo instructor, and engineer, to teach people how to "reconnect with their natural abilities to move, think, and feel."[3] It helps participants understand and utilize the connection between thought and movement. Training is rigorous, and practitioners are certified by the Feldenkrais Guild. Find experienced teachers and practitioners at the website.[4]

Continuum Movement: Developed as the life work of dancer, author, and healer Emilie Conrad, this profound method of authentic movement reconnects awareness of participants with the primordial, fluid self. In *Energy Medicine in Therapeutics and Human Performance,* James Oschman describes Continuum in this way:

> Continuum is at the same time a philosophical, scientific, artistic, musical, poetic, and spiritual concept, a cosmology, and an advanced state of consciousness. When applied to our affairs, Continuum leads us naturally to a saner and happier world. In other words, Continuum as an experience is a direct involvement in the harmony and congruence of our inner and outer realities. It enables us to live the real lives of our bodies.[5]

I have found Continuum Movement to be among the most helpful methods for persons with anxiety. It enhances physical, emotional, and spiritual clarity and ease. It helps participants access their inner wisdom through a natural and fluid understanding of movement. I would love to see this wonderful teaching available more widely. Classes and practitioners can be found on the Continuum website.[6]

Of course, these are just a few of the many types of exercise and movement available. The most important thing in choosing an exercise plan is to be playful and have fun! Discover ways of moving that you enjoy, and let exercise and movement become your friend and partner in relaxation.

Tools for Transformation: Forward and Backward Bending[7]

Safe for almost everyone, Forward and Backward Bending is a simple series of movements that can help improve sleep, mood, and focus. This gentle exercise is best done on an empty stomach. Do not continue Forward and Backward Bending if you feel tension, pain, discomfort, or dizziness while doing it. It should feel easy and gentle. Performed regularly, it can aid sleep and eliminate tension. Try it first thing after rising in the morning, and just before bed.

1. Start by standing comfortably with feet forward and parallel, about hip-width apart. Let your knees be slightly bent, as this eases pressure on the low back. If your legs are very tight, you may let the stance of the feet go wider—perhaps two hip-widths.

2. Let your arms hang easily by your side.

3. Direct your gaze forward. It is especially nice if you can view a natural vista or something beautiful.

4. Let the front part of your feet support most of your weight. This is your starting position.

5. Gently exhale, and with your exhalation slowly bend forward. Breathe in and out through your nose, or breathe in through your nose and out through your mouth. Bend your neck forward first, then your upper back, mid back, and lower back. Go only as far as is truly comfortable for you—even if this is only a slight bend. Do not strain!

6. When you have reached a comfortable resting place for you, take several refreshing breaths, perhaps thinking of a soothing word with each in and out breath. All the while, let your arms hang comfortably at your sides. This should all be comfortable and easy. If there is any strain, ease up.

7. Let yourself feel ease in your body with each of the breaths. Feel your back, legs, feet, neck, and head, breathing relaxation into them.

8. After three to five breaths, gently begin to rise up with your next exhalation. Rise out of bending in the opposite order that you went in—first raise your low back, then mid back, then upper back, then neck.

9. Stand again in the starting position with knees slightly bent. Feet should still be about hip-width apart.

10. Take a few more refreshing breaths. With each of these, expel as much air as possible during exhalation, without straining, by contracting your abdominal muscles.

11. After three to five breaths, inhale and begin to gently raise your arms in front of you. Let them dangle in front, at shoulder level. Take one or two breaths.

12. Inhale and slowly and gently raise your arms above your head, letting your neck and back extend in a mild backward stretch. Arch comfortably, but do not overdo this! Go only as far as is very comfortable for you. This should feel delicious!

13. Take three refreshing breaths in the stretch. Relish feeling a mild stretch in your abdomen, arms, and torso.

14. With the third exhalation, slowly let your arms come forward and down to your sides. Let them dangle comfortably there as you return to your starting position, with a calm gaze in the middle distance. The knees are again slightly bent, and your weight is slightly forward on your feet. This is one sequence.

Repeat the Forward and Backward Bending sequence more times as you become proficient. One to three repetitions are great at first. Work up to ten or more repetitions as this seems easier for you. It can calm and tone your whole system.

CHAPTER 7

~∽~

More Useful Tools

This chapter provides a valuable collection of assorted tools to help relieve anxiety. Each of them is potentially a gem that can give a great deal of relief. See which ones resonate with you!

Smile

While many people believe that their facial expressions are a result of their emotions, there is actually a two-way feedback. Your emotions will respond to your facial expression as well. So if you smile, even if you are not feeling joy, this action can lift your emotions. The act of smiling informs your brain that you are happy, whether or not you are feeling happy when you begin the smile, and your brain responds as if that is true.

One of my patients had a botox injection from a medical esthetician to clear her frown lines. To her amazement, she noticed that when her brow would not wrinkle up, and her mouth could no longer pucker into a grimace, she actually felt a lot happier. She found that the kind of thoughts that led to frowning were harder to access, and she began to smile more.

Smiling is a universal reflex of joy in humans. Even people in isolated tribes smile as a sign of pleasure. Fetuses smile in utero. Small children smile up to four hundred times per hour. Psychological researchers have found that adults who smile frequently are happier as ranked on personality tests, and are perceived as more intelligent and capable by others.

So, for a simple exercise, smile for one minute or longer, at least three times per day. Suggested times are when you awaken, at lunchtime, and before bed. Do this daily for a least a month. Notice any positive changes in your point of view.

Laugh It Up

I love to laugh, ha-ha ha-ha!

—UNCLE ALBERT IN *MARY POPPINS*

Laughter is a magical elixir of well-being. You cannot continue to feel anxious, depressed, irritated, or any other number of unpleasant emotions, while you are laughing. Laughter dissolves away anger, frustration, and worry. It helps us deal with life's challenges, allowing us to take ourselves and our current experiences less seriously. Laughter helps us take a fresh look at a situation, allowing more perspective and a new, more lighthearted understanding of our condition. It boosts our sense of well-being.

When there is a stressor, laughter can be cathartic, allowing a harmless release of emotion. During protracted difficult times, laughter can provide courage, comfort, and may even restore hope. The playful, whimsical energy of laughter can assist with release of painful memories. Laughter is also empowering. It is hard to feel helpless when one is laughing. Instead, it encourages a sense of optimism and a feeling that all is not lost.

Research on laughter has demonstrated that it can decrease our sense of physical pain, increasing the release of endorphins. Endorphins are our own internal opiates, so laughter is a potent pain reliever. Endorphins are also keys to immune function, so not surprisingly, it has been found that laughter enhances immune function. In addition, laughter has also been shown to increase levels of human growth hormone, another important immune system strengthener.[1]

It certainly decreases emotional pain as well. Laughter increases serotonin, the neurotransmitter of happiness and relaxation, and decreases levels of the stress hormones epinephrine, norepinephrine, and cortisol.[2] Physiologically, laughter has many other benefits. It lowers blood pressure and decreases the risk of heart disease. The shaking from laughter provides a gentle internal massage for all the organs and cells, enhancing the flow of lymph and supporting gentle detoxification. Laughter also aids sleep and can improve physical and emotional energy.[3]

A study done by David H. Rosen at Texas A&M University reported that humor supports greater self-worth, fosters hope, decreases anxiety, and lifts energy. Rosen believes that humor may "competitively inhibit negative thoughts." He observes that prior studies have found that as much as 94 percent of people believe that lightheartedness is necessary to effectively handle stressful life experiences.[4]

Studies have shown that children laugh around three hundred fifty times per day, but adults laugh an average of only fifteen times per day.[5] Children look at life as a game, usually approaching challenges by trying to have fun with them. Adults do well to mimic their attitude.

No wonder there is a yoga of laughter, which teaches people to laugh for no reason at all.[6] Psychologically, laughter helps improve optimism, self-confidence, resiliency, and hopefulness. It is good as a temporary coping mechanism as well as an oasis of joy during difficulties, even when there is chronic pain. I had a patient I'll call "Ben" with chronic severe pain in his legs. His condition, Reflex Sympathetic Dystrophy, was the result of a troubling workplace injury that eventually forced him to retire on full disability, although he was only in his mid-thirties. When I met him, Ben was anxious, depressed, and, at times, despairing. He was in constant pain despite a great deal of medication. He had almost no money, the disability check took care of only his basic survival needs, his marriage had dissolved with his health problems, and he tended to have a bleak outlook on his future prospects. He consulted me because he felt he could not live the rest of his life this way. He wanted to decrease or eliminate the pain and have a better, more hopeful attitude. He and I worked with many of the modalities in this book. One that really struck a chord with him and took hold was laughter yoga. He participated in a laughter group where people from all walks of life laughed together on the phone for thirty minutes each day. Eventually he began to lead one of these groups. Laughter was a critical step in helping Ben feel more hopeful and to gain a sense of control. His anxiety decreased as his optimism increased. Today Ben still has pain, but it is milder and much more manageable. He has found some part-time work with flexible hours that does not exacerbate his pain to supplement the disability check. Laughter has helped him to be freer in many ways.

Twelve-Step Recovery Programs

It is widely understood in psychological and recovery circles that many people who abuse substances such as drugs or alcohol, or engage in other addictive behaviors, are often self-medicating to alleviate painful emotions, including anxiety. One dear, very spiritual friend explained to me that twelve-step work was the main tool that resolved her lifelong anxiety. She said, "Though I have a vast amount of other influences, they were all theories I was unable to put to use until I had the entire psychic change that the twelve steps offer." She continued to explain that she has seen this work for many others as well: "One thing I see all the time in the twelve-step community is people who have been treated for anxiety disorders of all kinds who are finally able to have a complete and total release from their anxiety. They can eventually let go of all medications because they absolutely do not need them anymore."

As a physician, I have seen Twelve-Step programs be profoundly beneficial for patients with anxiety, especially those with substance-abuse issues or other addictions. Even if a patient does not suffer from addictions, if there is a family history of substance abuse, they can often be helped and soothed by Twelve-Step-related programs such as Alanon and Adult Children of Alcoholics (ACOA).

Twelve-Step programs are available for free, all over the United States, even in small towns. They are found in most other nations as well. The Twelve Steps help people find more constructive habits, greater inner resources, and a supportive, sympathetic community. The organization provides mentoring through sponsorship programs. I recommend the program highly.

Earthing and Electromagnetic Fields

Psychological and medical practitioners often advise clients to "get more grounded." *Grounding* is not just a fluffy New Age term. Grounding is significant for our physiology. Our bodies are electromagnetic and can build up charge. That is why when we walk on carpeted floors in the winter we build up static electricity, which makes our hair stand on end. We become aware of this electricity when it discharges with a crackling spark when we touch something metallic, like a doorknob, or even when we contact another person or animal, as each living being has an electromagnetic field.

For most of human history, people had much more contact with the earth than they do today. Most of us wear shoes that electrically insulate us from the earth, and many of us work in high-rise buildings, far from the Earth's surface. Many of us also stay indoors, working with electronic devices for hours each day. This has not always been the case. In fact, it is a very recent development. In 1800, 90 percent of the people in the United States lived on farms, in close contact with the land. Today, only one percent of Americans live on farms.[7] People currently living in developed nations have less contact with the earth than those in any other era, anywhere.

Building up electrical charge in our systems does not feel comfortable, and it can add to stress and anxiety, whether or not we are consciously aware of it. The concept of "Earthing" is elaborated by Clint Ober in his book *Earthing*. Ober lists a variety of methods for releasing pent-up charge. The simplest, available to nearly everyone, is to walk, stand, or sit outdoors, on the earth, without shoes. Even touching an ungloved hand to earth, or touching a tree or shrub growing in the earth (hugging a tree!), can be sufficient. Deliberately creating a direct connection between your body and the earth physiologically allows your bioelectric system to ground. I have found this free tool to greatly benefit my patients with anxiety.

Power Down Electronic Fields around You

I see many people do much better with less overall contact with electronic devices. Some people are quite sensitive to artificial electromagnetic fields. Many people who are agitated by electronic fields are not aware of the disturbance in their systems, largely because the devices are ubiquitous in our society, so it is rare that they are not around them. For this reason I encourage my patients, especially those with anxiety or sleep problems, to cease using all electronic devices, especially cell phones and computers, at least three hours before bedtime. I have personally observed, again and again, that if I stop using the computer and put away my phone three or four hours before bed, my sleep is much deeper and my sense of calm is greatly improved. This effect is enhanced if I spend five or more minutes outdoors, connecting with the earth, within two hours of bedtime. A nightly sojourn outdoors is a wonderful opportunity to appreciate the moon, the stars, and the serenity of the natural world. I will often, in pleasant weather, sit outside in the evening and meditate or do a breathing exercise.

I encourage people to turn off wifi (wireless devices) in the home overnight, to use screen filters on the computer, and to avoid sitting too close to a television. Red lights from LED clocks can also irritate sensitive persons. They have a strong EM field that can be disruptive, so they are not good in the bedroom, especially near the head. Unfortunately, electric blankets also have a substantial EM charge and can cause agitation in people who are sensitive to such effects. An old-fashioned stack of quilts and blankets is often much better. A lightweight down comforter is a good choice for holding heat close to the body, and this can be tried by people who have used electric blankets because they do not like much weight on them while sleeping.

Tone, Sound, and Music

Many people find that they enjoy working with sound as part of their journey to emotional well-being. Humanity has used sound and tone in cultural and healing arenas since the dawn of civilization. In every traditional civilization known, tones, peaceful rhythmic drumming, and chanting are time-honored tools for calming the mind, gentling emotions, and expanding consciousness. Sound and tone strengthen the connection among body, mind, and spirit.

The emotional response to certain sounds is universal. Some sounds, like the splash of waves lapping against the shore and the patter of a gentle rain, are soothing to just about everyone. Others, like the cry of a baby or the piercing wail of a siren, are almost always jarring.

Sound healing is an evolving, leading-edge field that promotes physical and emotional health and awareness through the use of sound, tone, and music. Hundreds of types of sound treatments are known, with more being developed all the time. Some, like chanting, tuning forks, and Tibetan singing bowls, have been used for many generations. Our organs respond to sound and tone and can become revitalized through simple techniques like resonant toning or application of tuning forks. Other valuable techniques are relatively recent—these include binaural beats and voice pattern analysis therapy.

Some psychologists work with Hemi-Sync[8] and other binaural beats to calm agitated clients. Monroe Institute's research indicates that patients who listen to soothing binaural beats and positive messages while undergoing surgery have quicker healing, require less pain medication after surgery,[9] and have fewer complications.[10] Physicians already use "ultrasound" therapeutically and diagnostically. This is a promising area of exploration. Research suggests that even serious illness may someday be treated with sound.[11] The California Institute of Integral Studies offers a certificate program in sound, voice, and healing music.

It is clear that sound can affect us profoundly. All physical matter vibrates at its own unique and specific frequency. Sound therapies can work directly with our vibratory nature at a level beyond that of our conscious mind. With the many wonderful advances in the area of sound and health, it's useful to remember that some of the most powerful tools for creating resonance in our bodies are some of the most basic, ancient, and easy to access: drumming, singing, overtone singing, and chanting. Try them for yourself.

More on Nature

Nature can be our greatest healer and our greatest teacher. By observing and learning from nature, we can develop greater peace and contentment. Through the years I advised many of my patients who find it difficult to meditate or do other exercises to merely spend more time in nature, and when they do, they usually find relief. Here is a collection of simple ways you can find greater harmony through the love and support of nature.

Look out the window. Go outside. Watch the sunrise or sunset. Breathe fresh air whenever you can. Walk in a natural area, when you are able, or just sit outdoors. Rest under a tree and lean against its sturdy trunk. Watch clouds and muse about their patterns. Sit by the ocean, or a lake, or a river. Feel sea spray and taste the salt in the air near the ocean. Observe the flight of birds. Learn to identify the birds of your area by sight and song. Pay attention to the sequence of blooms in your region. Smell some flowers and pick one or two.

Marvel at "Jack Frost" on your windows. Taste raindrops and snowflakes. Admire the changing colors of fall leaves. Appreciate a spring tree in blossom, then watch its tender green leaves unfurl. Observe a fruit growing through its stages, from a tender blossom to a sun-ripened wonder, and then enjoy eating the fruit. Watch ants and beetles doing their important work. Feel the breeze on your skin. Notice any scents wafting by. Admire how "weeds" can come up almost anywhere. Look up, at the day and night sky, and at the stars. Find a place to see the Milky Way. Observe the constellations and notice the colors of individual stars. Track the motion of planets over several nights. Touch the rough bark of a tree. Tickle yourself with the softness of a dandelion puff. Connect with nature, in any form, and let her soothe you, for soothe you she will if you but crack open the door to your heart and let her in.

Tools for Transformation: Soothing with Sound

1. Pay attention to the sounds around you. Notice how sounds in your environment affect you. Perhaps you do not always want the television or the news droning in the background.

2. What types of sounds are soothing to you? Do you have easy access to them? How can you include them more in your daily life?

3. What types of music support your calm peace of mind? Make sure you have plenty of soothing music available to you.

4. Try toning and humming. Vowel sounds—ah, eh, ii, oh, uu, y—are often beneficial. The tone OM can be marvelously healing when repeatedly chanted. Try it!

CHAPTER 8

⌒

Breathing and Pranayama

It might seem obvious that breathing is essential to well-being, but it is rarely discussed in conventional medical contexts. Breathing is taken for granted, unless, of course, there is some specific ailment like asthma, pneumonia, or emphysema that impairs it. Numerous spiritual and health traditions offer a variety of breathing techniques, both for spiritual enhancement and health. Breathing techniques are among the most revered tools for centering in the heart and dwelling in a state of inner peace. They help us to center our consciousness in the here and now, so that we can more fully explore and dwell in the life force nourishing us in each present moment. They also help us connect with greater forces and tides in physical and spiritual realms.

In the yogic tradition, there is an entire branch of practice called *pranayama* devoted to conscious breathing techniques. Breathing techniques are taught in almost all yoga classes. The ancient yogis taught that learning to control the breath can assist in regulating and calming the mind. Many martial arts incorporate breathing techniques into the training. Proper breathing enhances focus, concentration, relaxation, and energy.

I commonly teach specific breathing techniques to patients to help with their health concerns. There are many easy-to-learn techniques that can be helpful for anxiety relief. Experiment and see how these simple techniques feel to you, and focus on the ones that you enjoy and find calming, skipping any that seem overly challenging, uncomfortable, or jangling to you.

Breathing Techniques for Emotional Calm

Awareness of Breathing

Awareness of breathing is the most basic breathing technique for beginning meditation. I have utilized this one in several exercises earlier in this book. Awareness of breath simply employs focus. The natural rhythm of the breath is observed. No changes are made unless they occur spontaneously. Observe the inhalations and the exhalations. Observing breath can be powerfully calming on its own and is an important first step for any other breathing technique. Observing breath assists the mind in moving away from the chatter of thoughts, enhancing awareness of quiet in the present moment.

Deep Abdominal Breathing

Another basic technique for enhancing calm, deep abdominal breathing is one of my personal favorites, and it is easy to do at any time. For deep abdominal breathing, place your hands upon your lower abdomen, below your navel. Breathe in slowly, gently filling your lungs until you feel your hands and lower abdomen rise. Feel your breath filling your abdomen. With the exhalation, gently let the breath flow out, as you feel your abdomen relax and deflate.

There is no force involved with this type of breath, or with any of these exercises. Let your breathing be gentle and natural. Feel a gentle rising and filling of the abdomen with the inhalation, and a gentle falling and relaxation of it with the out-breath.

Deep abdominal breathing allows awareness to sink deep into the body. It helps free up the diaphragm and relax the belly, so is soothing for those who tend to hold tension in their gut. It is a good tool for releasing the grip of a swirl of thoughts. It can also be helpful for relieving asthma and some types of cough. Try a few deep abdominal breaths before any event that may provoke stress.

Conscious Breathing

This is a beginner's yoga breathing technique that links the breath with the heart. It is the breathing tool I used in the guided meditation at the end of chapter 5.

Conscious breathing begins with deep abdominal breathing. After a few deep abdominal breaths, let breath fill the belly and then flow, energetically, from the abdomen into the heart. Again, there is no force involved in this; it is a flow of awareness. With the exhalation, the breath flows out from the heart as the abdomen relaxes. Breaths are gentle and natural.

Conscious breathing brings awareness to the heart, and it can be used at any time to ground, center, and soothe jangled emotions. It helps connect us with the calm at our core. It can be wonderfully restorative to perform conscious breathing while sitting or lying on the earth.

Square Breathing

Square breathing is a simple technique that harmonizes and balances the excitatory and calming branches of the nervous system. When we are anxious, we are generally in a state of overdrive of the sympathetic (excitatory) nervous system. This is commonly known as "fight or flight." I learned this technique from the Ortho-Bionomy instructor Luann Overmyer. She has a nice description of square breathing in her book *Ortho-Bionomy: A Path to Self-Care.*

Square breathing can be done anywhere, at any time. It involves a little counting, done silently in the mind, as the breaths are taken. Breaths in square breathing can be any natural breath. To perform:

> Inhale for 4 counts
>
> Hold 4 counts
>
> Exhale for 4 counts
>
> Hold for 4 counts, and then repeat.
>
> Breathing should be gentle, relaxed, and natural.

Count, thinking to yourself as you observe your breath, calmly:

In–two, three, four

Hold–two, three, four

Out–two, three, four

Hold–two, three, four.

Repeat this sequence several times.

If four counts seem too long for you at first, then try three. Some people who are very anxious may find the second set of holds difficult to do. That is okay. The technique can be modified temporarily to omit the second hold, or it can be shortened until it can be done comfortably. Try to do at least three square breaths in a row, and observe whether you feel more balanced afterward.

Yogic Three-Part Breath

This is another calming, grounding breathing technique. It is usually done seated on a chair or in a cross-legged position but can also be done lying on your back. If possible, breathe in through your nose. You may breathe out through your nose or slightly part your lips to exhale.

Begin by closing your eyes and observing the breath. Then move on to deep abdominal breathing. After a few deep abdominal breaths, on your inhalation fill the lungs and abdomen as completely as possible. Do not strain.

With your next exhalation, expel the breath as completely as possible, while remaining gentle. Contract your abdominal muscles, slightly drawing your navel toward your spine to assist you. Repeat this pattern of inhalation and exhalation for three to five breaths.

The second series of breaths builds upon the prior pattern. Allow your breath to fill your abdomen with each inhalation. Then pause and breathe in a little more, expanding the lower ribs. With the exhalation, let the ribs contract and release the breath before the belly contracts to expel breath. Do this step three to five times. Do not force this. Open the chest and contract the abdomen with awareness.

The final, third part of yogic three-part breathing repeats the first two parts. Then, at the end of the inhalation, after a pause when the lower ribs have been expanded with breath, yet a little more air is allowed in, expanding the upper chest around the heart, all the way to the collar bones. To exhale, first release and exhale from the area of the upper chest, then the lower chest, and finally the abdomen, remembering to contract the abdominal muscles toward the spine to completely empty the breath.

Repeat this three to ten times. Never strain or force. If you need to take a "regular" breath at any time, do so. Yogic three-part breathing helps expand lung capacity and clears old stale air from deep in the lungs. It enhances calmness and feelings of vitality, grounding, and centering. As with any technique, it can be performed in association with Earthing for added benefit to the nervous and immune systems.

Alternate-Nostril Breathing

This is another simple, classic yogic breathing technique that is a part of Ayurvedic medicine. While many of us think that we breathe equally through each nostril, this is rarely so. Usually we have one nostril that is more dominant. Ayurveda recognizes a cycle of nostril dominance through the day; healthy individuals will predominantly breathe through one or the other nostril for about two hours at a time before automatically shifting. There has been some scientific research demonstrating that the opposite side of the brain from the more open nostril is electrically stimulated.[1] That is, if a person predominantly breathes though her left nostril, the right brain is more stimulated and vice versa.

Like square breathing, alternate-nostril breathing can balance the sympathetic and parasympathetic branches of the nervous system. It does this by helping activate the opposing hemispheres of the brain. For most of us, the left brain (dominated by the sympathetic nervous system) is the area of rational thought, language, and intellectual activity, while the right brain, dominated by the parasympathetic, is the area of emotion, creativity, and intuition. By going back and forth with alternating breaths, the technique aims to balance the two brain hemispheres. It also can stimulate the corpus callosum or "great road" between the brain hemispheres. This supports integration of brain function and communication between the hemispheres. Alternate-nostril breathing may assist whole-brain focus, integration, and concentration. Yoga teachers frequently encourage students to perform a few minutes of alternate-nostril breathing before important exams, public speeches, or interviews. The technique helps deepen one's practice when performed before meditation.

Alternate-nostril breathing also supports healthy detoxification of waste products that are released through the breath. It can be quite relaxing while simultaneously revitalizing the entire nervous system. I have found alternate-nostril breathing to be helpful for patients with a variety of anxiety disorders including generalized anxiety, phobias, and PTSD. This breathing technique may also calm the mind at night if there is anxiety-related insomnia.

Here are the steps for performing alternate-nostril breathing for a right-handed person. A left-handed person will substitute left finger/thumb.

1. Close right nostril with your right thumb. (Close right)
2. Slowly inhale through your left nostril. (In left)
3. Pause for a moment. (Pause)
4. Release thumb from right nostril and close your left nostril with your right forefinger or ring finger—whichever is more comfortable for you. (Release right, Close left)
5. Exhale through the right nostril. (Out right)
6. Pause briefly, then inhale through the right nostril. (Pause, then In right)
7. Pause again briefly, release finger from left nostril and close the right nostril with your thumb. (Pause, Release left, Close right)
8. Exhale through the left nostril. (Out left)

This completes one circuit. Continue in this manner for two to ten minutes. Always switch which nostril is closed or open after an inhalation. The basic breathing technique is performed at one's natural pace and rate. It can be combined with other breathing techniques such as square breathing or deep abdominal breathing as you develop proficiency. It is best to perform alternate-nostril breathing on an empty stomach. Skip it completely if you have a cold or if your nasal passages are blocked. Nor is this a good choice if you have a deviated septum with one airway significantly narrower than the other. Try the basic method a few times before moving on to any variations.

One variation of alternate-nostril breathing is to take slightly deeper breaths and exhale slightly more vigorously. This variation enhances the flow of vital force and is good for sluggishness and fatigue. But the difference between this and the basic technique should only be mild. No force should be used during any pranayama technique.

Yet another variation is to perform one-nostril breathing for more intensive relaxation. This is done by lying on the right side and closing the right nostril with the right thumb, while breathing solely through the left nostril. This variation is used to help induce sleep if alternate-nostril breathing was not sufficiently relaxing.

Heart-Centered Breathing Exercises

1. Basic Heart-Centered Breathing

One of my goals in writing *Freedom from Anxiety* is to help readers develop confidence allowing the heart to guide their decisions and actions, i.e., that they feel secure knowing their connection with intuition is a wise one. This series of exercises helps people to center in their hearts, facilitating improved communication between the heart and the mind. This is one way we can cultivate a "wise heart and a loving mind."[2]

The simplest form of heart-centered breathing is a variation of basic awareness of breath. It is very helpful for agitation. Begin with basic breath awareness. After a few relaxing breaths, bring your awareness to your heart. Now imagine, as you breathe normally, that your breath is flowing in and out through the heart or breastbone. Let your breath be relaxed, natural, and easy. Take several breaths energetically linking the flow of breath into the heart and out from the heart. Of course, you are physically breathing in and out through your nose or mouth. In these exercises, imagining breathing in through anatomical areas like the heart or the top of your head refers to an energetic flow that accompanies the breath.

You can do this technique with breath alone. A variation that is useful for any of the heart or chakra breathing exercises is to think of a soothing word such as *ease, calm, freedom, peace,* or *love.* Choose one word that you like, and with each inhalation and exhalation, breathe the soothing word into your heart, then breathe it out. Imagine the calming words flowing into and out from your heart with the tides of your breath. *Ease in, ease out, love in, love out, freedom in, freedom out, peace in, peace out, calm in, calm out.* Notice how this steadies and slows the heart rhythm when you are agitated, and strengthens feelings of centered well-being when you are happy.

2. Head/Heart Breathing

This is another technique that can help us release our focus upon the constant patter of thoughts, by relaxing into a quieter, heart-centered awareness. Begin with basic heart-centered breathing. After a few breaths, shift focus and imagine inhaling through the top of your head and exhaling through your heart or breastbone. Breaths can be normal, or slightly deeper than normal. Do at least three breaths this way, and as many more as you like.

3. Heart/Upper Abdomen Breathing

This technique can be excellent for quelling anxiety, especially "butterflies" in the stomach and nervous digestive disturbances. Begin with either of the heart-centered techniques above. Next imagine that your breath is flowing in through your heart and out through your solar plexus, the area of your stomach in your upper abdomen. All breaths are gentle and natural. Take several breaths in through the heart and out through the stomach.

As a variation, you can go back and forth between the stomach and the heart. Breathe in through your heart and out through your solar plexus, then in through the stomach and out through your heart. Do at least six breaths in this pattern. Many people find this very calming and relaxing and will preferentially perform a few repetitions of this breath when stress begins to mount. I often utilize this pattern when I feel tension or strain, including when I need to share potentially upsetting health diagnoses with my patients. Breathing in this manner helps me to stay centered and compassionate.

4. Heart/Lower Abdomen Breathing

Breathing between the heart and lower abdomen may help with feeling more grounded, embodied, and connected to the earth. This technique may be done after the previous heart-centered breaths, in a sequence, or performed alone.

When doing this as a stand-alone exercise, begin with a few basic heart-centered breaths. Next, breathe in through your heart and out through your lower abdomen, below the navel. Repeat at least three times.

When performing this in a sequence with other techniques, do each of the above breaths three to ten times, one after another. Follow this sequence with three to ten breaths in through your heart and out through your lower abdomen, below the navel. This last step may be performed along with deep abdominal breathing, or done as an energetic flow of normal breath. Relax and enjoy this sequence. If there are any types of breath that you do not like or find difficult, just skip them.

5. Heart/Health Breaths

You can breathe between your heart or a chakra and any anatomical area of concern or discomfort. For example, if you have a sore knee, a shoulder injury, or even a serious illness like breast or prostate cancer, imagine breathing love and light into the affected area and releasing this breath through the heart. Then reverse the flow to send the insight and love of the heart to the area that is exhibiting an imbalance. In this case, it is best not to think of your health concern as a "problem." Instead, you might reframe this and consider it an area where there is misunderstanding between the physical you and the emotional or spiritual you.

Many people find breathing between an area of misunderstanding and the heart very soothing. It may also help with insight that can expedite healing of the situation. If you try this technique and no insight comes right away, don't fret. These breaths can help you feel calmer and improve your self-awareness. By doing the breathing exercises, you are augmenting the energetic flow of communication between your heart and the affected region. The details of information or insight may come later.

Be creative and have fun with these techniques. Feel free to expand on any of them, perhaps including more than two areas. For example, if you have an unresolved hip pain, you might try breathing in a triangle between the hip and heart, heart and third eye, and third eye and hip. This connects the heart, area of concern, and the intuition and can be a wonderful catalyst for inspiration. If you do this, it may be helpful to pay attention to dreams and subtle impressions that you might perceive over the next few days.

6. Joy Breathing

In Traditional Chinese Medicine there is an emotion associated with each organ and meridian. The emotion of the heart is joy. I have found that joy breathing is wonderful for nourishing well-being, especially after a calming sequence of heart-centered breaths has cleared away mind chatter and worry.

To perform joy breathing, think of something that gives you pure joy. This can be a person, place, thing, memory, or expectation, but a mix of emotions should not encumber it. It can be a small vignette, or a single image or event. The thought should give you good feelings, like falling in love. For me, it is easy to think of my small niece and nephew and have those sorts of feelings. A moment of appreciation of my spouse, Star, can do it too. As an opera buff, I can also think of the "Flower Duet" from *Lakme* or several other sublime pieces of music and feel the love. Remembering a gorgeous sunset, the chevron flight of geese, or a waterfall can elicit a swell of joy. Think of whatever creates that feeling for you, after you have relaxed with a flow of heart-centered breathing. Breathe feelings of joy into your heart, and breathe them out. Bask in the well-being, enjoying several joy breaths.

Chakra Breathing

In the Ayurvedic tradition, there are seven major chakras or spiritual-emotional energy centers aligned over the physical body. They are not, themselves, physical structures. Each of these is associated with a color, emotions, and various tones. The major chakras are counted one through seven, from the base of the spine on the physical body to the crown of the head. I like to visualize them as luminous interconnected spheres, rather than single spots. Their energy extends in all directions, like small suns. Visualizing the energy flow this way is helpful when doing a chakra breathing exercise.

Any physical or emotional problem can be addressed on a vibrational level. Chakra techniques may be useful vibrationally for opening and supporting the flow of the spiritual and emotional energies. They may help us clear old road-blocks, without having to consciously focus on "issues."

For those who are not familiar with the chakras, I give more information about them below. But if you are not interested in chakras, it is fine to do these exercises anyway, like the heart-centered ones above, by merely focusing on the anatomical regions. You do not need to know anything about them, or even believe in chakras, for the exercises to be soothing and effective. If you prefer, just let the anatomical areas guide you.

Begin chakra breathing with several basic heart-centered breaths. As you feel your relaxation, shift to breathing in and out of the chakra area of interest to you. For example, if you want to enhance intuition, you might focus on the sixth chakra, the ajna center ("third eye"). Or if you want to enhance your grounding and sense of connection to your body, you might focus your breathing on your first or second chakra. We can "breathe" in and out of any of the chakras. This helps us support internal balance of that area.

We can also easily "breathe" between any two chakras, or any two anatomical regions of the body, to support physical and emotional health, and to potentially get information about our connection with that area or the relationship between two areas. I find that it is almost always soothing to practice breathing in through any area of concern or discomfort, and out through the heart center. You can also breathe back and forth between another chakra and the heart. For example, to enhance the connection between your intuitive capacity and your heart's wisdom, try breathing in through the heart and out through the third eye, and then reverse and breathe in through the third eye and out through the heart.

Some people may notice that it is difficult for them to breathe between two particular areas. This may indicate an imbalance between the two, or a region where energy is not flowing well—valuable information in supporting well-being. For example, one patient who was very cerebral and analytical, but who wanted to be more grounded and earthy, noticed that she had difficulty breathing between her heart and her pelvis, while she could easily breathe between the top of her head and her heart. She became quite intrigued, in a positive way, in developing the connection between her heart, her pelvis, and her lower chakras, believing this would help her in a number of ways. We evolved a program to gently open up the connection. It included "baby step" breathing exercises, massage, and some yoga movements to enhance the flow of energy. Over time, this program helped her in a number of ways. On a physical level, her menstrual cramps decreased. She also noted improved feelings of intimacy during contact with her partner, as well as less of a tendency to over-analyze her emotions.

If you are trying to breathe between two areas and find there is some difficulty, do not worry. This is merely useful information, not a problem. Make a mental note of the information, and notice what thoughts (if any) come up, and then let them go. It is best to do these practices with mindfulness, staying in the present moment. Try not to analyze the impressions that come while you are doing the breathing exercise. Let your experiences be. You can explore the content and its meaning to you later, when you are relaxed. As in meditation, if you start to over-think and notice that you are no longer focusing on the flow of your breath, gently return to focus on the breath alone.

It is possible that focusing breath on a particular area may temporarily increase anxiety or tension, especially if one is not conscious of an ongoing issue that relates to that region. If this happens, do not worry. Make note of the information, mentally bookmarking it to explore from a calm and peaceful state of mind, and shift back to a calm center in the heart with some basic heart-centered breathing or another technique that you find soothing. Again, in this case, you can explore your observations at a later time, when you can comfortably ponder the information. Always do chakra breathing in a manner to support calm, while noticing what you notice.

About the Chakras

The first chakra, also known as the root chakra, is located in the area of the perineum. Its color is red. In women the perineum is located between the vagina and the anus, and in men it is located between the scrotum and the anus. Energetically the first chakra roots us to the life force, helping us with grounding and connection to the Earth. I often meet people who have very little connection to their first chakra. These people can be ungrounded and spacey, and may also be quite fearful and lack confidence. When we are well connected in our root chakra, we are exuberant about our lives and feel full of energy and self-confidence. We take good care of our selves. If you notice that it is hard to breathe into your first chakra, try Earthing to support your breath work.

The second chakra is the realm of sexuality, libido, and power. It is located on the back in the area of the sacrum and on the front just above the pubic bone. In women, the uterus and ovaries sit in this area. In male embryos the testicles form in this region and descend later into the scrotum. The testicles as well as the ovaries are governed by the second chakra. The second chakra is also the center of "moving qi" in the body. In many martial arts including aikido and tai qi, students are encouraged to strengthen their connection with this energy center for balance, vitality, and strength. The color of the second chakra is orange. When the energy in the second chakra flows well, we are friendly and compassionate, have a healthy connection to our sexuality, good relationships with others, and a sense of belonging in the world.

The third chakra is sometimes referred to as the navel chakra, but it is actually located more in the region of the solar plexus. Anatomically, on the front, this is the area between the navel and the bottom of the breastbone. On the back, this area is in the region of the tenth through twelfth thoracic vertebrae. Its color is yellow. This area is responsible for processing emotional information, digesting our life experience, and physically digesting our food. The association of the third chakra with a central area of digestive function explains why so many people experience digestive upset when they are emotionally off balance. A healthy and balanced third chakra leads to hearty digestive health, a good appetite, emotional ease, and feelings of self-respect and calm. People well balanced in this area are able to take on new challenges with confidence. They can process their foods as well as their emotions.

The fourth chakra is the heart. On the front of the body this is in the center of the chest, in the area of the sternum or breastbone, and on the back it is roughly opposite that, around the level of the fourth through sixth thoracic vertebrae. Both rose and green are colors of the heart chakra. I like to combine the two colors in my visualizations. People who are vibrationally balanced in this area have access to an unshakable sense of inner peace. They are intuitively compassionate and able to release old hurts and patterns that no longer serve their higher good. The heart is considered a master key to all the chakras, and it can balance the entire emotional and physical body. That is one reason why so many of the tools of this book are methods that over time may improve balance, ease, and peace in the heart.

The fifth chakra is the throat. It is located in the front and back of the neck. Physically this chakra is associated with the thyroid gland, thymus gland, and lymphatic system, so it has a lot to do with the immune system, physical energy, and lymphatic flow. Emotionally, from this chakra, informed by the heart, we speak our truth in the world. This speaking does not have to be verbal; rather, the fifth chakra assists with any sort of authentic self-expression, including creative expression such as writing, music composition, choreography, etc. Its color is blue. People who are balanced in this area are good communicators and can speak with the courage of their convictions.

The sixth chakra is also known as the third eye, or ajna center. It is located around the area of the pineal gland, in the center of the brain. In the front of the body, it is referred to as the brow chakra, as it is located just above and between the eyebrows. There are many Hindu and Tibetan spiritual paintings depicting this energy center, in balance, as an open third eye. On the back of the body the exit point of the sixth chakra is located at the occiput and is called the "alta" center. The color of the sixth chakra is indigo. The sixth chakra is involved with intuitive knowledge, higher inspiration, and true wisdom.

The seventh chakra is located at the top of the head, where the posterior soft spot of an infant can be felt. This junction is where the frontal and parietal bones of the cranium form a cross. The crown chakra connects us to spiritual realms and is our gateway to even higher energy centers that are located beyond the body. Its color is violet in some traditions, gold in others, and the chakra is often depicted also as a luminous, white, thousand-petaled lotus.

There is also an eighth chakra (and some traditions observe many others) that is often called the soul star or transpersonal chakra, located six to twelve inches above the head.

Many minor chakras exist as well. These are found on the palms of the hands, the soles of the feet, most organs of the body, the tips of the fingers and toes, and various other locations. If you feel inspired to study more about the chakra system, multiple books, DVDs, and other resources are available.

In an esoteric understanding of the human energy field, the spherical chakras intersect like cogs and wheels, forming two primary flows. Each chakra spins in relationship to the others, especially in relationship to the ones immediately above and below it. This spin, when balanced, creates an energetic flow upward toward the heavens and downward toward the earth and the "underworlds." This constant flow centers the soul in physical reality, between heaven and earth. Mystics have seen this flow as infinitely ascending and infinitely descending realms of sacredness.

The mystery of this entire flow is contained in the structure of our bodies. In the Hindu tradition the three tracts that mediate this flow are called the Ida, Shushumna, and Pingali, and they are visualized overlying the spinal column. Working to develop and balance these energies is an alchemy of both ancient wisdom and ultra-modern science. When these tracts are fully open and balanced in their flow, we are enlightened, in total harmony with ourselves, nature, our inner wisdom, and the world around us. We are at peace and filled with joy. This is an admirable and worthwhile goal, and many of the tools of this chapter and book can assist in improving the balance, flow, and communication throughout the chakra system, moving us toward greater harmony and inner peace.

A good meditation for exploring more about the chakras is found in the book *Joy's Way* by Brugh Joy, MD. He describes a spiral meditation that traverses the chakras, opening each one on the outward spiral; then on the inward spiral, re-integrating each one into the physical plane.[3]

CHAPTER 9

Nutrition and Emotional Health

Most people accept that good nutrition is a cornerstone of health. But what is good nutrition? There are lots of ideas regarding what constitutes nourishment. Some are in total opposition to others. Various experts cry, "Eat this!" while others shout, "Don't eat this, eat that." Avoid fats, eat lots of healthy fats, avoid carbohydrates, have more whole grains, protein is essential, Americans eat too much protein, dairy is pure nutrition, cow's milk is only good for calves. Eat raw, eat cooked, eat vegan, eat a nutrient-dense, animal-based diet. Sound familiar?

Food means many things to people. So how do we sort this all out in order to find a diet that is right for us—one that will support our own best emotional and physical health? What part does nutrition play in well-being? This chapter attempts to answer these questions, and others, by giving *you* back the power in your life. I recommend several tools, as well as commonsense advice, that can help you get past the chorus of external opinions by developing and enhancing your own body's awareness.

Listening to Your Body

I used to be fairly dogmatic about diet, believing there was a right way to eat. In my twenties, this right way was vegetarianism. I was an ethical vegetarian and felt sanctimonious about it. I deplored the idea of killing animals for food. I loved the works of writer Frances Moore Lappé and would quote her to anyone vaguely interested. But, as I discuss below, my body did not agree with my mind's choice. In my early forties, I discovered the work of the nutrition-oriented dentist, Weston A. Price, then read Sally Fallon's book *Nourishing Traditions* and fell in love with the idea of a "right diet" all over again. In contrast, this diet incorporated lots of animal fats and animal protein. While I still respect these works and remain influenced by them, I have since come to an even broader understanding of health and nutrition.

Simply put, there is no one right diet for everyone. One person may actually feel fine on a vegetarian diet, while another may thrive with an abundance of saturated fats and animal protein. One person may do very well with wheat and whole grains, and another may not tolerate gluten, or grains. One person may feel best eating predominantly salads and light fare; another may flourish eating mostly cooked food. All of these, and more, are viable and appropriate for various people. An individual body may have changing needs over a lifetime, and that is fine too. A woman who is menstruating might crave meats, including liver, and want them daily, while the same woman post-menopause might find herself less interested in such foods.

There are many reasons why our dietary needs vary. Early nutritional factors, ethnicity, genetics, taste preferences, metabolic type, stress level, work load, allergies, environmental exposures, and phase of life all play a part. Not everyone can digest or metabolize certain foods. We have all heard that everyone needs to eat more fiber, but for many people, fiber aggravates existing bowel conditions. If your body cannot utilize or assimilate the six servings of fibrous "healthy whole grains" currently "recommended" per day, why on Earth would you eat them?

As simplistic as it might sound, the best way to find out what is right for you, at any moment, is to consult your own body. Consult your cells. Consult your organs. I found this out the hard way. As I mentioned above, when I was in my early twenties I was a vegetarian for about seven years. I was well intentioned, but my body had no part in the decision to become a vegetarian. I stopped eating meat from a place of youthful idealism, and the naive belief that this was the best way to be kind to animals. My body had other plans. I thought I was eating healthfully, having salads, vegetables, legumes, whole grains, and soy products like tofu. But over a few years, I grew tired and sluggish. Since I would not allow myself to eat meat, I developed a voracious need for eggs, cheese, and other dairy products. Eventually I was consuming large amounts of these daily, yet I still felt constantly hungry. I found myself craving sweets galore and gained a lot of weight on my supposedly "healthy" vegetarian diet. I also developed large uterine fibroids that may have been caused by the excessive soy consumption, and struggled with anemia.

Five years into my vegetarianism, I found my thoughts drifting frequently to meat, fish, or poultry. Sometimes I would catch myself staring at people in restaurants, vicariously enjoying their meaty dishes. The smell of bacon cooking became physically uncomfortable and confusing. A deeper part of me craved it, and yet I deplored these urges. I dismissed these cravings as "low consciousness" thoughts as I continued to sanctimoniously tout the spiritual benefits of a vegetarian diet. Interestingly, this was not what I would now regard as a particularly spiritually connected period of my life. I made whole-wheat bread from scratch but struggled with low self-esteem, frequent anxiety, and occasional panic attacks. I knew fifteen different tofu recipes and shopped exclusively at a food coop, but I meditated rarely, and I tried to please everyone in order to get them to like me. I had difficulty ending a relationship that had become stressful and, at times, abusive. Once we finally did part ways, I endured my ex calling daily for months after the break-up and verbally berating me. Around the time I began eating meat again, I had the brilliant and empowered realization that I could just hang up the phone. While I do not blame my emotional turmoil on the vegetarian diet, I think not listening to myself in one important area of my life and overriding my instincts had a resonating effect in other areas. It had become commonplace for me to ignore my natural inclinations, to the point that I even felt virtuous about doing so. In retrospect, I am thankful that veganism wasn't a common practice, or my health might have plummeted even faster and farther, since at this point I understand that a vegan diet is utterly wrong for my constitution.

In the seventh year of vegetarianism I found myself dreaming about eating meat almost nightly, visiting steakhouses and rib joints in those dreams and enjoyably dining on meaty delights. After about three months of this, I took a gentle but firm look at myself and asked some tough questions. I began with "What am I doing to myself?" and proceeded with "Why am I doing this and for whom?" and "Could I love animals and still eat them?" I realized that my opinions could not just railroad my body. I understood that I was doing my body a disservice by deciding what I would eat based upon a programmatic ideology. So I sought and found a different direction. I made the radical decision to include my body in the conversation about what to eat, by listening to what my body was asking for. My dreams were obviously indicating that meat was on my body's menu, so somehow I needed to make peace with that. At the same time, I easily found evidence of spiritual and moral people who ate meat. I discovered that even the Dalai Lama eats meat, because after two years of vegetarianism, he developed jaundice.[1] His body, too, asked for something different. Eventually I went out to a local restaurant and ordered ribs. An hour after eating them, I felt a deep flush of physical well-being, a feeling I had forgotten knowing. It was an almost religious experience of nutrition. I understood, viscerally, that the body itself must be consulted about its needs.

This is not meant to be an argument for or against vegetarianism or veganism. I know healthy vegetarians, and I have known others who could not get past their mental constructs when their body clearly had a different idea of what it needed. Many people stop listening within, as I did, based on ideology and opinion. As a society, we are obsessed with eating properly, yet many of us are poorly nourished. We cannot rely on external "experts" to guide us. "Experts" differ widely, and by listening to them instead of ourselves, we relinquish our power to notice, choose, and decide what is right for us.

Instead, I suggest that you feel your own way forward. You can learn to listen to your body, because your body is wise. It knows what it needs and wants. This is an opportunity for further self-exploration. The more you are able to tune in to your body, the less the question of what you "should" eat will occupy your conscious thought.

You might begin by examining any preconceived notions. Do you have beliefs about what is healthy for you? About what you should eat? About what is a more "spiritual" way to eat? About what is a more "healthy" way to eat? Where do these beliefs come from? Do you feel healthy? Do you feel spiritually connected? Do you feel vibrant? If not, do you recall feeling strong and fit in your life? When was that? What was your life like then?

A Technique for Dialogue with the Body about Specific Foods

This simple technique works well for many people who want to feel more in harmony with what they eat. The key is to ask, and then to listen for the answer. The body can respond in a variety of ways. You might feel something physically, like comfort or discomfort, or experience an emotion such as well-being or disgust. If you are someone whose tension manifests in the digestive tract, a food that is good for you in the moment will feel good emotionally. It will feel comfortable in your stomach when you think of it, while a food or nutritional supplement that is not right for you might cause a cramp, an "off" feeling, or a slight tensing. The more you practice this awareness, the easier it becomes to notice subtle cues. Another advantage of this practice is improved self-awareness. With greater attention to one's body/mind/spirit connection, emotionally related physical symptoms can diminish and even disappear through listening to one's inner wisdom.

When you are interested in a particular food but are not certain it is right for you, simply ask your body. You might start with doing some of the heart-centered breathing exercises I discuss in chapter 8. Then move to breathing between your heart and an area of concern. This can be a specific area of the body or just a general query. For example, if you have joint stiffness, think of or hold a particular food that you are wondering about and feel for it in your joints, breathing between your heart and your joints. Ask your joints, will this food nourish and support you at this time?

Consulting just the mouth or taste buds can, unfortunately, be unreliable. Our whole self is sometimes not in alignment with something our taste buds find appealing. One reason our mouth and taste buds can be out of sync with our overall well-being has to

(continued on next page)

do with our thoughts. Our taste buds can be influenced by culture, beliefs, and peer pressure, overriding our inner wisdom. We might associate the taste of a particular food with comfort, or relief, or happiness, even if it does not provide nourishment to the body. For many, the mouth's desires for sweets, in particular, has associations with soothing that do not apply to the rest of the body/mind/ spirit. Bringing the mouth and taste buds into alignment involves finding other healthful ways to soothe the emotions so that better overall alignment can be achieved.

Food for Thought

Our thoughts regarding our food are just as important as what we are eating. We eat not only our foods but also our thoughts about them. It is our thoughts around our choices and actions that influence the subconscious mind, directing it toward future outcomes. If we think as we eat a slice of cake, "I should not eat this, sweets are not good for me" or "this will undoubtedly cause me to gain weight," then we are eating a lot of negative expectations along with our dessert. We have an assumption about eating the cake that is not in alignment with our desire for health. Too often people eat what they believe is "bad" for them. Our bodies have no choice but to reflect this.

For example, Jennifer is a forty-three-year-old woman with a big sweet tooth. But she believes sweets are bad for her. She has collected a lot of experiential evidence to back up this belief. Nonetheless, Jennifer often feels that she "cannot help herself around sweets." She admits that she can eat a whole bag of cookies, half a pie, or a whole carton of ice cream in one sitting. Her usual strategy is to avoid buying them. Jennifer's whole process of eating sweets is furtive and guilt-ridden. She acknowledges that though she craves sweets, she can rarely even enjoy them while she is eating them.

Jennifer worked to shift many self-hating beliefs, including her feelings about foods. She wanted to be true to herself and find a path of balance. She believed it was possible to cultivate a new self-aware attitude, where she could occasionally enjoy sweets and feel truly good about eating them. She asked herself a number of questions like those in the "Tools for Transformation" section of this chapter (below) and came up with several affirmations that felt good to her. Among these were: "Food is good for me." "What I eat nourishes me." "I choose foods that cause my body to flourish, that make my mind healthy and strong." "I am clear-headed after I eat." "I enjoy foods that are delicious and nutritious." She chose to eat sweets only when she felt good about them, and when they resonated with her self-affirming thoughts. It took consistency and practice, but eventually Jennifer found that she could feel in alignment with small portions of desserts. Over time, she shifted many of her prevailing attitudes and beliefs. She now enjoys sweets a couple of times per week, without bingeing. She feels great knowing that she is once again in control of her thoughts around food.

Emotional Eating

Emotional eating is a tendency to eat when stressed, anxious, or blue. This would not be a bad thing, but it often dovetails with negative self-talk, as in the example above about Jennifer's way of eating sweets. When we eat in an effort to push aside, bury, or stuff down negative emotions, and then feel bad about what we've consumed, the strategy often backfires. Soon we feel bad about what was originally upsetting us, as well as about the emotional eating. This is a variation on "digging oneself further into a hole" with one's thoughts.

Once you begin to notice that you are eating emotionally, try sitting with your feelings. Do your best not to criticize, mock, judge, or belittle yourself. It does not matter, at this moment, if the story you are telling yourself is "true." What does matter is that you can begin to be true to yourself. A good first step is to acknowledge, without judgment, where you are emotionally. Gently be with your feelings, free of condemnation. It is okay to have emotions, no matter what they are. Many people eat emotionally in order to push away powerful feelings, and yet the only power our emotions have is what we give to them. So allow yourself to feel your feelings: lonely, anxious, or scared, or whatever else you are feeling when you notice that you are drawn to emotional eating. Then decide that you want to feel better, and claim it. If you have already eaten something and are regretting it, start by simply noticing that feeling, without judgment. Freedom from anxiety is always about compassion and kindness for yourself. It is a road that leads to inner peace and balance. You are okay just as you are. If you are prone to emotional eating, you might review and practice the techniques in chapters 3 and 4, and work with your breath, centering in your heart, as discussed in chapter 8.

Mealtime Peace

It may seem obvious, but eating in a peaceful manner is healthful both emotionally and physically. This is often overlooked but easily remedied. Anyone can and will benefit by eating meals calmly and mindfully. Digestion is a process of the parasympathetic nervous system, the calm and relaxed portion of the nervous system. Activation of the fight-or-flight portion of the nervous system, the sympathetic branch, actually shuts down digestion. So if you eat when upset, you literally cannot digest your food or your experience. Here are a few suggestions for cultivating mealtime peace to ease anxiety and enhance digestion.

1. Turn off media news broadcasts while eating. Instead, perhaps, listen to pleasant music or watch something funny or lighthearted.

2. Refrain from difficult conversations. Mealtimes are an ideal time to share with others, but complaining about your day is likely to increase anxiety and spoil digestion by activating your fight-or-flight response.

3. Eat at a slow pace that feels good, chewing and savoring your food. Enjoy the flavors, textures, and smells. Be aware of what you notice while eating, and perhaps talk about or think about what you enjoy about each meal.

4. Many people enjoy saying grace or giving thanks to set a nice tone for a meal or snack. Gratitude can activate the calm portion of the nervous system, thus improving digestion. Thanks can be in any form you prefer, from traditional prayer at the beginning of the meal to silent words of appreciation for the farmers, ranchers, and

farm workers who raise the food, the markets and distribution channels that bring the food to you, the cook (even if it is yourself), and,
of course, the plants and animals whose life force nourishes yours,
as a part of the web of life that holds us all.

5. Refrain from electronic stimulation at mealtimes, including texting,
video games, and reviewing emails. Try to let yourself really relax
and appreciate your food, your surroundings and/or your dining
companions.

6. Eat only the foods that you are enjoying at your meal. If there is
something you do not like, you do not have to eat it. Eat only as
much as you want and resist the compulsion to "clean your plate" if
you are already full.

Foods for Calming Nourishment

There are many nourishing foods that over the years have gotten a "bad rap"
and have been wrongly vilified in our contemporary society. The reasons these
have been rejected are complex but have surprisingly little to do with nutrition.
Other, more dubious foods, including processed foods containing coloring
agents and chemicals, are widely accepted but may trigger anxiety and mood
swings. As you consider your thoughts, beliefs, and attitudes toward various
foods and food groups, it might be helpful to look at our traditional cultural
understanding of nourishment and its connection to inner peace and harmony.

Traditional Fats

Prior to the late twentieth century, traditional fats were prized above almost
all other foods. Culturally we have embedded phrases associating fat with
well-being, such as "living off the fat of the land" and "fat and happy." In
the wild, carnivorous animals will always first eat the fattiest tissues and the
nutrient-rich organs of their prey. They instinctively understand, without any
advanced degrees, that these parts are the most nutritious and life-sustaining.
Some species, like wolves, will not eat lean meat at all. They leave lean muscle
meat for scavengers.

Advertisers and the media have associated fat, an essential nutrient, with physical fatness and obesity. This association is not correct, and many researchers have discovered just the opposite.[2] Saturated fats are essential for brain and nervous system function, including calmness, as well as absorption of minerals and production of hormones. The fat content of a meal is what signals satiety to the brain, which is why some people overeat carbohydrates until they are stuffed before they feel a sense of fullness. Their brain is simply not getting enough fat to trigger satiety.

In my experience, many anxiety sufferers get relief by simply incorporating more traditional fats into their diet. This finding is supported by a Belgian study that infused either fatty acids or saline into the veins of volunteers. They then exposed them to sad music, interviewed them, and performed MRIs to ascertain which areas of the brain were activated. In those who received the fatty acids, the areas of the brain that regulate emotional calm were highlighted, and feelings of sadness were only half as prominent as in those who received the saline.[3]

The term "traditional fats" refers to those that existed before approximately 1900, prior to the advent of industrial farming and food production and before most domestic animals raised for slaughter were forced to live indoors while being fed food unnatural to them. So, for example, margarine of any sort (even if it has "balance" or "smart" in its name) is not a traditional fat. Products are named by advertisers in order to create a perception of wholesomeness and health that the products themselves may lack.

The industrially produced oils like safflower, canola, soy, and corn oil are not traditional fats, either. But lard from pastured pigs, butter from pastured cows, virgin coconut oil and palm oil,[4] extra virgin olive oil, and tallow from pastured cattle are all traditional fats. Pastured animals are raised outdoors in a traditional manner. For example, pastured cattle eat grass and hay, and pastured chickens eat insects and seeds.

I recommend that people who are experiencing anxiety incorporate into their diet more traditional fats like organic butter, ghee, coconut oil, and healthy fats from pastured animals. Eating foods and fats from animals that are raised in a respectful, traditional manner that honors the sanctity of their lives helps many ethical people who were formerly avoiding animal foods, whose bodies are craving fats and animal products, to come to terms with a new choice.

When adding fat back into the diet (if you have avoided it), it is best to begin slowly. Those who have avoided fat for a long time may, ironically, be starving for fat and yet unable to digest it well. Reintroducing it slowly, taking bitters before meals, and adding lacto-fermented foods can help enhance digestion. There are many nutritionists and resources that can help with this journey. Consult the Weston A. Price Foundation for more information and a list of resources in your area, including nutritionists who understand this philosophy.[5]

Cholesterol

Cholesterol is another essential nutrient of well-being that has been vilified by some modern and industrial food scientists. The human brain and nervous system are actually made up of a great deal of cholesterol. About 25 percent of the total cholesterol in the body is found in brain tissue,[6] and cholesterol is a major essential component of myelin, the protective sheath that covers nerves and comprises much of the white matter of the brain. In fact, every cell not only contains cholesterol, it has the capacity to make cholesterol. Most of the cholesterol in your body is formed in the liver, but any cell can manufacture cholesterol when necessary. When I learned this in medical school, it was my first clue that something was amiss in our knowledge. As a naturalist with a deeply spiritual understanding, I know that nature does not make enormous mistakes. It does not base life on a molecule that is "bad" for us. Cholesterol is, in fact, a fundamental molecule of life on this planet. It is essential in cell membranes, the envelopes around each living cell, and is essential to the nervous system for nerve impulse conduction in humans, animals, and most insects. Cholesterol is a necessary building block for hormones such as estrogen, progesterone, testosterone, DHEA, cortisol, and anti-diuretic hormone. Cholesterol is also what your skin uses to make vitamin D from sunlight.

Another important indicator of a misunderstanding that I picked up in medical school is the fact that when cholesterol is very low, below 140 mg/dl, patients are prone to depression and anxiety. Very low cholesterol impairs brain function and can contribute to mental dullness and dementia.

Low cholesterol is further correlated with immune dysfunction, fatigue, and increased risk of illness. In AIDS patients, very low cholesterol denotes a poor prognosis.

For these reasons, I encourage depressed or anxious people to include more cholesterol-rich foods in their diet. These foods, which are all from animal sources, ideally should be raised in a natural, traditional manner. Eggs, for example, should be from hens that are actually outside, pecking in a yard, and ideally fed a diet of organic grains and food scraps to supplement their foraged intake. Meats and animal products such as dairy foods should ideally be from animals raised in a traditional manner. I find it easiest to shop for these foods directly from farmers, at the farmer's market and through community-supported agriculture. Then I can truly understand how the animals are raised and know they are likely to be nutritious and health-supporting.

The issues regarding the dangers of high cholesterol are complex, but there is plenty of evidence supporting the healthfulness of a cholesterol-rich diet. My favorite resources are the books of Uffe Ravnskov, MD: *Fat and Cholesterol Are Good for You* and *Ignore the Awkward: How the Cholesterol Myths Are Kept Alive.* He reports many facts that have been ignored by mainstream media, including over twenty-five studies demonstrating that elderly people with the highest cholesterol live the longest. In his books, Dr. Ravnskov explains clearly how we arrived at this misunderstanding, and how it is has been perpetuated.

The Weston A. Price Foundation website offers a great deal of useful information about revising our understanding of cholesterol, as does Greenmedicineinfo.com. The prestigious Framingham study, which was supposed to prove the cholesterol diet/heart hypothesis, did nothing of the sort. In 1992, the director of the Framingham study, Dr. William Castelli, wrote in an editorial: "in Framingham, Mass., the more saturated fat one ate, the more cholesterol one ate, the more calories one ate, the lower the person's serum cholesterol."[7] Dr. Castelli goes on to explain that "we found that the people who ate the most cholesterol, ate the most saturated fat, ate the most calories weighed the least and were the most physically active."

The study did not address the relationship between emotional health and levels of cholesterol consumption. That is for future researchers. But I am confident that studies eventually will prove that increased cholesterol consumption helps in lowering anxiety, and that low-cholesterol diets contribute to anxiety. The writer Chris Masterjohn published an article in 2005, "My Experience with Vegetarianism," in which he candidly discussed how his lifelong anxiety was severely exacerbated after he adopted a low-cholesterol, high-soy vegan diet.[8] We know that stress and anxiety may raise serum cholesterol levels, and that generalized anxiety disorder may elevate overall cholesterol.[9] Perhaps that rise is a healthy body compensatory mechanism, with the cholesterol increasing to support the anxious individual in developing greater calm, rather than a pathologic process. I think this is likely, as I believe in the wisdom of our bodies. Left to their own devices and offered healthy choices, they will naturally gravitate toward balance.

So, if you are anxious, you may want to consider adding more cholesterol-rich traditional foods to your diet to help nourish and calm your nervous system. These foods are also rich sources of healthy, calming, traditional saturated fats. Examples include butter, lard, cheese, meats, and egg yolks, all ideally from pastured and organically raised animals. If you feel nervous about doing this because of all the negative publicity about cholesterol, consider doing a little review of some of the above resources, and it is likely you will feel reassured.

Protein

Our bodies are about 16 percent protein, mostly concentrated in the muscles, connective tissue, and skin. But every cell of the human body contains some protein. Adequate protein in the diet supports a calm and healthy nervous system, since protein is essential for the production of neurotransmitters, hormones, and enzymes involved in tranquility, and for repair of DNA and RNA. The amount of protein an individual requires is related to many factors, including their age, overall health, amount of carbohydrate consumption, level of exercise, body composition, rate of growth and repair, and lean body weight. Adult women typically need 40–60 grams of protein per day while adult men require 50–70 grams per day. Endurance and elite athletes who exercise more than two hours a day may need significantly more than this.

There is a recommended range for protein consumption. But there is no need to log grams of protein or measure your food to determine what is right for you. Once again, simply pay attention to what your body is requesting. Many patients tell me that they feel best when they have some animal protein at every meal, while others observe that large amounts of protein at one meal seem to irritate their system. To help determine what is best for you, use the tools we have already discussed. These can help you notice how you feel when considering what to eat.

Pay attention after eating as well. How do you feel after a breakfast of bacon and eggs as opposed to a bowl of oatmeal? How do you feel after a fruit and yogurt smoothie? It can be illuminating to keep a log of food and mood. In it, write down what you eat, the time of day, and the approximate amount consumed. Later note how you felt emotionally over the next few hours, when you felt hungry again, and whether any food cravings developed. Here is a sample entry from one patient: "Breakfast 8 AM: 2 eggs scrambled in one teaspoon butter with one ounce cheddar, one slice rye toast with thin layer of honey. Felt happy after the meal for about an hour, then began to notice some irritability. Distracted at work. Hungry again 10 AM, craving sweets with rising anxiety, feelings of overwhelm and sense of alarm. Had snack of soaked raw then roasted nuts and a raw carrot and felt myself smooth out emotionally over the next hour." The next day she ate again at 8 AM, skipping the toast and honey and substituting a half cup of leftover broccoli and a little more butter (2 teaspoons) in her eggs. She reported "feelings of well-being throughout the morning, with a steady calm mood and good ability to concentrate on my work. Feeling of mild hunger, without cravings, began around noon."

Chocolate

Chocolate has many health benefits, especially in its raw state. (Actually, it is the raw cacao that has the most benefits, and they are lessened by the addition of sugar and milk in conventional chocolate. But to keep things simple, I will refer to chocolate generally.) Many people with anxiety and depression crave chocolate. That is easy to understand when we learn that chocolate has a number of nutritional components that support emotional health. One is l-phenylalanine, a chemical that slows the breakdown of endorphins, our internal feel-good chemicals. Another is phenylethyl-amine, also called PEA, which supports the sense of bliss and gives the feeling of "falling in love." No food has higher levels of PEA than chocolate. Chocolate is an excellent source of another important calm-mood nutrient, magnesium, a mineral that is greatly diminished in our current food supply, largely because it is reduced in soils since the advent of industrial farming practices that strip soils of many minerals, while replacing just nitrogen, potassium, and phosphorus. Raw chocolate is also extremely high in anti-oxidants, making it generally good for detoxification and cellular repair. Chocolate does contain natural stimulants: PEA can be one, and theobro-mines can mimic the activity of caffeine. Still, a small amount of chocolate is fine for most people, and a little is all it takes to get a mild, pleasant lift from this nutritious food. The best chocolate for mood support is high in cacao, organically grown or wild-crafted, and rich in cacao butter, as the fat helps assimilation of minerals. My personal favorites are the Chocolove organic 73 percent cocoa content bar, which is also fair-trade certified, and the products of a local California raw chocolatier, Coracao Confections, which makes various types of raw chocolate bars.

Sugar-Free Raw Chocolate Confection

I came up with a completely sugar-free recipe that is so delicious I have to share it:

1/2 cup softened raw coconut butter—this contains some coconut meat and is not the same as the oil (I use either Artisana brand or Nutiva brand)

1/4 cup raw organic cacao

1/4 cup shaved organic coconut (unsweetened)

1 tablespoon chopped almonds or pecans (pre-soaked then roasted)

1 tablespoon cacao nibs

1 tablespoon softened or sun-melted organic butter

I like to soften both the coconut butter and dairy butter on a sunny windowsill for a few hours. When both butters are soft, I blend all ingredients together, spread the dough out on an environmentally friendly parchment paper or cookie sheet, and then put it in a moderately cool place (not the refrigerator) overnight until it hardens. The natural sweetness of the coconut butter makes this very tasty, without any added sweeteners. One patient substituted regular organic cocoa powder for the raw cacao, and added in some cocoa butter. Her variation was delicious as well.

If you include chocolate, remember to see how you feel when you eat it. Only consume foods that support your personal well-being. If chocolate triggers excessive food cravings or emotional upset, then you may want to avoid it.

Traditional Food Preparation

Soaking Grains and Beans

Many agricultural food products such as grains, beans, and nuts are actually seeds that the plant produces for its own reproduction. Most have a skin or seed coat that can contain many "anti-nutrients" such as phytates, which can block mineral and nutrient absorption in the gastrointestinal tract. Some grains and most legumes have naturally occurring goitrogens that can impair the function of the thyroid gland, causing fatigue. Traditional methods of food preparation addressed these issues by soaking, sprouting, or leaching many foods. These time-honored techniques for enhancing the nutritive value and absorbability of foods have been lost in the industrial food-delivery system.

It is easy to return to these healthy food-preparation techniques. They improve the digestibility, taste, and nutritive value of many of our common plant foods. For example, the protein content of raw nuts that have been soaked and sprouted is doubled in some cases, while the indigestible seed coating is rinsed away. Ideally nuts should be purchased raw, not irradiated or pasteurized, and soaked overnight. Similarly, instead of purchasing canned beans or legumes, buy fresh, organic ones and soak them until plump, discarding the soak water. Also soak grains overnight, and pour off soak water.

Lacto Fermentation

Pre-industrial food preservation involved salting, pickling, curing, and other lacto fermentation processes. Consuming these naturally preserved and fermented foods encourages the growth of healthy probiotic bacteria that support a flourishing gastrointestinal (GI) tract and mucous membranes. These products of natural fermentation also help harmonize individuals with the dominant microflora of their bioregion. In traditional cultures, lacto-fermented foods were consumed daily, sometimes at every meal. For example, in the Swiss highlands, cultured dairy products were consumed at each meal, all year long.

In Japan, a wide variety of pickled vegetables, long-fermented soy products, and fermented seafood was consumed daily. In Korea, kim chi is still eaten with every meal. One of the greatest changes in our diets in the last hundred years has been the disappearance of these health-giving foods from our plates. Over the years, I have observed that many otherwise health-conscious individuals consume no lacto-fermented foods. This is especially true for people who avoid dairy products.

Emotional health is interwoven with the health of the GI tract. Most of the neurotransmitters of well-being are synthesized here, rather than in the brain, and thriving healthy intestinal bacterial colonies support emotional health in a number of other ways. Adequate levels of GI flora can mitigate systemic stress responses and support feelings of calm well-being.[10] For example, a recent study at UCLA found that volunteers who ate yogurt twice daily for a month exhibited decreased activity in the areas of the brain associated with emotional distress and pain, and enhanced brain activity in the area associated with decision-making.[11] Friendly lactobacilli may also decrease levels of stress-induced glucocorticoid hormones, and increase levels of the calming neurotransmitter GABA.[12] Lacto-fermented foods are high in enzymes, which can assist digestion. Many health practitioners today, including conventionally trained physicians, are coming to understand the importance of healthy bacteria.

If you have not previously consumed lacto-fermented foods, there are many delicious choices. There is a resurgence in their availability and popularity. If you are so inclined, it's relatively simple to learn to make your own ferments. Sandor Katz's book *Wild Fermentation* is a great resource for getting started. If your body is not used to consuming lacto-fermented foods, begin with small amounts and see how they affect your digestive tract. If you do well with dairy products, then yogurt, raw milk cheeses, cultured butter, kefir, natural buttermilk, and sour cream are all good choices. Non-dairy choices include raw sauerkraut (not the pasteurized stuff on the supermarket shelf), traditional kim chi, miso paste, tamari and shoyu, kombucha, fermented Thai fish sauce, and fermented/naturally preserved vegetables. As always, try to get veggies, sauces, and animal products that were produced and raised in accordance with time-honored principles. If necessary, work with a nutritionist or healthcare provider in learning ways to help your body flourish with more lacto-fermented foods. Sometimes a probiotic supplement is helpful in building a vibrant internal microflora, and many professionals can advise you about this as well.

Common Foods That Can Trigger Anxiety

Gluten and Grains

I personally find that I do well without gluten. For the most part, I stopped eating gluten fifteen years ago, during a period of time when I was experiencing gastrointestinal disturbances including irritable bowel syndrome, heartburn, and daily stomach aches. Though I test "negative" for celiac disease, these symptoms and others (such as mental fogginess, skin rashes, and excessive moodiness) cleared up in a few weeks off of gluten grains, including wheat. Nowadays I can occasionally have a little gluten without too many negative consequences. But if I think that this means I can regularly consume wheat and gluten again, my body swiftly reminds me with several types of gastrointestinal upset, including heartburn, that this is not a good choice for me.

What is gluten? There are many types of glutens and glutenin. They are proteins present in many grains, and one of their qualities is that they provide elasticity in breads and pastries. These proteins are predominantly found in wheat, rye, and barley, as well as in ancient forms of wheat like einkorn, kamut, and spelt. Corn and oats do not technically contain gluten, though they have similar molecules that can cause sensitivity.

Eighty percent of the protein in breads is actually glutenin, although there are currently no medical tests available for glutenin sensitivity. Since discovering the connection between my symptoms and gluten, I found evidence and science that confirm the connection between gluten grains and a host of emotional and physical health problems in people with allergy or sensitivity. I now see celiac disease as an extreme tip of the iceberg, the far end of a range of problems that can be caused by these difficult-to-digest foods.

Even in the best of circumstances, gluten is a challenging molecule to digest. Its structure consists of a protein core tightly wrapped by a large amount of loose, fluffy carbohydrates. Gluten digestion requires many enzymatic processes, and these are found only in a healthy, vibrant intestinal tract. There are even more problems with modern wheat hybrids than ancient varieties. Modern wheat contains novel glutens that never previously existed in the human diet, which can contribute to a great deal of digestive dysfunction.

There are still more links between emotional well-being and the health of the digestive tract. First, most of our neurotransmitters are produced in the gut, and not the brain.[13] Second, the gut is where we absorb (or fail to absorb) important nutrients like minerals and amino acids that form the building blocks of health. When gastrointestinal function is impaired, we can manifest conditions such as mineral deficiencies and leaky gut syndrome, where toxins and waste products are absorbed back into the blood stream. Persons who consume a lot of grains may have low levels of the essential amino acid L-tryptophan, which is more prevalent in animal foods. Low levels of tryptophan have been associated with development of serotonin deficiency syndromes including anxiety, depression, and related disorders such as forms of ADD/ADHD. Metabolism of carbohydrates in grains depletes serotonin, as well as B vitamins needed to convert amino acids to neurotransmitters.[14]

I suggest that anxious patients try eating a gluten-free diet for three months, to see how they feel. Gluten grains also contain gluteomorphans, which act as opiates in the body. Many individuals with anxiety, brain fog, or fatigue find that they have better moods and increased mental clarity when they eliminate gluten and reduce overall consumption of grains.

Sugar, Alcohol, Caffeine, Chemical Food Additives

Alcohol, sugar, and caffeine are popularly known as common anxiety-trigger foods. They all may cause elevated lactic acid. In persons with anxiety, high levels of lactic acid may trigger worsening of symptoms, including panic attacks. Deficiencies of other nutrients can elevate lactic acid as well, causing a cascading anxiety effect. This is especially true of B-vitamin deficiencies, magnesium deficiency, and calcium deficiency. B vitamins are utilized in metabolizing of stress hormones and are easily depleted if anxiety or stress is chronic, setting up a negative biochemical feedback loop. Consuming an excess of cold foods and drinks also depletes B vitamins. Alcohol can decrease B vitamins and magnesium, exacerbating deficiencies of those nutrients.

Likewise, excessive amounts of sugar are associated, in many ways, with increased anxiety. This may be, in part, because people believe sugar is bad for them. But it is also because sugar creates acid in our system, allowing imbalanced flora to proliferate. Sugar also taxes the adrenal glands by causing alarm in the neurochemical system. Especially when there is already a blood sugar disturbance, the body can perceive large doses of sugar as an emergency. Fructose, a component of high-fructose corn syrup, found in many sodas, can be especially difficult for the insulin/leptin/blood sugar cycle, triggering a state of fight or flight in sensitive persons.

I recommend decreasing or eliminating caffeine, alcohol, and sugar for those attempting to quiet their nervous system and decrease anxiety. Likewise, artificial sweeteners such as aspartame should be avoided. Many studies indicate that these are excitotoxins that irritate the nervous system and exacerbate mood disturbances.

Artificial sweeteners and food colorings, chemical preservatives, "conditioning agents," and pesticide and herbicide residues are all newfangled products of modern food production. None of them were found in the traditional foods consumed throughout human history. In my opinion, none of these serve our health. Our bodies cannot easily process them; and they can lead to toxic overload. Avoid them as much as possible, choosing natural, whole, unprocessed foods for greater emotional calm. If most organically produced foods are not in your budget, try to get natural foods from local farmers and producers. Also consider looking at lists like the Environmental Working Group's "Dirty Dozen" and "Clean Fifteen" to determine foods that are most important to choose organic. The current (2012) fruit and vegetable "Dirty Dozen" list includes apples, celery, strawberries, peaches, spinach, green beans, nectarines, grapes (and wine), sweet bell peppers, potatoes, blueberries, lettuce, kale, collard greens, chocolate, and coffee.[15] The list for animal products includes butter, fatty meats, and milk. In 2012 the Environmental Working Group noted the following "Clean Fifteen" fruits and vegetables to be the least contaminated by problematic pesticides and herbicides: onions, sweet corn, pineapple, avocado, asparagus, sweet peas, mango, eggplant, cantaloupe (domestic), kiwi, cabbage, watermelon, sweet potatoes, grapefruit, and mushrooms.[16] However, they note that sweet corn could be genetically modified, so persons wanting to avoid GMOs will want to buy only organically grown sweet corn.

It is noteworthy to mention certain other modern foods that are almost always laden with herbicides and pesticides. One of the most notorious of these is cottonseed oil. Cotton is regulated as a fiber plant but not as a food, so tremendous amounts of pesticides and herbicides can be used on cotton fields, including ones that are banned in normal food production. These chemicals, unfortunately, can concentrate in the seed oil. For this reason, I advise avoiding all foods with cottonseed oil.

Food Allergies

Undiagnosed food allergies and sensitivities can increase anxiety. While "anything can cause anything in anyone," some foods are more common causes for allergies, while others are rarely triggers. The most common foods causing allergy include: wheat, gluten, and wheat products, corn and corn products including corn oil and high-fructose corn syrup, soy and soy products including soy protein and soy oil, cow's milk and milk products like yogurt and cheese, eggs and egg products, strawberries, peanuts, tree nuts especially almonds, Brazil nuts, cashews, filberts (hazelnuts), pecans, and macadamia nuts, fish, shellfish and mollusks, sesame seeds, and mustard seed.

Foods that are rarely allergenic include lamb, rabbit, wild game, ghee (clarified butter), butter, carrots (organic only), quinoa, amaranth, sago (arrowroot), pears, blueberries, cassava, tapioca, beef, turkey, veal, broccoli, beets, goat and sheep milk yogurt, and buttermilk. If you suspect food allergies, consider consulting with a knowledgeable nutrition or medical practitioner, and consider trying an allergy elimination diet under their supervision.

Tools for Transformation:
Nutrition and Happiness, or "Letting Go of Dogma and Consulting Your Body"

Freedom from Anxiety is a path of self-examination and improving self-awareness in many facets of one's life in order to find greater equilibrium and overall health. This can be exemplified by improving communication with one's physical body. In order to begin to dialogue with the body, start by asking yourself some basic questions. It is all right if you do not initially know the answers. Remember, this is a tool for transformation. Awareness that we do not know something can be very useful information. One of the fundamental principles in both spiritual growth and psychological expansion is uncovering our "blind spots" and our rote misconceptions about ourselves. Only when these are illuminated can we establish new thoughts and beliefs that are maximally supportive of our overall health and wholeness.

Below are some questions for self-exploration about food and diet. They are useful on their own, or they can be used to evaluate a food/mood/well-being journal like the one explained above (page 108).

1. What foods do I find most satisfying?
2. Why, or in what ways, are these satisfying?
3. Do I feel good when I think about eating these foods?
4. Do I actually feel good when and after I eat them?
5. Do I have ideas about what is "good" for me to eat? In what ways do I believe that certain foods are good for me? From when and where did those ideas come? Do I actually experience well-being when I eat those foods?
6. Do I have ideas about what is "bad" for me to eat? In what ways do I believe that certain foods are "bad" for me? From when and where did those ideas come? Do I eat foods that I believe are "bad" for me? Under what circumstances? How do I feel emotionally and physically when I eat foods that I believe are "bad" for me?

7. Do I believe that some foods or ways of eating are more spiritual or enlightened? From when and where did those ideas come? Do I eat in that way? Do I feel spiritually connected and fulfilled? Do I know others who eat differently yet seem spiritually in tune?

8. Do I want to continue to hold these beliefs? Are they in harmony with who I am right now, and with the calm, centered, and self-actualized person I am becoming?

CHAPTER 10

⚜

Nutrients and Amino Acids

Nutritional supplements are frequently used as part of a program for improving emotional well-being. While it is ideal to meet one's nutritional needs by consuming a healthy, nutrient-dense diet, some people, including many with anxiety, have higher nutritional requirements of certain nutrients than "average" persons. Those who suffer from anxiety can be deficient in specific nutrients, either for constitutional reasons or because they utilize more of these nutrients as their bodies attempt to reestablish balance. These persons may find judiciously chosen nutritional supplements to be of great benefit as restoratives for quieting anxiety.

In this chapter I introduce a variety of individual nutrients that are potentially of benefit in persons with anxiety. Nutritional supplements should be selected carefully, with good reasoning, and with a gut sense that they are correct. Ideally they are used to correct imbalances, so they may not need to be taken for extended periods of time. It is a good idea, when possible, to consult with a trained practitioner who can advise about supplementation.

Discussed below are some of the most beneficial nutrients for relieving anxiety. For each one, some rich food sources are listed, as well as notes about supplementation including which forms are most bioavailable.

B-Complex Vitamins

B vitamins are essential for many chemical processes in the body. They support healthy neurotransmitter levels, a calm and serene nervous system, and balanced energy production. Physiologically, our bodies most often utilize them synergistically; we need a balance of B vitamins for healthy biochemistry. While there are certain circumstances for which higher levels of individual B vitamins are required, it is usually best to take them as a group, or complex.

Emotional and physical stress, including chronic anxiety, can raise overall nutritional requirements for B vitamins. Metabolizing stress neurochemicals and clearing them from the body requires a lot of B vitamins. Some supplementation of B vitamins is frequently of benefit when chronic stress has been or is present. B supplementation can benefit adrenal fatigue, a condition that may result from stress. Many chronically anxious persons have some amount of adrenal fatigue.

The common modern practice of chewing on ice is detrimental to B-vitamin absorption and can create B deficiencies independent of stress levels. It is just not a good idea to chew on ice. Even drinking lots of iced drinks can deplete B vitamins. Our bodies most easily process foods consumed at room temperature, or better still, at body temperature.

Most B vitamins are water-soluble and are safe in larger than physiologic doses, as long as they are in balance with each other. A few B vitamins, mentioned below, have upper limits for safety. If you choose to take a B-complex vitamin, it is often best to choose a co-enzymated B, since this is the form of the vitamins the body utilizes most easily. Also choose a B complex that is balanced, meaning that relative amounts of each nutrient vary with how much is typically used by most people, rather than selecting a "B50" or "B100," which simply means there are 50 mg or 100 mg of each B vitamin.

Rich Food Sources of B-complex Vitamins: Many foods are rich in a variety of B-complex nutrients. Whole grains are good food sources of many B's. The B vitamins are found in the outer layers of the grain, so refined products like white flour and white rice are depleted of these nutrients. Whole grains are especially rich in B1. Ideally, grains should be pre-soaked for several hours to improve digestibility. The soak water should be discarded, as it contains anti-nutrients. Green leafy vegetables are rich in some B's, as are beans and legumes, though, like the grains, they should be pre-soaked and the soak water discarded.

Among animal foods, organ meats (especially liver) are rich in many B vitamins, as are fish, shellfish, meat, and poultry. Eggs, especially the yolks, are a good source of several B's, as are dairy products. For optimal nutritional value, as well as for ethical considerations, animal foods should be raised in a truly natural manner, with ruminant animals grazing on grass, and poultry pecking in yards. The words "all natural" on packaging are often a marketing gimmick that is essentially meaningless. When possible, purchase from farmer's markets or directly from local farmers and ranchers, whose practices you understand and agree with.

Yeast Products and B-Complex

Many of the B vitamins sold in capsule and tablet form are derived from nutritional yeast. It has a nutty or cheesy flavor and is a rich source of B vitamins and protein. Often incorrectly called "brewer's yeast," the most common type used is deactivated *Saccharomyces cereviseae* yeast that is cultured with molasses and sugar cane, which is more correctly named "nutritional yeast." Most nutritional yeast is fortified with B12 (usually cyanocobalamin, a less desirable but cheap form of B12). Nutritional yeast is widely available in natural food stores, sold in bulk.

Some individuals with yeast sensitivities or a history of candida may not do well with this supplemental product, or with commercial B vitamins. Furthermore, nutritional yeast is somewhat high in the excitatory neurotransmitter free glutamic acid, which the body uses to make the calming neurotransmitter GABA. Glutamic acid may convert to the excitotoxin glutamate when the yeast is processed at high temperatures, potentially causing a reaction similar to monosodium glutamate (MSG). If you use nutritional yeast, do not cook with it at high temperatures.

True brewer's yeast, as opposed to nutritional yeast, is not gluten-free, so I do not recommend it. Nor do I recommend torula yeast, which is a strain of candida called *Candida utilis* that is used in manufacturing many packaged "natural" foods, including spicy or barbecue chips and veggie burgers. It is used as a flavor enhancer instead of MSG. Torula can be grown on sugar from paper mills (a by-product of the paper industry), on cane sugar, fruit sugar, or on sulfite liquors. Like MSG, torula yeast is quite high in glutamic acid and can act as a nervous system stimulant in a manner similar to MSG. Torula yeast "looks better" on the label to many consumers who are aware of the endocrine and nervous system problems associated with MSG, but it is not really an improvement. I advise people with anxiety to steer clear of products that have any glutamic acid-rich excitotoxins listed on the label, including torula yeast, MSG, and autolyzed yeast extract, and to use nutritional yeast with circumspection. Torula also is potentially highly allergenic, and persons sensitive to *Candida albicans* will frequently cross-react with this. Torula can colonize the body, especially the bladder, causing discomfort and bladder irritability. Unfortunately, it is found in many dietary supplements because of its high protein content, and it is fed to farmed fish. The take-home point for anxiety relief here is: avoid torula yeast in food and supplements, as well as true brewer's yeast. If desired, use *Saccharomyces cereviseae* nutritional yeast cautiously, especially at first, to be sure you tolerate it well. Many vegetarians rely on nutritional yeast for B vitamins since they don't eat animal products.

There is evidence linking OCD with excessively high glutamic acid levels in the brain.[1] Persons with OCD should avoid nutritional yeast as well as brewer's yeast and torula yeast products.

Vitamins for Soothing Anxiety

B1—Thiamine

Active form (coenzyme): Thiamine Pyrophosphate (TPP)

RDA: 1.1–1.4 mg. Optimal: 25–100 mg per day

Rich food sources of thiamine include liver, nutritional yeast, beef, pork, whole grains (especially those which have been soaked before cooking), green peas, asparagus, spinach, beans, nuts (especially Brazil nuts), peanuts, and bananas.

Discussion: Thiamine is a water-soluble vitamin that is not stored in the body, so it must be derived from the diet. It is essential in many biochemical processes, including metabolization of carbohydrates and fats for energy, proper functioning of the heart, brain, muscles, nervous system, and gastrointestinal tract, and proper growth and development.

Emotionally, low thiamine is associated with obsessive and negative thoughts and feelings of impending doom. Adequate levels of this vitamin are important for resolution of anxiety. Thiamine can be an important factor in good sleep. When thiamine is deficient, sleep can be interrupted, or a person may fall asleep only to waken shortly afterwards and have difficulty returning to sleep.

Many foods and drinks affect our levels of thiamine. Most notably, thiamine is depleted by alcohol. In chronic alcoholism, the depletion of thiamine can cause Wernicke-Korsakoff syndrome, which is marked by degeneration in the nervous system.

Thiamine can also be opposed by consumption of large amounts of foods that contain thiaminase, an enzyme that breaks it down. The enzyme is most plentiful in raw fish and shellfish. Tea, coffee, and betel nuts contain other anti-thiamine factors. Diets high in processed foods can contribute to thiamine deficiency, and some medications will deplete this nutrient as well.

Precautions: None known.

B3—Niacin

Active form: Niacinamide

RDA: 16–18 mg per day. Optimal, varies with situation: 100–1000 mg three times daily.

Rich food sources: Bacon, wheat and rice bran, beets, nutritional yeast, organ meats (especially liver and kidney), fish (especially anchovies, salmon, swordfish, halibut, and tuna), meats (including chicken, turkey, veal, beef, venison, and lamb), turnips, sunflower seeds, potatoes, lima beans, peanuts, sun-dried tomatoes, and paprika. Our bodies can convert the amino acid tryptophan into niacin. Foods high in tryptophan include meat, poultry, eggs, and dairy products.

Discussion: Niacin is an essential B vitamin that is a valuable anti-inflammatory and also of potential therapeutic benefit in normalizing blood sugar. It is used as a pharmaceutical in treatment of cholesterol imbalances. It is sometimes used in treatment of anxiety, usually under medical guidance, to quell anxiety and help patients discontinue or taper benzodiazepine medications.[2] Some research suggests that high doses of niacinamide (but not other forms of niacin) may calm anxiety in a manner similar to benzodiazepines,[3] though more research is certainly needed. Many types of anxiety symptoms, including social anxiety, generalized anxiety, PTSD, and panic attacks, may be improved with this nutrient.

Precautions: 1. Avoid using high doses of niacin in gout, or in known liver disease. 2. May cause flushing of the skin, especially if deficient. 3. May aggravate peptic ulcers. Avoid if an ulcer is present or suspected.

B5—Pantothenic Acid

Active form: Pantethine or calcium pantothenate

RDA: 5–7 mg/day. Optimal: For anxiety or stress, 200–400 mg/day, higher in some conditions such as inflammatory bowel disease.

Rich food sources: Liver, eggs, dairy products such as milk and yogurt, many nuts, ocean fish, many green vegetables, legumes, tomatoes, avocado, mushrooms, nutritional yeast, whole wheat and whole rye.

Discussion: B5 or pantothenic acid is well known as a stress-busting vitamin. It is essential for the body's production of stress-modulating adrenal hormones, and for formation of immune system antibodies. The name derives from the Greek word *pantos,* which means "everywhere." Indeed, pantothenic acid is found in every cell of the body. It has a host of important functions: metabolism of foods, enzyme production, energy production, bile production, regulation of healthy lipids and triglyceride levels, detoxification, and biosynthesis of hormones, hemoglobin, and neurotransmitters.

Pantothenic acid can be especially helpful for anxiety relief. It is an essential co-factor for increasing production of the calming neurotransmitter serotonin. It offers extra benefits to anxious persons with adrenal fatigue, migraines (often associated with low serotonin), chronic fatigue, and lipid abnormalities, since it is necessary for proper fatty acid metabolism, and stress is known to change serum lipid concentrations. It is frequently used to support the body in smoking cessation and alcohol recovery.

Precautions: Avoid in hemophilia as pantethine may increase bleeding time; otherwise it is considered safe.

B6—Pyridoxine

Preferred forms: pyridoxal 5' phosphate (PLP or P5P) and pyridoxamine 5' phosphate (PMP)

RDA (adults): 1.3–1.7 mg. Optimal: 25–50 mg. Despite its importance, there is an upper limit for this B vitamin, as high doses can cause neurotoxicity. Avoid ongoing supplemental use of more than 100 mg per day.

Rich food sources: Beef, chicken, fish, organ meats (especially liver), avocado, bananas, cabbage including fermented sauerkraut and kim chi, chickpeas, potatoes, winter squash.

Discussion: B6 is an extremely important nutrient, used in more than a hundred physiologic pathways, and it is key for mental and emotional health. Low B6 has been linked to many chronic inflammatory problems.[4] It is important for good sleep, proper nervous system function, feelings of well-being, metabolization of proteins, lipids, and sugars, immune function, and metabolism of neurotransmitters. Along with B5, it is required in the conversion of the amino acid tryptophan to serotonin, and is essential as well for conversion of serotonin to melatonin. It is required in the brain for making GABA from glutamic acid.[5] With anxiety and/or insomnia, some supplementation of this nutrient may be helpful. It may be deficient in individuals who have autoimmune problems, chronic bowel disease, alcoholism, or kidney disease.[6]

Precautions: 1. May affect blood sugar. 2. May increase risk of bleeding. Discontinue supplemental B6 one week prior to surgery. 3. May lower blood pressure, so avoid if blood pressure is already too low. 4. Neurotoxic with prolonged high-dose use. Avoid more than 100 mg/day.

B12—Cobalamin

Active form: Methylcobalamin, which is highly preferred to cyano-cobalamin, as the latter contains cyanide, a known toxin

RDA (adults): 2.4–2.8 mcg/day. Optimal: 500–1000 mcg/day.

Rich food sources: Liver and other organ meats, beef, lamb, egg yolk, chicken (dark meat), turkey, clams, tuna, cheese, milk, yogurt. A minuscule amount of B12 is made in tempeh, and cyanocobalamin is often added to nutritional yeast.

Discussion: B12 is essential for proper nervous system function and is important for maintaining good mood and good sleep. There is evidence suggesting that B12 assists the body in resetting circadian rhythms in the presence of bright light.[7] B12 may improve the time it takes to fall asleep and the quality of sleep.[8] Deficiency of B12 can lead to neuropathy, depression, fatigue, and even dementia, as well as many of the symptoms of anxiety, including heart palpitations, irritability, and forgetfulness. B12 is also important in the body's synthesis of SAM-e, a significant biochemical for happy mood, joint health, and lowered inflammation.

B12 is almost exclusively found in animal foods. Long-term vegans frequently develop a deficiency of this nutrient, unless they take it supplementally. B12 in animal foods is generally absorbed via a co-factor called "intrinsic factor" that is made in the stomach. Persons who do not eat meat for several years may lose the ability to make intrinsic factor, and then they cannot absorb oral B12 supplements. For these people B12 shots can be required for a healthy nervous system. B12 levels can easily be tested in the blood. A frank deficiency is less than 200 pg/ml,[9] while a relative deficiency is less than 400 pg/ml. Ideal levels are 600–1200 pg/ml. An excess of folate or supplemental synthetic folic acid can lead to a deficiency of B12.

Precautions: Safe, except with Leber's disease, a rare hereditary eye disease, or allergy to cobalamin.

Inositol

Preferred sources: Myo-inositol, or inositol

RDA: None. The average diet supplies about 1000 mg per day. Optimal: varies widely, with 2000–8000 mg commonly used in anxiety.

Rich food sources: Cantaloupe, oranges, other fruits, nuts. A form of inositol, inositol hexaphosphate, is found in many foods, including legumes and whole grains, in conjunction with the phytates, but it is not very useable because phytates in these same foods block nutrient absorption. Soaking grains and legumes, and discarding the soak water, makes the inositol more bio-available.

Discussion: Inositol is a carbohydrate that is sometimes mentioned as part of the B-complex group. It modulates the effects of serotonin, making it more available to cells, and is vital in supporting cell-to-cell communication and signaling. It deserves special mention as an anti-anxiety nutrient, since it is often of great value for persons with anxiety, OCD,[10] PTSD, panic disorder, phobias including claustrophobia, social anxiety, insomnia, and intrusive or recurrent negative thoughts.[11] For patients who struggle with anxiety, I frequently advise a trial of inositol. Some people find that this simple, relatively inexpensive supplement changes their life for the better.

Inositol has many other non-anxiety-related uses, including helping normalize cholesterol and triglyceride levels, decreasing polycystic ovarian syndrome (the D-chiro-inositol form), and decreasing nerve pain in diabetics.[12]

There have been many promising positive studies of inositol for support of positive mood. In one small study, it was shown to be as effective for OCD as SSRIs (selective serotonin reuptake inhibitor pharmaceuticals), but without significant side effects.[13] A different, double-blind study of inositol in panic attacks found a substantial benefit as compared with SSRIs.[14]

Dosage in anxiety: A wide range can be effective, but it is good to increase dose gradually, starting with 250–500 mg once or twice a day. Increase every few days, until a desired level of relief is achieved. Commonly 750–1000 mg three or four times per day, before meals and at bedtime, is helpful for most types of anxiety, but higher doses, perhaps 1500–2000 mg three or four times per day, are sometimes used in OCD, PTSD, and panic attacks. While inositol is safe for adults in large amounts, up to 20 grams (20,000 mg) per day, most people see improvement with much lower amounts, in the range of 2–10 grams (2000–10,000 mg) per day.

Precautions: 1. Can cause loose stools at higher doses, resolved with lowering dose or discontinuation of the supplement. 2. Dizziness has been reported in the literature.

Vitamin C

Preferred form: C ascorbate

RDA: Adults, 75–120 mg/day[15]

Suggested dose: 500 mg–3 grams daily, in divided doses

Rich food sources: Camu camu, rose hips, goji berries, acerola, black currants, cayenne, chili peppers, bell peppers, strawberries, elderberries, oranges, grapefruit, lemons, kiwifruit, tomato juice, cantaloupe, Brussels sprouts, broccoli, collard greens, raw oysters, and liver (all sorts).

Discussion: Vitamin C is a water-soluble antioxidant nutrient, essential in many areas of health including immune function, wound repair, skin and joint health, energy production, metabolism of cortisol, and production of the neurotransmitters norepinephrine and serotonin. It is plentiful in many fruits and vegetables.

In times of stress, extra vitamin C can help the body to clear excess cortisol. It also supports the body's ability to remove other stored toxins that may be associated with anxiety symptoms. For example, vitamin C is effective and safe in helping support the body to clear mercury and other heavy metals. Vitamin C is also essential in the biosynthesis of the calming neurotransmitter serotonin. Serotonin, in turn, helps with positive mood, good sleep, a healthy sex drive, and increasing the pain threshold.

Of note, if you are trying to avoid corn and/or other genetically modified foods and supplements, it is useful to know that virtually all vitamin C supplements are made from genetically modified corn, unless the packaging says otherwise. There are beet, tapioca, and non-GMO corn-sourced vitamin C products available, but you need to request them. As more consumers do so, more non-GMO products will become available.

Precautions: 1. Safe, though large oral doses can trigger loose stools. 2. Avoid with kidney stones.

Vitamin D

Preferred forms: Ideal is D3 cholecalciferol—it is the human form of the vitamin, the type our bodies manufacture from sunlight on the skin. D2 is a synthetic plant form that some researchers believe may actually exacerbate vitamin-D deficiencies.

RDA: Adults, 400–600 iu (international units) daily. Optimal: 1000–2000 iu per day, and sometimes more. If using higher doses, consult a physician and monitor blood levels.

Rich food sources: Egg yolks, cod liver oil, fish liver (monk fish liver is a delicacy served in many Japanese restaurants), many fatty fish including salmon, mackerel, canned sardines, herring, and shrimp.

Discussion: Vitamin D is a fat-soluble nutrient with many essential functions. It is required for calcium and mineral absorption and is necessary for healthy bones, immune system, and muscles. It is also essential for support of healthy mood. Many psychiatrists now regularly recommend supplemental D3 for patients with anxiety and depression. Low vitamin-D levels may increase anxiety.

The common blood test for levels is 25 hydroxy vitamin D, and it measures the stored vitamin D. D deficiency is below 30 ng/ml (nanograms per milliliter). Optimal blood levels for persons with anxiety or depression are around 50 ng/ml. If supplementation is taken but blood levels fail to rise as expected, ask your physician to check 1,25 dihydroxy vitamin-D levels as well, especially if you suffer from inflammation. This test measures circulating vitamin D, which can be elevated even when stored D levels are normal or low. Also carry out this test if high-dose supplementation is undertaken.

Occasionally, supplementing vitamin D increases anxiety. In these cases there is usually a deficiency of magnesium, and supplementing magnesium will help eliminate the disturbance.

Precautions: While generally safe under 400 iu per day, supplemental D should be used under medical advice if you have sarcoidosis, kidney disease, kidney stones, hyperparathyroidism, or histoplasmosis.

Minerals

Calcium

Preferred forms: Calcium citrate or food-based calcium

RDA: Adults, 1000–1300 mg. Optimal: RDA levels are
appropriate.

Rich food sources: Dairy products (milk, cheese, yogurt, cottage
cheese). Full-fat dairy products are preferred, since fats are key to
the absorption of minerals, including calcium. Consuming raw
dairy products, including raw milk when it is available from a
certified raw-milk dairy, can enhance mineral availability. Other
rich sources include bones cooked in soups and stews, bone
broths, sardines, salmon, oysters, Brazil nuts, hazelnuts, sesame
seeds, hard water, collards, kale, chard, beet greens, cabbage,
mustard greens, broccoli, rutabagas, green beans, lima beans,
okra, sea vegetables, oranges, rhubarb, blackstrap molasses, ban-
cha tea, and many culinary and medicinal herbs.

Discussion: Calcium is found in every tissue in the body. It is essential for healthy bones and skeletal structure, proper function of
the heart, nerve conduction, muscle contraction and function,
strong teeth, acid/base balance, blood clotting, and coordination
of function. In our bodies, calcium exists in a balance with magnesium. Most of the calcium is outside of cells, while magnesium
is inside of cells. Nerves and muscles fire based upon calcium/
magnesium ion-exchange channels.

Calcium is absorbed in the intestinal tract, and persons with
chronic bowel problems may have difficulty absorbing it. Phytic
acid in grains and some veggies binds calcium in the GI tract.
Excess sugar and carbohydrates will pull calcium from bones to
buffer acid and base biochemical reactions.

Calcium deficiency can contribute to anxiety and anxiety-
related problems including insomnia, panic attacks, irritability,
and heart palpitations, but all of these problems may also be

related to magnesium deficiency. In fact, deficiency of calcium is a less likely cause of anxiety than deficiency of magnesium. Usually, with a healthy diet and sufficient magnesium, calcium supplementation is not required, as it can be easily absorbed from foods. Sometimes calcium and magnesium are taken together, particularly at bedtime, to promote restful sleep.

Precautions: Safe except in kidney disease, sarcoidosis, and other diseases of calcium metabolism. For osteoporosis, the chemistry is a bit more complicated, so consult with a nutritionally oriented physician regarding calcium vs. magnesium supplementation for this condition.

Lithium

Preferred form: Lithium orotate (lithium bound to orotic acid). This is considered by many to be an ideal form, as orotic acid may have independent benefits for heart, liver, and muscle health. It is efficiently absorbed.[16] (Lithium carbonate is another familiar form, available only by prescription, used as a mood stabilizer in bipolar disorder.)

RDA: None. Ideal: 1000 mcg/day is good for an average adult,[17] and this level has been provisionally suggested as an RDA.[18]

Rich food sources: Certain drinking waters, mustard, cheese and milk, kelp, potatoes, peppers, tomatoes, seafood, sardines, chamomile tea, whole grains.

Discussion: Many people think of lithium as a drug, but it is a mineral found in varying amounts in drinking water and soils around the world. The pharmaceutical drug lithium is used for treatment of bipolar depression, but it tends to be physically harsh and requires careful monitoring of levels.

Naturally occurring lithium, however, is typically soothing and gentle, and does not require monitoring if taken in small amounts, like the amounts naturally occurring in some water supplies. Our bodies do require a little lithium. It is naturally calming and balancing, helping the body metabolize and clear the fight-or-flight hormones epinephrine (adrenaline) and nor-epinephrine (noradrenaline).

Dosage: A standard dose of lithium orotate in lowering anxiety is 10–20 mg once daily.

Precautions: 1. Lithium is excreted almost entirely by the kidneys. Therefore, in pre-existing kidney disease, do not use lithium, even as a low-dose naturally occurring salt, unless advised to by a physician with levels monitored. 2. Over time, high doses of lithium may damage the thyroid. Acute lithium excess can cause muscle weakness, fatigue, diarrhea, vomiting and/or ringing in the ears. These problems are currently seen exclusively in persons who are taking pharmaceutical doses of lithium. 3. Side effects from low doses are rare, but consider using even low-dose over-the-counter lithium under the guidance of a physician, especially if using it for more than a few weeks.

Magnesium

Preferred form: Varies, see below for fuller discussion

RDA: Adults, 300–400 mg/day. Optimal: 500–800 mg/day, possibly more.

Rich food sources: Green leafy vegetables, chlorella, wheat and barley grass juices (the chlorophyll molecule has magnesium in the center just as hemoglobin has iron in its center); certain fish, especially halibut, sea bass, oysters, salmon, and raw tuna (sashimi); dairy products including milk and yogurt; whole grains; legumes including peas, beans, peanuts, and peanut butter; nuts, especially almonds and cashews; white potatoes eaten with the skin; and chocolate, especially raw with a high cacao content, is a rich source. Hard water is another major source of magnesium.

Discussion: Magnesium is the fourth most abundant mineral in
the body and the one many experts consider most likely to be
deficient. Important in more than three hundred biochemical
processes including those in the bones, muscles, nervous system,
immune system, and cardiovascular system, it is present in every
cell of the body. It is essential for keeping blood pressure and
blood sugar in a normal range, and for cellular energy and protein production.

Magnesium is absorbed in the intestinal tract. Persons with
chronic bowel problems may have difficulty absorbing magnesium, while acute or chronic vomiting and diarrhea can deplete
the body of magnesium. Absorption of dietary magnesium may
decline with age, so senior citizens may be especially low in this
essential mineral. Several nutrients, including calcium, may block
magnesium absorption. Teens and pregnant women need especially high levels of magnesium. In pregnancy, adequate magnesium levels decrease the risk of pre-eclampsia and eclampsia.

The kidneys excrete extra magnesium to remove it from the
body. Certain medications, as well as poorly controlled diabetes
and alcoholism, can result in excess excretion of magnesium
in the urine. Alcoholics who are actively drinking and those
in recovery from alcoholism usually benefit from magnesium
supplementation.

Physically, suboptimal magnesium can cause fatigue, tinnitus,
muscle weakness and aches, and nausea. The most common sign
of magnesium deficiency is muscle spasms.

Emotionally, magnesium is calming, and it is widely used in
anxiety disorders. It quiets heart palpitations and soothes frayed
nerves. It is very important for lowering stress hormones. Magnesium also promotes sleep, so while it does not necessarily cause
drowsiness, it is often used at bedtime.

Magnesium is very helpful as a muscle relaxant. Many people
with anxiety have a mass of tight muscles. Magnesium works
directly on the nerve cells to regulate how much calcium is

taken up by the cell, and it can calm muscles that are tight from nervous tension. If muscle tension is a frequent anxiety-related problem, a topical magnesium cream can be extremely effective for relief.

A typical oral dose of supplemental magnesium is 100–600 mg per day. But the maximum recommended dose of supplemental magnesium is 300 mg/day, unless blood levels are regularly checked once or twice a year to make sure the level of magnesium is not getting too high.

To accurately test the body's level of magnesium, it is important to check red blood cell (RBC) magnesium and not serum magnesium. Over 99 percent of magnesium is stored in cells, and the amount in serum generally remains stable unless there is catastrophic loss of the element. Most doctors, I have noticed, unfortunately order the wrong test unless (gently) reminded that RBC magnesium is more accurate.

Oral supplements of magnesium are usually combinations of the mineral and another substance. The combination forms a salt or chloride. Some of these are better absorbed; some are more laxative and others less so. Enteric coating of magnesium supplements is not advised, as it can decrease bioavailability. If orally taken magnesium is extremely laxative in an individual, this may be an indication that body stores are quite low in that person. When oral magnesium is not tolerated, use topical magnesium chloride oils and creams.

Magnesium chloride: Well absorbed orally and transdermally. It is laxative when taken orally but not transdermally.

Magnesium glycinate (oral): Bound to the calming amino acid glycine, this is the form I most often recommend in anxiety. It is less laxative than many other forms.

Magnesium malate (oral): Used often for treatment of fibromyalgia, it is a less laxative form of magnesium and is fine for persons with anxiety. It also helps with detoxification of aluminum.

Magnesium taurate (oral): Bound to taurine, this form of magnesium includes an important amino acid for the heart. I suggest this often for anxiety with panic attacks or nervous palpitations.

Magnesium aspartate (oral): Avoid, as aspartate can increase anxiety.

Magnesium citrate (oral): Quite laxative, thus great for persons with anxiety who also have constipation.

Magnesium lactate (oral): Very well absorbed, fine for anxiety, a less laxative form.

Magnesium oxide (oral): This is cheap, widely available, but less well absorbed and more laxative than other forms of magnesium. Will tend to form caprylates in the intestinal tract and can be detoxifying, so I advise it only for brief periods of time, or to address candida overgrowth.

Magnesium sulfate (oral and topical): Very widely available as Epsom salts, and quite inexpensive. Generally well absorbed and moderately laxative when taken orally. Used commonly in baths.

Precautions: 1. Because magnesium is excreted via the kidneys, supplemental magnesium (including magnesium laxatives) are not recommended for people with any amount of kidney failure, unless advised by a physician. 2. Excessive supplementation with magnesium should be avoided, unless under medical guidance.

Drug interactions: 1. Many drugs cause the kidneys to excrete magnesium, resulting in low levels of this mineral. These include the diuretics hydrochlorothiazide (HCTZ), lasix, bumex, the pain reliever Excedrin, antibiotics including gentamycin and amphotericin, and the cancer drug cisplatin, all of which cause wasting of magnesium. 2. Supplemental magnesium may decrease the effectiveness of tetracycline.

Amino Acids and Their Derivatives

GABA—Gamma amino butyric acid

Natural food sources: GABA itself is found in tea and a few
foods—fermented foods like kim chi, yogurt, and some raw-
milk cheeses, especially those with molds; brains of animals;
potatoes and cherry tomatoes—but many more foods contain
the GABA precursors glutamic acid and glutamine that increase
biosynthesis of this important amino acid. These include many
fish (especially mackerel, cod, and halibut), lentils, almonds,
walnuts, citrus fruits, bananas, nutritional yeast, cheeses (especially hard types like parmesan, cheddar, gouda, and provo-
lone), and whole grains such as whole wheat, whole oats, and
brown rice. L-glutamine supplements can also boost GABA
production.

Discussion: The amino acid gamma amino butyric acid, or GABA,
is the principal calming neurotransmitter in the brain, synthesized in the body from glutamine. As a supplement, it is used
widely in reducing anxiety, decreasing frequency and severity of
panic attacks, and improving well-being in PTSD.

   GABA is calming on its own, decreasing nervousness and
anxiety and elevating mood. It also assists in production of
endorphins (natural opiates that provide feelings of well-being)
and increases levels of serotonin. GABA reduces concentrations
of the fight-or-flight hormones norepinephrine and epinephrine.
GABA also assists production of calming alpha-state brain waves,
helping relaxation, happy mood, and good sleep. It can cause
some drowsiness when used as a supplement, particularly at first
and with higher doses, so it is good to try it initially at bedtime.

   GABA can be reduced by chronic stress and low levels of B
vitamins, zinc, and manganese, all of which are required for
its formation. Low levels of the hormone progesterone can
also affect GABA production. Low progesterone is a common

occurrence in perimenopausal women who are experiencing some increase in anxiety. The heavy metals mercury and lead can also block synthesis of GABA.

Dosage: Typical dose is 250–1000 mg once or twice a day.

Precautions: 1. Avoid if also taking drugs involved in GABA pathways, particularly the benzodiazepines and barbiturates, unless under medical supervision 2. High doses can cause a number of unpleasant side effects: changes in blood pressure, racing heart, nausea, flushing, and increased anxiety. Do not exceed recommended doses.

Glycine

Rich food sources: Animal proteins such as eggs, fish, shellfish, meat, poultry, and dairy products, as well as legumes including peanuts and various beans, spirulina, and seaweeds, especially nori (laver).

Discussion: Found in many foods and in relatively high concentrations in the brain and spinal cord, glycine is an amino acid that acts as a neurotransmitter. It is important for the brain, musculoskeletal system, digestive tract, growth and development, skin, and prostate gland and helps calm a number of forms of anxiety including generalized anxiety. At higher doses, glycine may improve symptoms of OCD.[19] One way glycine may calm anxiety is by decreasing secretion of norepinephrine.[20] Along with magnesium, it helps tense muscles to relax and can be very helpful for calming nervous tension associated with muscle spasms in the neck, back, and abdomen. It may also help improve the REM (rapid eye movement) stage of sleep.[21]

Dosage: 500–1000 mg once or twice a day. Bedtime is an excellent time to take glycine, as it can help sleep to be more deep and restful.[22]

Precautions: Exert caution when supplementing with any amino acids if there is kidney disease.

5-HTP—5-hydroxy-L-tryptophan

Food sources: There are trace amounts of free 5-HTP in poultry and cheese, but chicken, turkey, and red meat are rich sources of L-tryptophan that the body converts first into 5-HTP and then serotonin.

Discussion: 5-HTP is a naturally occurring intermediate biochemical, mostly made in the intestinal tract during the body's synthesis of the hormone serotonin from the amino acid L-tryptophan in foods. Taking 5-HTP as a supplement, along with adequate intake of vitamin B6, can increase the body's stores of serotonin, a neurotransmitter of calm well-being.

Serotonin is utilized in the brain and tissues to support normal appetite, diminished food cravings, good moods, impulse control, decreased worry, and healthy sleep. At night, some serotonin is converted in the pineal gland to melatonin, a hormone important for healthy sleep. When serotonin is low, as is often the case with depression and anxiety, melatonin is usually low too. Low serotonin and melatonin may be one cause of sleep difficulties in people who are depressed or anxious. Supplemental 5-HTP is often used beneficially for improved sleep.

Many people with addictive and compulsive behaviors such as gambling, food addictions, and drug and alcohol addictions are actually quite low in serotonin.[23] Increasing serotonin via 5-HTP can help with impulse control. It also can decrease negative thinking and reduce obtrusive and repetitive thoughts.

Receptors for serotonin are found in the brain, GI tract, and blood cells that circulate throughout the body. It is often claimed that 5-HTP helps reduce appetite. Others believe, though, that it normalizes appetite, so appetite is lowered in compulsive overeaters but improved in anorexics. This is not surprising, as studies have shown serotonin depletion in anorexics.[24] It can also help, in some cases, to decrease the compulsion that anorexics have to deny food and may decrease other addictive behaviors as well.

Through increasing serotonin, 5-HTP helps mental clarity and well-being. Higher serotonin levels can also prevent panic attacks. Studies have shown beneficial results, including fewer and less severe attacks in participants who used 5-HTP.[25] Increased serotonin is also helpful for decreasing obsessive thinking in OCD.

Commercially available supplements of 5-HTP are usually extracted from the seed of *Griffonia simplicifolia,* a tree native to Western Africa. It takes a lot of griffonia seed to extract 5-HTP; therefore taking the seed alone will not give appreciable amounts of 5-HTP. It can be synthesized in a laboratory as well. The molecules, in both cases, are identical to the naturally occurring compound that the body makes from L-tryptophan in foods.

Other conditions where 5-HTP has been beneficial include fibromyalgia, PMS (including moodiness associated with PMS migraines), and recurrent headaches. 5-HTP and serotonin can also help people with chronic pain by improving pain tolerance.

5-HTP is not for everyone. People with depression or anxiety are not always deficient in serotonin. Currently there are no good blood tests to determine serotonin levels. So most people who are interested in it just give 5-HTP a try to see if it will help in their situation.

Precautions: 1. Potential side effects of 5-HTP include the common ones: rashes, nausea, diarrhea, constipation, and headaches. These are the most commonly reported side effects from any drug or natural product and are not unique to 5-HTP. 5-HTP does often cause drowsiness, thus its use as a sleep aid, and it is therefore best taken at night. In my experience, however, a small percentage, perhaps up to 5 percent of individuals, will actually get some stimulation or alertness from 5-HTP, in which case it is best taken in the morning. There are reports on the Internet of side effects such as palpitations and shortness of breath, but so far, I have not observed these in my patients. Discontinue 5-HTP if anxiety worsens with use, a rare side effect. 2.

Nightmares are another rare side effect and usually will cease or not occur at very low doses (10–50 mg). Often nightmares go away on their own after a few days on 5-HTP. Vivid dreams may also occur, probably because of increased production of melatonin. 3. The sexual side effects associated with selective serotonin reuptake inhibitor pharmaceuticals (SSRIs), including decreased libido, have been reported with 5-HTP. Decreased libido and delayed orgasm may result from higher serotonin levels, which can be a benefit in premature ejaculation. However, most healthcare practitioners observe far fewer problems with loss of libido with 5-HTP than with SSRIs. Some people even report improved libido with the supplement. 4. As of 2013, there have been no reports of serious or life-threatening side effects from 5-HTP. Still, there is no long-term research regarding its safety. 5. 5-HTP is not recommended in pregnancy or breast feeding, as there have been no data collected regarding safety for the fetus or baby. Serotonin does cross the blood-brain barrier.

Dosage: Most capsules are 50 or 100 mg. Patients take 50–300 mg per day, and occasionally higher doses. High doses are best administered with medical supervision. For faster results, patients can take higher doses initially and then lower this as their mood improves and serotonin metabolism normalizes. Highly sensitive people often require lower doses; for them 10–20 mg may be effective, while more might be likely to cause unpleasant side effects. Lower doses are also needed if the 5-HTP is taken sublingually.

Average starting dose is 50 mg at bedtime for adults under 200 pounds, and 100 mg at bedtime for adults who weight over 200 pounds. Increase, if needed, in 50-mg increments up to 100–300 mg, as long as there is no daytime drowsiness. A typical an ongoing daily dose for several months is 50–150 mg.

Most people do not need to endlessly take 5-HTP. Often patients will taper up to a comfortable dose, and taper down a few months later, noticing improvements in the first few weeks. If ongoing supplementation is helpful, usually lower doses of 50–100 mg are best. This being said, I have seen several people who took a longer time (1–2 months) before noticing improvements in mood after starting 5-HTP. If people are not seeing any benefit early on, but are not having unpleasant side effects either, I encourage them to stick with it for at least 2 months because the anxiety may be slow to improve.

Drug interactions: 1. Because 5-HTP increases the body's stores of serotonin, and SSRI drugs keep serotonin from breaking down, taking both together can theoretically result in excessive levels of serotonin. This is called the "serotonin syndrome," marked in its early stages by mental confusion, headache, shivering and sweating, nausea, diarrhea, agitation, and muscle twitches. In late stages coma or death may result. While this sounds, and is, alarming, there have actually been no published reports as of this writing (late 2013) linking use of 5-HTP supplements to serotonin syndrome. Most recorded cases of the syndrome involve interactions of two or more pharmaceutical drugs (not including 5-HTP, which is an over-the-counter supplement).

In practice, I sometimes advise using 5-HTP and SSRIs together while a patient is tapering off the SSRIs, since increasing serotonin levels can be essential in successfully tapering off SSRIs. Nonetheless, persons interested in combining 5-HTP and a SSRI are advised to undertake the combination *only* under knowledgeable medical supervision.

2. It is advisable to have medical supervision when combining any psychoactive nutrient and a pharmaceutical drug. 3. Avoid using 5-HTP when using triptan-class medications for migraines, as there is a potential for drug interactions that might include serotonin syndrome. (These include Zolmitriptan-Zomig, Sumatriptan-Imitrex, and Rizatriptan-Maxalt.)

L-tryptophan

Rich food sources: L-tryptophan is a component of most protein-rich foods, especially chicken, turkey, other poultry, red meat including beef and lamb, pork, venison, fish, eggs, and dairy products including cheese, milk, yogurt, and cottage cheese. Good vegetable sources include cacao, chickpeas, peanuts, oats, sesame, pumpkin and sunflower seeds, dates, bananas, and spirulina.

Discussion: L-tryptophan is a naturally occurring amino acid found in many foods, especially in meats and dairy products. Like 5-HTP, it is a precursor of both serotonin and melatonin. It is an essential amino acid, meaning our bodies cannot synthesize it from other nutrients; it must be taken in directly through dietary protein consumption.

The body manufactures 5-HTP from L-tryptophan, and then uses it to make both serotonin and melatonin, so the benefits of using L-tryptophan are essentially the same as those of 5-HTP. By increasing serotonin, L-tryptophan is useful for supporting healthy mood, well-being, and hopefulness, and in decreasing symptoms of anxiety and depression as well as moodiness associated with PMS. Increased serotonin and melatonin promotes restful sleep and can prevent or minimize jet lag. It may help pharmaceutical antidepressants to be effective at lower doses. Other potential benefits include a decrease in the incidence and severity of panic attacks and decreases in carbohydrate cravings.

The supplement L-tryptophan was widely used throughout the 1980s as a sleep aid. But in 1991, it was removed from the market, after an outbreak of illnesses in some persons using the supplements. Eventually the problem was traced to a contaminant from a genetically modified organism in one manufacturer's (Showa Denko's) product. After this matter was clarified, it still took many years for L-tryptophan to return to wider distribution, though it continued to be used in all infant formula manufactured in the U.S., and remained available by prescription through compounding pharmacies. In 2005, L-tryptophan was fully exonerated by regulatory agencies, and importation was reinstated. Showa Denko, the company that produced the tainted supplements, ceased all manufacture of L-tryptophan after the 1989 outbreak.

Dosage: L-tryptophan is generally found in 250- or 500-mg capsules. A standard bedtime dose is 250–1000 mg. I have seen patients who do better with 5-HTP and others who improve more easily with L-tryptophan, though I cannot explain why this is so. Still if a person has not seen improvement with one of these, it may be worthwhile to try the other. I generally advise 5-HTP before suggesting L-tryptophan, simply because L-tryptophan is more expensive.

Precautions and drug interactions: Same as with 5-HTP.

Melatonin

Food sources: Olive oil, grapes, tomatoes, wine, beer, walnuts, many fruits (especially tart cherries), bananas, oats, barley, brown rice, and milk and other dairy products. However, none of these foods have the levels found in supplements.

Discussion: Melatonin, an important hormone for sleep, is the primary hormone of the pineal gland, a small, light-sensitive, pinecone-shaped structure in the center of the human brain. The pineal gland stores and secretes other unique biochemicals, including the cannabinoid anandamide, a neurotransmitter with many functions, one of them being an association with states of bliss. The peak of secretion of melatonin is during the nighttime hours of normal sleep. Melatonin improves restful rejuvenation and resynchronizes our circadian rhythms (biological clock) with the light cycle. It is a potent antioxidant and anti-inflammatory as well, and supplements are used frequently as part of alternative cancer-treatment protocols and in natural therapies for reflux esophagitis and macular degeneration. Melatonin is also believed by many to have "anti-aging" benefits, no doubt because of improvements in rest and antioxidant activity. In the body, melatonin is made from L-tryptophan via serotonin.

Dosage: Supplements of melatonin are available in a variety of strengths. A normal dose range for support of sleep is 0.5–3.0 mg, taken a half hour before bedtime. Larger doses up to 10 mg are considered safe but are rarely required. The body can habituate to supplemental melatonin. While this is not considered dangerous, melatonin works best as a sleep aid for most people if used three or fewer times per week.

Precautions: 1. Excess supplementation can decrease sperm count in men and may decrease fertility in women. 2. Side effects may include headaches, GI upset, dizziness, nightmares, irritability, and daytime drowsiness. Side effects are temporary and will resolve after melatonin is discontinued. 3. Avoid in pregnancy and breast-feeding. 4. Avoid with hypertension, diabetes, seizures, or depression, unless under medical supervision.

Drug interactions: 1. May decrease efficacy of immunosuppressive drugs, steroids, and antidepressants. 2. Diuretic drugs may decrease the secretion of melatonin in the body, and decrease the effect of melatonin supplements. 3. Can interact with blood pressure medications. 4. Avoid if taking oral contraceptives, unless blood pressure is monitored regularly. 5. Avoid if using pharmaceutical blood thinners.

Taurine

Rich food sources: Meats and seafood, dairy products, and eggs; also breast milk. Vegan and some vegetarian diets are often chronically deficient in taurine.[26]

Discussion: Taurine, a semi-essential amino-sulfonic acid with many important roles, is one of the most prevalent compounds in the body, especially in muscle. It is required for proper cardiac function, is a main fuel for the heart, protects and nourishes the liver, and may lower blood pressure in essential hypertension. It is also a key constituent of bile, so is critical for detoxification, and is important as an antioxidant and for healthy blood lipids. It is essential for development and maintenance of skeletal muscles, the retina of the eye, and cell membranes.[27] It is considered "semi-essential" because the pancreas can synthesize some taurine from the amino acid cysteine, but we utilize taurine from animal foods most easily.

Taurine has important functions in the central nervous system, many of which contribute to its value in calming anxiety.[28] Taurine acts synergistically with magnesium, GABA, and glycine, enhancing the benefits of each, and it can protect the central nervous system from the excitotoxin glutamate. Taurine is often used successfully to calm nervous heart palpitations, especially in combination with magnesium. The combination also helps support sound and restful sleep and is often used at bedtime. Taurine mimics and amplifies the activity of GABA in quieting anxiety.[29] Taurine also can help regulate excesses of the stress hormone cortisol. Persons low in taurine may be hyperresponsive to stress. In addition to its calming properties, taurine helps improve overall energy and stamina.

Dosage: Typically, persons with anxiety use 500–1000 mg two to three times daily, between or before meals.

Precautions: 1. Taurine is quite safe, and it is found in many energy drinks in doses of 1000–2000 mg.[30] 2. Persons with bipolar disorder should only use taurine under medical supervision, as there is one anecdotal report of it possibly causing an exacerbation,[31] though it is also under investigation as a treatment for relief of bipolar disorder. 3. There is some question of whether taurine might temporarily exacerbate psoriasis, so use with caution or avoid it with this skin condition. 4. Interacts with the pharmaceutical drug lithium. Consult a doctor before combining taurine and lithium.[32]

Essential Fatty Acids

Omega-3 Fatty Acids

RDA: None in the US, though there are standards in other countries. A typical range is 300–500 mg per day. Optimal: For anxiety, 400–600 mg DHA, possibly up to 1000 mg per day, and half as much EPA.

Food sources: Omega-3s are found in fish, fish oils, egg yolks from pasture-raised poultry and those fed flax seed, and in the fats of grass-fed animals, particularly cattle. DHA is found in some algae. The true omega-3s are EPA and DHA (not DHEA, which is a hormone produced by the adrenal glands). Both are present in fish oils such as cod liver oil, generally in a ratio of three parts EPA to two parts DHA. There are no ideal vegan sources of both these essential oils. There is a supplement with the brand name of Neuromins, which is a DHA extracted from algae. It is quite expensive, though, and may not be as beneficial as DHA from fish, but it is useful for vegetarians and people who do not tolerate seafood. There are some vegetable sources of omega-3s, like alpha linolenic acid, discussed below, that can serve as a reservoir for EPA production in the cells.

Discussion: Omega-3s are essential in the diet because we cannot synthesize them. DHA, or docosahexaenoic acid, is a fatty acid that is essential for brain function, nervous system function, sperm production, development and health of the retina of the eye, child development, and maintaining a healthy heart. It is the most abundant omega-3 fatty acid in the brain and in neurons. Breast milk is very high in this nutrient, even if the mother does not eat fish.

EPA, or eicosapentaenoic acid, is a precursor for several anti-inflammatory prostaglandins. It is important for maintaining healthy blood pressure and blood lipids. It also helps reduce menstrual cramps, and may help reduce symptoms in asthma, allergies, eczema, psoriasis, diabetes, and many other health problems.

Omega-3s offer many benefits in support of positive mood. A simple but essentially correct characterization is that EPA predominantly raises low mood, while DHA principally reduces anxiety. Some studies have shown that high-dose omega-3 supplementation can be as effective as pharmaceuticals for treating anxiety and depression.[33] For anxiety relief, use more DHA than EPA, or even use DHA alone.

Precautions: Fish oils are blood thinners. People using very high doses of them may experience easy bruising. They should only be combined with prescription blood thinners like warfarin (Coumadin) under medical guidance.

Alpha-Linolenic Acid

RDA: None

Food sources: Kiwi, flax seed, chia seed, perilla leaf, lingonberry, purslane, sea buckthorn, hemp seed, walnuts

Discussion: Alpha-linolenic acid, or ALA, is another omega-3 fatty acid. ALA may be cardio-protective and can serve as a precursor for cellular production of EPA but not DHA. ALA may help with anxiety by lowering excess levels of the stress hormone cortisol, by lowering systemic inflammation, and by increasing levels of calming neurotransmitters.[34]

Precautions: Though safe, ALA-rich oils like flax oil oxidize very quickly and the oxidized (rancid) oils are unhealthy. To prevent oxidation, they should never be used in cooking, only taken raw, and even then, prepared and utilized in small batches. Shelf life matters with this oil. Toss any ALA-rich oils or supplements, including flax oil, that are past their expiration date, and store flax and chia seeds in the freezer or refrigerator.

Other Nutrients

Theanine, L-theanine

Food sources: Green and black tea, boletus mushrooms

Discussion: Theanine is an amino acid commonly found in tea, in which it modulates the caffeine, producing calming effects. Theanine has a chemical structure similar to glutamate, an amino acid used in the biosynthesis of the calming neurotransmitter GABA. Theanine supplementation can increase levels of GABA in the brain. In anxious persons, theanine can quell nervousness and improve ability to focus.

Dosage: Typical dose in anxiety is 100–200 mg one to three times daily or as needed.[35] A typical cup of green tea has 8–25 mg of theanine.

Precautions: Safe in normal doses; may lower blood pressure.[36]

Lactium

Discussion: Lactium is a protein hydrolysate isolated from milk. In the marketplace, it is found alone and in a number of stress-reducing and slimming products. Lactium contains a biologically active peptide that is relaxing and stress-reducing. Lactium can help anxious and stressed persons fall asleep and stay asleep, though it is not sedative.[37] It assists sleep by reducing physiologic stress response.[38] It can mimic the activity of GABA and act on GABA receptors.[39] (GABA is a natural neurotransmitter of calm.) Lactium can also decrease excess cortisol production in times of stress, including chronic stress.[40]

Incidentally, lactium is used in weight-loss products because heightened response to stress is strongly associated with weight gain and difficulty losing weight. By increasing calm well-being, lactium may help people achieve their desired weight.

Dosage: Used once or twice daily, or as needed. A typical dose is 150–200 mg per day, and it is often taken at bedtime. It can be used every 12 hours for added benefit.

Precautions: Safe. In persons with milk allergies, lactium is usually tolerated. It is a hydrolysate of casein (a part of the molecule), but it does not contain the whole protein, casein, or any lactose. Those are the two common sensitizing agents in dairy. Nonetheless, persons with dairy allergies, especially casein sensitivity, may react to this product so should use caution when trying it.

CHAPTER 11

꩜

Herbs for Natural Well-Being

I serendipitously began my journey with herbs at age twelve. One fine spring morning, I had a magical, life-transforming experience while on a day-long bike trip in the countryside. While riding, I spied a field of wild flowers, resplendent with thousands of dancing blossoms. I parked my bike and sat there to rest and appreciate all the colors and life. There were flowers of many hues and shapes, and so much activity—bees hummed, beetles crawled, roly-poly bugs inched along, butterflies fluttered, and humming-birds sipped nectar. Sitting there amidst all the life, with warm sunlight on my skin and a gentle breeze rustling, I felt deep peace and contentment. Then I thought about how I would describe this pastoral harmony to my parents, and I felt a moment of sadness when I realized I did not know the names of any of the flowers there except for dandelions. The fleeting sadness left me with a strong surge of desire to really know the plants, their names, their natures, and their personalities.

At that moment I had what I now understand to be a spontaneous shift of consciousness, to a more expanded state of awareness. I felt the oneness of all creation, and the love that underlies it. I knew that I am fundamentally interconnected with the plants, insects, animals, and even the rocks and soil. I understood that all of us are linked, and that in some significant way, we are all one. In that state of consciousness, I understood from the plants that they were willing to be my teachers. They would guide my growth through feelings of love, delight, and wholeness. I accepted their offer, and have cherished our fellowship since.

I continue to have a great reverence and respect for the assistance that plants offer us. In the context of this book, herbs can be wonderful, willing participants in positive support of mood. This chapter provides a general overview of the properties and applications of many of the commonly used herbs that aid emotional well-being.

Notes for Co-creation with Herbs

Throughout this book, I encourage readers to develop informed intuition. As I learned from the wildflowers that magnificent spring day, cultivating inner wisdom includes following a trail of love, delight, and wholeness. So if you are choosing to utilize herbs therapeutically, align with inner guidance by selecting the herbs that are most pleasing or fascinating to you from amongst those that are appropriate for your situation.

While dose ranges are suggested, these ranges can be broad. Each person is unique. Regardless of how most people respond to a remedy, there will always be a few individuals who will have a different experience or even respond in an opposite fashion to the typical pattern. I have known people who drink coffee to help themselves fall asleep, and others who feel anxious when they utilize the usually calming herb valerian. While these are unusual responses, working with herbs or any substance can provide a lesson in honoring our individuality and deepening appreciation of our unique ways of being.

I urge those who are considering using botanicals as part of their treatment program to be aware of ecological and ethical considerations in the application of plant medicine. It is always good to work with organically grown herbs, and even better to choose ones that are biodynamically cultivated. Wild-crafted herbs may seem like a good choice, and often are, but many plants are over-harvested in the wild. Often the most responsible choice is to utilize herbs that are ecologically farmed, unless you are certain that they are abundant in the wild and respectfully harvested. If you are not familiar with any of these terms, you might take a moment to look them up.

I also encourage people working with any botanical medicines, whether they are herbal, homeopathic, or essence, to appreciate and give thanks to the plants for their medicine. Herbs and plants are living beings, with some sort of consciousness. As I understood that spring day in the field, the same life force that flows through us flows through them. There is a unity within all creation, and at the heart we are all interconnected and interdependent. Quantum physics has come to understand that consciousness is present in every particle. The concept of consciousness in the natural world is presented more extensively in my first book, *Transforming the Nature of Health*. I offer suggestions for plant-spirit communication and appreciation for the medicine they provide at the end of this chapter, in the section "Tools for Transformation."

I begin this chapter with an overview of herbs frequently used for various symptoms found in persons with anxiety. The herbs are listed by their common names. I have grouped them according to their predominant emotional benefits, so it will be an easy way to begin, whether or not you are familiar with herbs. Several herbs appear in more than one category. I end this section with a quick reference table of key indications. The next section is a materia medica, or examination of the medicinal properties of plants, in alphabetical order. It provides an expanded discussion of each of the herbs mentioned in this chapter. Both common and botanical names are indicated here. A third section explains common preparations like teas, tinctures, and herbal baths. The final section, "Tools for Transformation," includes meditative tools for communicating with plant spirits to assist in healing and suggestions for enhancing your intuitive connection with plants. Working with plants as flower essences and aromatherapy is discussed in upcoming chapters.

At the end of the materia medica presentation, I discuss "spirit" uses. Throughout my life, even before my transformative experience in the wild-flower field, plant spirits have shared information with me about emotional and spiritual wholeness. I refer to this connection as spirit medicine or spirit communication, with profound appreciation and respect for the Native American traditions who also use these (or similar) terms. I have not, except briefly, studied Native American plant-spirit traditions, though I did attend three excellent weekend courses several years ago with Karyn Sanders, a well-known Bay Area herbalist and radio personality of Native American ancestry. If I have not had a direct spirit communication with a particular plant, I do not discuss it in that manner in my writing, so all I relate is from my own personal experience. If you want to work with the spiritual properties of these or any plants, use only low dosages or flower essences. Larger doses tend to elicit more of the herb's physiologic effects.

Herbal Support by Symptoms

Herbs for Anxiety

Anxiolytics is a relatively modern term for herbs that are traditionally used to help decrease anxiety and nervousness. They soothe jangled nerves, helping us to calm down. Some are also sleep aids, so they are listed in the sedative category as well. Other herbs are relaxing but not particularly sleep-inducing. There is a lot of overlap between sedatives and anxiolytics, so many herbs are listed in both categories. The list here is, of course, not exhaustive. Instead, it reflects plant allies with whom I have collaborated for many years. Herbal anxiolytics I discuss in more detail in the next section include Bacopa, Balm, California Poppy, Cannabis, Catnip, Chamomile, Holy Basil, Kava-kava, Lavender, Linden Flower, Longan Fruit, Oat Straw, Passion Flower, Peach leaf and twig, Red Clover, Rhodiola, Skullcap, Valerian, Vanilla, Vervain, and Wood Betony.

Herbal Stimulants

Herbal stimulants support wakefulness and mild mood elevation. They can enhance feelings of well-being and thus support overall harmony of mood. The milder ones mentioned here rarely contribute to anxiety, but always trust your own experience over the advice of others, including mine. Avoid using any herbs that increase your anxiety. Mild herbal stimulants include cinnamon, licorice, and the mints. Mints are a special case since they are mildly stimulating if drunk cold, and calming if taken warm or hot. Different properties of the mint plants are activated by temperature. Mints used for calming or uplifting include catnip, lemon balm, holy basil, and wood betony.

Moderate and strong herbal stimulants may more commonly contribute to anxiety, and it is generally a good idea to avoid or minimize using them if you are working to decrease anxiety. These stimulants include plants containing caffeine such as coffee, yerba mate, guarana, and even green or black tea. However, the caffeine in tea is modulated by the presence of theanine, a compound that is soothing, so green or black tea is often a better choice than coffee for anxious individuals who want some sort of caffeinated beverage. Nonetheless, small amounts are advised. Guarana has twice the caffeine of coffee and is best avoided, as are caffeine-laden "energy" beverages.

Herbal Sedatives for Insomnia or Agitation

Sedatives are plants with relaxing properties that are often used for insomnia or deeper agitation. There is a lot of overlap between sedatives and herbs for anxiety. Various mild herbal sedative plants are found in assorted commercial herbal sleep blends and teas. Most will help us feel mellower or a bit more like sleeping, but they will not affect our ability to drive or operate machinery. The mild sedatives, in normal amounts, are usually safe for children, healthy adults, and the elderly, unless of course one is allergic to the specific herb or there is a listed contraindication. The stronger herbs may have contraindications or might affect one's ability to drive or operate machinery, so employ caution and common sense when trying those. Many moderate or stronger sedatives will not be appropriate for children. Mild herbal sedatives include Ashwagandha, Balm (also called lemon balm, taken hot), Chamomile, Lavender, Linden Flower, Longan Fruit, Oat Straw, Red Clover, Peach Leaf, Vanilla, and Wood Betony (taken hot). Moderate and strong herbal sedatives include California Poppy, Cannabis, Catnip, Hops, Kava-kava, Passion Flower, Scute, Skullcap, Valerian, and Vervain.

Adaptogenic Herbs

Adaptogens are tonic herbs that over time help minimize the stress response. They are generally used in low doses over months or years to increase resilience and build emotional and physical stamina and vigor. Many also help support the immune system. Adaptogens are well known to herbalists worldwide and are found in virtually every medicine tradition. They are among the most revered of remedies. But most are not well understood by the scientific medical community, since they have broad but general (and sometimes immaterial) effects on supporting health. Adaptogens often help those who have experienced chronic stress, chronic anxiety, or PTSD. Adaptogenic herbs discussed here include Ashwagandha, Bacopa, Holy Basil, Licorice, Red Clover, Rhodiola, and Wood Betony. Ginseng and Siberian Ginseng are other well-known adaptogens that will not be discussed in this book, simply because they tend to be more stimulating, which is not the best route for anxious persons.

Herbs for Depression

I include a brief discussion of selected herbs often used for depression because anxiety is often accompanied by depression. But I want to say that treatment of depression is a vast topic, certainly worthy of its own book, so the herbs mentioned here are meant as an adjunct only in support of people with combined anxiety and mild depression. Some of the most commonly used herbs in this category include Holy Basil, Wood Betony, Kava-kava, Oat Straw, Passion Flower, Rhodiola, and St. John's Wort.

HERB	TYPE(S)	KEY INDICATIONS FOR SOOTHING
Ashwagandha	Mild sedative, adaptogen	Improves sleep, nourishing, calming, stabilizing, adrenal support, relief for "tired and wired"
Bacopa	Calming, stress-reducing, brain tonic	Memory improvement, reduces anxiety
Balm	Anxiety, mild sedative, calming, mild stimulant	Mild, pleasant taste, calming, helps relieve insomnia, cheerful
California Poppy	Anxiety, strong sedative	Improves sleep, helps relieve insomnia, deep relaxation, soothes jumpiness and agitation, pain relief
Cannabis	Anxiety, strong sedative	Improves sleep, calming, expansive, hypnotic

(continued on next page)

HERB	TYPE(S)	KEY INDICATIONS FOR SOOTHING
Catnip	Anxiety, calming, mild stimulant, strong sedative	Decreases worry and ruminations, relaxes smooth muscles, decreases crampiness, sleep-inducing, reduces tension and tension headaches
Chamomile	Anxiety, mild sedative	Improves sleep, settles digestion including nervous stomach, comforting
Cinnamon	Mild stimulant	Comforting, stabilizing, warming, energizing, improves well-being
Holy Basil	Anxiety, calming, mild stimulant, adaptogen, depression	Nervine, tonic
Hops	Strong sedative	Improves sleep, soothes upset stomach, calming, stabilizing, relaxing, decreases jitters
Kava-Kava	Anxiety, strong sedative, depression	Improves sleep (at higher doses); decreases social anxiety, nervous stomach and anxious heart palpitations; calming; enhances cheerfulness, friendliness, tranquility, sociability
Lavender	Anxiety, mild sedative	Calms nervous stomach, comforting, soothing, uplifting
Licorice	Mild stimulant, adaptogen	Eases nervous exhaustion and fatigue, aids digestion
Linden Flower	Anxiety, mild sedative	Good for children, eases nervous stomach and aids digestion, calming, easygoing
Logan Fruit	Anxiety, mild sedative	Calming, soothes nervous heart palpitations
Oat Straw	Anxiety, mild sedative, depression	Calming, nutritive, replenishing; a nervine that relaxes – "why was I so worried about that?"

(continued on next page)

HERB	TYPE(S)	KEY INDICATIONS FOR SOOTHING
Peach Leaf and Twig	Anxiety, mild sedative	Calms nervous stomach, calms panic attacks especially if centered on digestive symptoms
Red Clover	Anxiety, mild sedative, adaptogen	Gentle, mildly calming, soothing, nourishing, grounding, centering
Rhodiola	Anxiety, adaptogen, depression	Helps with PTSD and GAD; eases fatigue; offers adrenal support; calming; enhances self-expression
Skullcap	Anxiety, moderate sedative	Supports restful sleep; calming, nourishing, tonic
St John's Wort	Anxiety, depression	Anti-inflammatory
Valerian	Anxiety, moderate sedative	Improves sleep; calming, eases jumpiness and worry; relaxes tight muscles
Vanilla	Anxiety, mild sedative	Great for children, gentle and pleasant; calming, soothing, comforting, nourishing
Vervain	Anxiety, strong sedative	Softens rigidity
Wood Betony	Anxiety, mild sedative, calming, mild stimulant, adaptogen, depression	Restorative, eases nervous stomach, helps clear stagnation and softens chronic tension

Materia Medica (alphabetized)

Ashwagandha—Withania somnifera (Solanaceae)

Anxiety Uses: Relaxing, mild sedative for nervous exhaustion, confusion, brain fog, support of the adrenals

Other Oral Uses: Anti-aging, anti-stress, adrenal support, lowers blood pressure, tonic, nourishing, low back pain, fibromyalgia, possible anti-tumor effects;[1] anti-inflammatory, immune-enhancing, fever-reducing

Discussion: Ashwagandha is the most distinguished adaptogenic tonic of the Ayurvedic medical system, widely used and revered. Also known as "India's ginseng," the name *ashwagandha* refers to the strength, smell, and power of a horse. The medicinal parts are the root, leaves, and berries of this common Western Indian shrub. In India ashwagandha is used, along with milk and ghee, for children who are not growing well, and as a strengthener for the elderly and persons with emaciation. As an adaptogen, it is similar in potency to ginseng.[2] A proprietary extract of ashwagandha called Sensoril has been found to be quite relaxing, and several studies have shown it to be beneficial for stamina and support of restful sleep.[3]

Spiritually, ashwagandha supports a grounded sense of well-being and improved *joie de vivre.*

Dosage: With the unextracted herb, the powdered root is most effective. A customary adult dose range is 3–6 grams per day in tea form. A typical tincture dose is 10–25 drops three times daily. Dose range of Sensoril is 125–250 mg per day.

Precautions: 1. Can have narcotic effects at high doses, especially if leaves are used. 2. May lower body temperature. 3. Is anabolic, potentially promoting weight gain. 4. Is controversial in use with hypothyroid and autoimmune disorders, so avoid using it with these conditions unless under medical supervision.

Bacopa monnieri, also known as Brahmi (Scrophulariaceae)

Anxiety Uses: Anti-anxiety, calming, stress reduction, brain and nervous system tonic, sedative (very mild)

Other Oral Uses: As a brain tonic, it inhibits memory loss, ADHD, Alzheimer's; also used for joint pains, epilepsy.

Discussion: Bacopa is a safe, widely used tonic herb from the Ayurvedic tradition and has been employed for centuries to improve memory and decrease anxiety. In recent years it has been studied in human volunteers and was found to significantly decrease anxiety symptoms while improving mental concentration and focus.[4] A different twelve-week study of elderly persons with memory loss, depression, and anxiety noted significant improvement in all areas.[5] This is in contrast to benzodiazapene drugs, which are known to impair memory and focus. As a calming tonic, bacopa can be used by people with all types of anxiety.

Promising studies of bacopa used as a brain tonic appear to confirm its traditional use as a memory enhancer and its benefits in children with ADHD.[6]

Dosage: Varies with effects desired. Bacopa is considered a safe herb. It is used traditionally as a powder, syrup, and tincture and is not standardized to a particular constituent. Typical adult doses are 5 grams of powder daily, one teaspoon tincture, or 20 ml syrup, all taken as divided doses two to three times daily. Standardized products are also available. A study of memory and anxiety reduction in children in India used a syrup that contained 350 mg and was given three times per day.[7]

Precautions: No significant side effects have been noted to date in studies of bacopa on humans, though mild stomach upset (which resolves after discontinuation of the herb) was noticed in a few volunteers.[8]

Balm, Lemon Balm, *Melissa officinalis* (Labiatae)

Anxiety Uses: Anti-anxiety, calming, antidepressant (mild), sedative (mild), sleep-enhancing

Other Oral Uses: Allergies, anti-spasmodic, eczema, emmenagogue (encourages menses—mild), eases flatulence, headache, *Herpes simplex* type I (cold sores of the mouth area)

Discussion: Lemon balm has a pleasant lemony taste and fragrance and is commonly found in many commercial herbal tea blends. It grows exuberantly in home gardens. Lemon balm has been used for anxiety and nervous disorders, as well as inflammation, for at least two thousand years. The ancient Greeks used it in tonic formulas for longevity. Its main contemporary uses include alleviating agitation, anxiety, and depression as well as providing digestive support and decreasing inflammation.

Lemon balm's volatile essential oils are primarily responsible for its antidepressant, sedative, and anti-anxiety effects. It is delightful as a tea or in an herbal bath, and can be used frequently. It is safe for babies' baths and in teas or baths for children.

Spiritually, lemon balm is steadying and serene, while sunny and cheerful too. Her energy is like a smile from a trusted friend.

Dosage: Most often used as tea or infusion. Be sure to steep covered, as the medicinal components are volatile oils that will escape with steam. Typical dose is 1/3–1/2 cup infusion or 1 cup tea, two to three times per day. For anxiety or depression, smaller doses are usually effective. See also its aromatherapy applications.

Precautions: 1. Not recommended for pregnant women in the first trimester (encourages menses), but it is probably fine in small amounts, such as in commercial herbal tea blends. 2. Recent research has shown that lemon balm mildly inhibits the effects of Thyroid-Stimulating Hormone (TSH) in the laboratory. It is questionable whether this effect occurs in people, because many have consumed this herb daily for years without ill effects. Still, if you suspect or observe any problem with the thyroid gland, avoid daily use of lemon balm.

California Poppy, *Eschscholzia californica* (Papaveraceae)

Anxiety Relief Uses: Insomnia, lowers agitation

Other Oral Uses: Pain relief, fibromyalgia

Discussion: California poppy, the state flower of California, is a magnificent orange-flowered plant with dainty pink frills around the cup. It is in the same family as opium poppies but much milder in its effects. As member of the poppy family, it is a relatively strong herbal sedative, with a calming yet cheerful energy. It is commonly used as a sleep aid and also helps quell agitation, restlessness, irritability, and severe anxiety.

Spiritually, California poppy enhances the ability to quiet the mind and find inner silence. It can help restore a comfortable tempo during times of rapid spiritual growth, rejuvenating *joie de vivre* and optimism when they are flagging due to prolonged or excessive stress. In spirit doses or as a flower essence, the plant offers particular support to persons who have suffered trauma or PTSD.

Dosage: Usually used in tincture form, 5–30 drops at bedtime or two to three times daily, if agitated. Spirit dose is 1 drop of tincture in a glass of water. Tea can also be used.

Precautions: 1. Poppy and poppy seed can show up as a positive on drug tests for narcotics. 2. Avoid high doses. 3. Avoid in pregnancy and while breast-feeding. 4. Avoid with sedative pharmaceutical medications.

Cannabis (Marijuana), *Cannabis sativa* or *indica* (Cannabinaceae)

Anxiety Uses: Anti-anxiety, moderate euphoric, anti-insomnia (promotes sleep), decreases nervous tics including Tourette's, PTSD

Other Oral Uses: Asthma, nausea (anti-emetic), glaucoma (lowers intra-ocular pressure), multiple sclerosis, neuropathy, lupus, HIV wasting, migraines, pain, among dozens of medical indications[9]

Topically (infused oil or lotion): Pain relief (anodyne), possible anti-cancer activities

Discussion: Despite its current illegal status in some states and many countries, cannabis is a safe and tremendously useful medicinal plant. Generations of marijuana smokers, as well as contemporary cancer researchers, can attest to its efficacy as an anti-nausea, calming, and generally uplifting herb. In many states, including California, it is legal to obtain medical cannabis with a physician recommendation, for a number of health indications.

Marijuana, especially cannabadiol (CBD)-rich strains (as opposed to THC-rich strains), is typically moderately relaxing. In the cannabis literature, the indica varieties are known for their calming and sleep-inducing effects, and many anxious persons self-medicate with this herb. The herb has demonstrated efficacy in decreasing nervous tics and outbursts in Tourette's syndrome.[10] It has been used successfully for insomnia, and in the mid-nineteenth century that was one of its main prescriptive indications.[11] It has also been successfully used to address several mood disorders: panic attacks, depression anxiety, PTSD, phobias, and stress reactions. Israeli cannabinoid researcher Dr. Raphael Mechoulam "hypothesizes that THC can relieve flashbacks of traumatic battle incidents by helping suppress unwanted memories."[12]

Other people, however, may have increased anxiety with marijuana use, especially with some sativa strains, so those who have not previously used it and decide to try it should initially experiment with very small amounts to test how their systems might respond. It is best, if it is medically available in your state, to try a variety that is known to be suitable for calming anxiety.

Many physicians, nurse practitioners, and even cannabis dispensary staff personnel are educated about which varieties are most useful for anxiety, chronic pain, etc., and many can share studies that have been done, substantiating the soothing medical benefits of this herb. The anxiety-relieving cultivars tend to be the same varieties that will aid sleep and soothe nervous tics. Small amounts are often effective for anxiety relief and give less of the "high" feeling that some find disconcerting. CBD does not significantly contribute to a high feeling; in fact, it appears to have mitigating effects, dampening a "high," but is often excellent for soothing anxiety. Some dispensaries sell CBD tinctures, and some research groups are focusing on enhancing concentrations of this cannabinoid.

Other medical indications include bronchodilating effects on asthma, appetite stimulation in cancer patients and AIDS wasting syndrome, nausea relief, and relief of chronic or severe physical pain, as in fibromyalgia, disc disease, and neuropathic pain. Marijuana is used especially for the nausea related to chemotherapy. It can help pain sufferers reduce dependence upon narcotic pain medications, and it can substantially lower intraocular pressure in glaucoma. Cannabis (a.k.a. hemp) seeds are considered to be one of the best tonics in Chinese medicine for moistening the colon in cases of chronic constipation, and they have many nutritional properties.

Spiritually, marijuana could be characterized as spacey, mystical, expansive, calming, or slightly agitating (tends to depend on the variety and amount consumed), loving (think of Rastafarians and reggae music), and it enhances creativity. "Can do" attitude, as epitomized by the many medicinal, fiber, and product uses. The plant spirit is very interested in helping humanity.

Dosage: Cannabis can be smoked, vaporized, or taken as tea, tincture, butter or oil extract, or fresh juice. Most of the medicinally active constituents are lipid-soluble, so inhalation (utilizing the lipid layer in alveoli to assist absorption) or cooking the herb in some butter or other fat (and then usually eaten as a food) are reportedly preferred methods of usage among medical cannabis patients. Dosage will depend upon the strength of the herb and the level of effect desired.

Precautions: 1. If you are unfamiliar with marijuana and you choose to utilize it where you are able to legally obtain it, go slow! Less is often better. Be especially cautious with ingesting cannabis products, since the effects are delayed in onset and can be overly strong, especially when people eat too much of the product too quickly because they don't feel anything (yet).

Catnip, *Nepeta cataria* (Labiatae)

Mood Enhancement: Calms anxiety (taken hot), helps sleep and quells insomnia (hot), mild sedative (taken hot), mild stimulant (taken cool), supports alertness and focus (cool)

Other Oral Uses: Headache relief (especially tension headaches), eases menstrual cramps (taken hot), calms flatulence

Discussion: Catnip is an herb with a very long tradition of use. It is, of course, most famous as a stimulant/sedative for cats; give a cat a pinch and she will exult in ecstatic frenzy for around 30 minutes, then fall asleep. Catnip is *not* intoxicating or addictive in humans, but the tea does cause mild stimulation or sedation in people, based upon the temperature of the catnip tea when it is consumed. A cup of iced catnip tea is a mild stimulant that provides a pleasant temporary lift without caffeine jumpiness, while hot catnip tea or infusion, which has been steeped covered, is a mild to moderate sedative and antispasmodic. Hot catnip preparations will relax the uterine smooth muscle, relieving painful menstrual cramps. It might *slightly* increase menstrual flow, though, so if flow is already heavy, choose other herbs for cramp relief.

For most people hot catnip is gently calming and sedating. A few of my elderly patients have told me that hot catnip is "just too strong for them" and it really knocks them out, while other patients, particularly recovering drug addicts, report that catnip "does nothing for them" and is too weak to bother with. Generally, catnip is excellent for people having trouble falling asleep, especially if they are anxious, stressed, or "wired." It is calming and sleep-inducing, helping individuals let go of worries and rumination that disrupt falling asleep. However, a caveat is in order here. About 1 in 100 people will *always* have a mild stimulant effect with catnip, even if it is taken hot, so if you want to experiment with it for insomnia, I suggest doing so first on a lazy afternoon when you could afford to fall asleep or get a mild lift, whichever occurs. Finally, catnip can alleviate tension headaches, and a cup of tea taken for a headache may result in a refreshing nap.

Dosage: One to two cups of half- or full-strength infusion, as desired. Tea as desired. Dosage varies with age/strength of herb. Tincture, 1/2–2 full droppers or 15–60 drops.

Precautions: 1. Catnip tea may make some people (especially elderly and babies) very sleepy, so start with a small dose. 2. Herb must be steeped *covered* and never boiled, since the active components are the volatile oils that will escape with the steam. 3. Crosses into breast milk, so use cautiously with breast-feeding. 4. Avoid giving tea directly to babies.

Chamomile, *Matricaria chamomilla, Matricaria recutita,* or, *Anthemis nobilis* (Compositae)

Anxiety Uses: Anti-agitation, calming, comforting, helps sleep, can prevent nightmares, mild sedative, fine for adults and children

Other Oral Uses: Antiviral, colds, digestive aid, flu, infant colic, nausea, flatulence

Discussion: Chamomile is a familiar herb loved throughout the world by both children and adults. It has a distinguished history of continuous medicinal use, spanning more than two thousand years. Chamomile is a traditional medieval "strewing herb" that was spread in living quarters and straw bedding to keep it fresh and sweet. It is also planted in walkways and is a widely beneficial plant in companion planting, encouraging health in the plants surrounding it, just as it encourages health in people.

Chamomile has a pleasant, sweet taste that most children like but some adults find cloying. It is one of the most versatile of the gentle herbs, with a wide range of beneficial actions. Chamomile tea is frequently taken as a digestive aid after meals in European and North African cultures.

Chamomile is a pleasant, mild sedative, gently relaxing but not aggressive in its actions. It calms anxiety, soothes agitation, and settles frayed nerves. A cup of chamomile tea can be the perfect antidote to a stressful day and is a delightful wind-down tea at night. It can also be used to settle and soothe teething babies.

Physically, chamomile is a mild antiviral, and safe for all sorts of viral conditions in adults and children. It also settles upset stomach and is often combined as a tea with ginger or lavender for further digestive benefits.

Spiritually chamomile is comforting and protective against illness as well as "bad vibes." Chamomile induces pleasant dreams and feelings of safety and security, and prevents nightmares. Chamomile has a loving, balancing energy and happily cooperates with humans and assists us in finding balance in our lives. The herb asked me to mention that she is especially fond of children and has a gentle, playful energy. She helps the timid to be more curious, and the clingy to be more independent and courageous. Chamomile would like more people to plant her in their gardens, and thinks babies and children especially will love to crawl on the ground with her. She encourages those who are beginning to study plant-spirit medicine to explore communication with her. She can enhance communication with other plants because she is widely beloved, in the human world as well as the world of nature.

Dosage: Because most of the medicinal components of the flowers are concentrated in the essential-oil fraction, it is important to steep the flowers by the infusion method. They should never be directly boiled or decocted. Typically taken as a tea or infusion, chamomile can be enjoyed as desired. Tinctures are also useful; the dose for adults is 1/2–2 cc two to four times daily, or 15–60 drops two to four times daily.

Precautions: 1. Pregnancy: Chamomile is not contraindicated, but limit use to no more than two cups tea per day. 2. Somewhat high rate of allergies, compared with other plants. Some allergies can be severe. Use judiciously first few times, particularly *Anthemis nobilis.*

Cinnamon, *Cinnamomun zeylanicum* or *Cinnamon cassia* (Lauraceae)

Anxiety Uses: Comforting, calm, imparts cheerfulness and positivity, reduces fear, mildly stimulating, stabilizing

Other Oral Uses: Antifungal, balances blood sugar, contributes to healthy lipid balance, warming, supports adrenals, antiseptic

Discussion: The beloved spice cinnamon is also an excellent medicinal herb. It has a warm and homey energy that is mood-elevating and mildly energizing, but still comforting and calming. The fragrance of cinnamon is often used by realtors to make a house feel "homey," and many people associate the scent and taste with feelings of love and well-being. It decreases fatigue without overstimulation, and so is used in many adrenal tonic blends.

Physically, cinnamon is warming and antiseptic. It is often used in cold remedies. It is frequently used in herbal blends at the first sign of a cold, to warm and nourish. It is an excellent antifungal, used frequently for chronic yeast infections, and also has powerful effects in balancing blood sugar.

Spiritually, cinnamon has an earthy, comforting energy of well-being. It is grounding and stabilizing. It helps people feel greater self-esteem and self-confidence.

Dosage: Used as a spice, and in teas and tea blends, tinctures, or capsules. There is wide dose variation. Larger amounts are more stimulating, and just a little can be very comforting. Use common sense.

Precautions: 1. Potentiates methergine, a hormone of labor, so do not use it medicinally in pregnancy, though it certainly can be used as a spice throughout pregnancy.

Holy Basil (Tulsi), *Ocimum tenuiflorum* or *Ocimum sanctum* (Labiatae)

Anxiety Uses: Nervine, adaptogen, tonic, insomnia, stress reducer, calming

Other Oral Uses: Fatigue, antiviral, antibacterial, antifungal, flu, colds, anti-inflammatory, gastritis and gastroenteritis, headache, antioxidant, immune tonic, children

Discussion: Holy basil or tulsi is an important Ayurvedic tonic and nervine that has been used medicinally and ceremonially for thousands of years. Hindus consider it a sacred plant; the name *Tulsi* means "the incomparable one." It is associated with certain Hindu deities, especially the goddess Lakshmi and the god Hanuman, and it is often planted in or near temples and in the courtyards of private homes. Holy basil is a medicinal herb, related to the popular spice basil, and has a somewhat spicier and hotter flavor than culinary varieties. The main part used medicinally is the leaves, though essential oils and seeds are also employed.

Emotionally, holy basil is a nervine tonic. It works gently over time, as an adaptogen, to mitigate the effects of stress. It enhances resilience, calms frayed nerves, and settles the emotions. It combines well with other nervine tonics such as rhodiola, ginseng, and wood betony. It also helps with nervous digestive problems. It is useful acutely and chronically for tension headaches and migraines. Studies have shown that holy basil lowers excessive levels of stress hormones, including cortisol.[13]

Physically, holy basil is an excellent antiviral, useful at the first sign of colds and the flu. It can be used as a mouth rinse for apthous ulcers and for chronic dental problems. Safe for older children (not babies or toddlers), tulsi is used in India for a variety of ailments, including gastrointestinal upset, coughs, and fevers. In Ayurvedic medicine, holy basil is also employed for more chronic and severe viral problems, such as herpes and hepatitis. It can be mixed into stored grains to repel insects.

Dosage: Tincture, tea, and capsules of the leaf are most commonly used in the West, though tulsi is an excellent garden plant and the fresh herb is delicious. In both India and the West, the juice of fresh leaves is used; small daily doses once or twice a day are often the most useful for tonic purposes. Typical doses are tincture, 5–30 drops one to three times daily; tea, one cup, once or twice daily; and capsules, approximately 500 mg once or twice daily. Or try growing it at home and chewing a few fresh leaves daily.

Precautions: 1. May slow blood clotting. Do not use if taking pharmaceutical anticoagulants, and cease using two weeks prior to surgery. 2. Avoid in pregnancy and when planning pregnancy in the near future, as tulsi may have some anti-fertility effects.

Hops, *Humulus lupulus* (Cannabinaceae)

Anxiety Uses: Calming, relaxing, stabilizing, mild to moderate sedative, can help relieve insomnia

Other Oral Uses: Bitter, estrogenic, increasing lactation, anti-nausea

Discussion: Hops flowers, which grow in dense mats like a blanket, are best known for their significance to the brewing trade, but they are also quite valuable medicinal herbs. Originally added to brews as a preservative, hops gives beer its bitter or "hoppy" flavor. Hops has been used medicinally for about two thousand years and was well known to the ancient Greeks as a bitter tonic and a safe, effective sedative. Medicinally, it is one of the best herbs for occasional insomnia, helping a person to relax and feel drowsy about 20 minutes after it is taken, but usually without residual sleepiness the next morning. It is also good in quelling anxiety, alone or in formulas. It can be helpful alone or in blends during recovery, for drug or alcohol detox jitters.

Physically, in folk medicine hops is used effectively for enriching breast milk and increasing flow of milk. It is also used as a digestive bitter, stimulating the flow of bile and the secretion of stomach acid to aid digestion.

Spiritually, hops has a bitter, earthy side. It is grounding, calming, and connects people with a greater comfort within their body and with its physical function. It can help people who have shame or disgust about their body to feel greater ease. It also has a bit of a sexy energy and is a little playful, but not pushy.

Dosage: Usually taken as a tincture, 5–30 drops once to three times daily. As a tea, for sleep or anxiety, hops can be used alone or in combinations, occasionally. If hops is used on an ongoing basis, tea blends that include other herbs are best, in order to minimize the cumulative estrogenic effects found in a strong concentration of hops. Or, for sleep and relaxation, many people simply enjoy a hoppy beer now and then.

Precautions: 1. Because of the significant phytoestrogens present in the plant, large amounts of hops may not be healthy. Female farm workers who pick hops frequently notice cessation of menstrual periods; this is thought to be because of the high exposure to estrogens. 2. Hops may decrease sex drive in men, especially when consumed in larger amounts, though it often increases it in women. 3. Like valerian, hops can increase underlying depression if administered on a frequent basis. Avoid regular use of hops if you suffer from depression.

Kava-Kava, *Piper methysticum* (Piperaceae)

Anxiety Uses: Antidepressant, anxiolytic, calming, insomnia relief, improves sociability, helpful in social anxiety, eases some phobias, improves tranquility

Other Oral Uses: Restless legs, muscle relaxant, mild anesthetic, pain reliever, reduces menopausal symptoms including hot flashes and heart palpitations

Discussion: Kava-kava is an herb native to the South Pacific, where it is traditionally used to make an intoxicating beverage. A member of the pepper family, kava-kava grows from a moderate to large perennial shrub. The root, and only the root, is traditionally used medicinally.

When traditionally prepared, small pieces of fibrous kava root are chewed by indigenous people, who masticate it for about a minute then spit it into a communal bowl. Usually in New Guinea, women chew and spit the kava, while men drink the prepared drink. This is a group activity; several people participate in chewing and spitting kava into a common bowl. Coconut milk is then poured over it, and the masticated pulp plus coconut milk is strained and then drunk. Although missionaries tried to discourage this preparation method and advocated grating instead, natives resisted this change, feeling that the kava drink was not as effective when made by the new, more sanitary method. Recent chemical analysis does indicate that tribesmen are correct in their perceptions, particularly if kavanolactones are the primary medicinally active constituent. Saliva activates these compounds, making them significantly more bioavailable. Perhaps a more hygienic preparation would be to chew and spit one's own kava root.

Kava can help with many symptoms of anxiety. In addition to increasing feelings of calmness and overall well-being, it decreases unpleasant anxiety-related symptoms such as sweaty palms, nervous heart palpitations, headaches, dizziness, and nervous stomach. Kavanolactones, concentrated in the fat-soluble portion of the kava root, are considered to be pharmacologically active constituents. However, kavanolactones may not be the only medicinally active constituents. Studies indicate that the whole, crude herb is more effective for relieving anxiety than are isolated kavanolactones.

Traditionally, and in at least two studies I have reviewed, kava does not impair coordination. Although it is in some ways intoxicating, kava can be consumed in low doses and a person can still drive and operate machinery without clumsiness. It actually improves mental function, including word recognition, but decreases anxiety. It has been shown clinically to be helpful in decreasing social anxiety.[14]

Kavanolactones differ from pharmaceutical anxiolytics in their mechanism of action. Most sedatives, particularly the benzodiazepines such as lorazepam (Ativan), diazepam (Valium), or alprazolam (Xanax), work by binding to specific receptors, such as GABA receptors in the brain. This leads to potentiation, or enhanced activation of these receptors to promote sedation. However, kavanolactones have a nontraditional mechanism of action whereby they appear to modify the whole field around the receptors, rather than binding to specific receptor sites. Also, some studies have indicated that kavanolactones have some direct effects upon the limbic system, the emotional processing area of the brain. One theory is that kava may promote sleep by changing the way the limbic system processes emotional inputs.

People who use kava on an ongoing basis do not seem to require higher doses over time, nor do they experience diminishment of its beneficial effects. In numerous studies, no physical addiction to kava has been observed.

At low doses kava increases a sense of tranquility, well-being, and social grace. Kava stimulates appreciation of subtle natural phenomena, like sounds and colors. At high doses (one half coconut shell by traditional preparation, or 300–400 mg kavanolactones in the current model), kava is a moderate to strong sedative, generally causing a person to sleep, usually within 30 minutes. Sleep is deep and dreamless. At those doses it is a moderately strong muscle relaxant as well. Unlike alcohol, kava produces no hangover.

Spiritually, it is not surprising that kava has many attributes, similar to its mood-enhancing effects. It can increase a person's feelings of contentment and well-being, and allows one to be in the present moment more easily. It is a social plant, offering assistance to people who struggle with feelings of loneliness and isolation, especially if due to social anxiety or phobia. Kava can heighten the senses, particularly vision and hearing, while increasing the desire to experience and create a calm, tranquil environment, while being with others. It helps with finding serenity and balance. There may be a certain timelessness to the experience, as if coming into the present moment brings one into relationship with the eternal now.

Dosage: Varies depending on the effects wanted. For help with anxiety, 30–75 mg kavanolactones can be used two to three times per day. For sedative effects, to help sleep, around 150–300 mg one hour before bedtime is typical. More is safe, but of course, circumspection is always advised. With tinctured root: 5–30 drops one to three times daily is commonly used. In the Oceanic cultures, several bowls per person might be consumed in an evening, each containing 100–400 mg of kavanolactones, but this would not happen every night. For spirit doses, 1–3 drops of kava tincture are utilized.

Precautions: 1. Never combine kava with any benzodiazepine drugs such as Valium (diazepam) or Xanax (alprazolam). Nor is it advised with common sleep prescriptions like Ambien (zolipidem). Their interaction is potentially dangerous and has landed people in intensive-care units! If you are not sure if your medication is a benzodiazepine or modified benzodiazepine, check with a pharmacist or a physician before using kava. 2. Kava can cause a type of dermatitis (skin rash). This occurs most frequently in people who use a lot, usually more than 400 mg per day, for longer than one year. The skin becomes scaly and dry and there can be abnormalities in the blood and urine chemistries, such as low serum protein and low serum urea as well as decreased platelets and white blood cells. Some people have also noted blood in the urine. All these symptoms stop within a few days or weeks after kava is discontinued. Please, use common sense when working with this and any other herb. 3. Only kava root preparations should be used. Whole plant or leaf preparations, despite high kavanolactones, can be toxic.

Lavender, *Lavandula angustifolia* or *officinalis* (synonyms) (Labiatae)

Anxiety Uses: Calming, comforting, antidepressant, mild sedative, relieves stress, soothes nervous stomach, uplifting

Other Oral Uses: Antiseptic, asthma, digestion, headache, menstrual cramps, migraine

Discussion: Fresh, clean-smelling lavender is soothing and relaxing, and most people love its fragrance. Lavender was grown in medieval herbal gardens and was loved by Queen Elizabeth I, who drank it in tea to treat her migraine headaches. Lavender is native to Southern Europe and North Africa but has been naturalized in other Mediterranean climates such as Northern California. It has long been widely cultivated throughout the world.

Lavender is usually used as an essential oil for aromatherapy, or in baths or steams, but it can be used in teas as well. Lavender tea is very tannic so is usually combined with other herbs. It is too tannic to be used alone as an herbal infusion. The tannins in lavender can help dry dampness in the intestinal tract, and in low doses of tea or tincture lavender promotes digestion.

People spray lavender water or hydrosols on bed linens to perk up the senses. Emotionally, lavender lifts spirits and promotes a sense of calm and well-being. Lavender reminds us in any season of a bright summer day. Deeply calming, lavender also renews, refreshes, and enlivens.

Spiritually, lavender increases courage, fortitude, and a sense of purpose. Stabilizing and soothing, its energy is positive and uplifting. Lavender is about gentleness, friendliness, comfort, and love. Lavender is used often in dream pillows and sachets.

Dosage: Tea, one or two cups daily, usually blended with other herbs, especially chamomile. Tincture, 3–15 drops once or twice daily. Spirit doses, 1–2 drops once or twice daily. See also aromatherapy uses in chapter 13.

Precautions: Tannic, can upset digestion at high doses. However, small amounts usually ease digestive upsets.

Licorice Root, *Glycyrrhiza glabra* or *Glycyrrhiza uralenis* (Leguminosae)

Anxiety Uses: Nervine, supports adrenals, decreases fatigue, helps recovery in nervous exhaustion, stabilizing

Other Oral Uses: Adrenal insufficiency, anti-inflammatory, apthous and other ulcers, asthma, bronchitis, blood circulation, cough, heartburn, hepatitis, herpes,[15] laxative, liver disease[16] (hepatoprotective), pharyngitis

Discussion: Licorice is one of the most widely studied herbs in the world. It has been used in China for more than three thousand years, and all its major components have proven efficacy. A main component, glycyrrhizin, is fifty times sweeter than sugar and is also effective in suppressing coughs. Another constituent, glycyrrhetic acid, is molecularly very similar in structure to adrenal cortical hormones. Thus the herb is useful in recovering from nervous exhaustion or adrenal fatigue.

Emotionally, licorice is both stabilizing and energizing. It helps people heal when they are run down from having acute or ongoing stress. A small amount can be very supportive, without stimulation.

Glycyrrhizin has affinity for kidney aldosterone receptors, thus long-term moderate to high dosage may lead to retention of sodium and elevation of blood pressure. However, this affinity is weak, and generally high doses of licorice are necessary for these effects to manifest. Licorice is used traditionally in China for harmonizing herbal formulas. It is believed to balance the individual herbs and is found in small amounts in more than half of the common Chinese medicinal formulas.

Dosage: Tincture, tea, and capsules are commonly used, and licorice is often combined with other herbs. For fatigue due to stress or anxiety, a tincture or tea is usually selected. For nervous exhaustion, a cup of tea, alone or blended with other supportive herbs like cinnamon and cardamom, is often used in the morning and/or early to mid afternoon. Tincture can be used in the range of 5–30 drops one to three times per day. DGL (deglycyrrhizinated licorice) capsules are used for digestive purposes but not for relief of fatigue.

Precautions: Generally regarded as safe (USDA-GRAS). 1. A chemical constituent of licorice, glycyrrhetic acid, may raise blood pressure or cause fluid retention in higher doses. Avoid high doses or do not use this herb in hypertension, borderline hypertension, and renal disease. These effects are reversible with discontinuation of the herb. 2. Avoid in pregnancy. 3. Interacts with many medications. Consult an herbally trained physician or naturopath before combining licorice with pharmaceuticals. 4. Tiny amounts, as are used as a harmonizer in many traditional Chinese herbal formulas, are unlikely to be cause for concern and are probably safe for longer-term use. If higher doses are needed, two weeks on, two weeks off as a dosing schedule is recommended.

Linden Flower, *Tilia cordata* or *europea* (Tiliaceae)

Anxiety Uses: Insomnia relief, relaxation, eases nervous stomach, calming and soothing, easygoing and cheerful

Other Oral Uses: Diaphoretic (mild), hoarseness, lipid balance, laryngitis

Discussion: Linden flower, also commonly called "lime blossom," is the flower of a common European tree. In persons with anxiety, this safe herb is useful for relaxation, calming, and support of sleep. The taste of the tea is pleasant, and adults and children often enjoy drinking it.

There is no known addictive potential with this herb. Taken hot, linden flowers are mildly diaphoretic (promote sweating) and can be used for colds or the flu. It is taken in Europe after meals as a popular digestive aid.

Spiritually, linden flower has a light, kind, and easygoing energy. It is a "fairy" flower, with a soft, soothing fragrance and a pleasant, harmonious energy. It is good for people who need more kindness and grace in their lives.

Dosage: Usually taken as tea, but do not steep more than a half hour or it turns bitter (although it is still safe to use). Can also be used as a tincture: 15–60 drops two or three times daily as desired.

Precautions: Safe

Longan Fruit, *Dimocarpus* or *Euphoria longan* (Sapindaceae)

Anxiety Uses: Insomnia relief, nervous heart palpitations, forgetfulness, self-expression, anxiety, calming

Other Oral Uses: Emaciation, anti-inflammatory, colds and flu, bleeding and blood loss, fatigue, convalescence

Discussion: This Chinese herb is actually a tropical fruit. Dried longan fruit is sold in boxes and cans in many Chinese grocery stores. The dried fruit looks like a large raisin and tastes like a hickory-smoked raisin. The tree is in the same botanical family as lychee fruit, and when fresh it actually looks like a lychee fruit. The Chinese name means "dragon's eye."

In Chinese medicine, longan is used to nourish, calm, reduce anxiety, and help with sleep. It is a common remedy for insomnia and heart palpitations. Nutritionally, it is used for rebuilding people who have lost a lot of blood or who are convalescing. It is also considered a "weight loss" herb.

In the *Shen Nun Bun Cao*, an ancient Chinese medical text, this herb is spoken of as "penetrating divine illumination." Spiritually, it helps people to be more in the present moment, with more awareness and equanimity. It also enhances psychic expression, but only in people who are otherwise prepared for it.

Dosage: Usually taken as a dried fruit, longan can be added to cooked foods like oatmeal, or enjoyed as a tea. It is safe, so use as much as desired. For sleep or anxiety, 2–6 dried fruits are commonly used.

Precautions: Safe

Oat Straw, *Avena sativa* (Graminaceae)

Anxiety Uses: Drug and alcohol recovery, insomnia, nervine, calming

Other Oral Uses: Convalescence, eczema, exhaustion, skin rashes, smoking cessation

Discussion: Oat straw is the green milky seed and hay from the common grain, wild oat, before the mature grain forms a head. It is a wonderfully gentle nutritive herb with a broad range of benefits. It is calming and relaxing but not sedating, and is useful for a wide variety of anxiety-related nervous disorders. Oat straw is naturally high in bioavailable silica, which nourishes the nerves, helping to soothe anxiety and relieve insomnia. It may help chronic insomnia that is related to nervous tension or depression by supporting relaxation. Often when I have given or advised oat straw, I notice that people relax with a new, improved attitude. They start to think about their problems differently, saying things like "Why was I so worried about that anyway?"

Oat straw is quite helpful for the jitters associated with drug and alcohol withdrawal and smoking cessation. It is safe and non-addictive, and useful in sleep-promoting blends because it is calming and gently helps stimulate sleepiness. Oat straw is also useful for a wide variety of skin rashes, again probably because of its high silica content. A bath of oat straw infusion is less drying to eczematous skin than colloidal oatmeal and is quite soothing. Topically it is used for sore, dry skin, often mixed with comfrey leaf.

Spiritually, oat straw is grounding but flexible. A field of wild oats, fluttering and bending in the breeze, is a magnificent sight. Oat straw promotes gentle resilience, trust in nature, and an awareness of our natural ability to connect with health. It helps us reframe our problems from the perspective of a larger current of love.

Dosage: Infusion 1/4–1/3 cup two to five times per day, or 1–3 cups of tea daily. Also available in tinctures; a typical dose is 15–60 drops two or three times daily.

Precautions: 1. Avoid excessive ongoing doses (more than 2 cups of infusion or more than 5 cups of tea per day for more than three months) because a high silica content in large amounts, over time, could irritate the kidneys. 2. Use only under medical supervision with chronic kidney disease. Otherwise, oat straw is safe to consume on a regular basis in normal doses, including most blends, and is safe in pregnancy and for children. 3. Oat straw is mildly diuretic.

Passion Flower, also called Maypop, *Passiflora incarnata* or *edulis* (Passifloraceae)

Anxiety Uses: Panic attacks, generalized anxiety disorder, nervous stomach, palpitations (especially from nervousness or panic), antidepressant

Other Oral Uses: Antispasmodic, upset stomach, asthma, cough, menopausal symptoms, ADHD

Topical Uses: Soothes hemorrhoids, burns, and inflammation

Discussion: Passion flower is a fast-growing perennial climbing vine, native to the forests of North and South America. It produces showy and enchanting blooms that are popular with gardeners worldwide. There are passion flowers in a variety of colors, but the one used medicinally has blue/purple blooms. Passion flower produces a fragrant and delicious fruit that is a main food for several species of caterpillar. The whole aboveground herb is used medicinally for calming frayed nerves, easing anxiety and stress, and assisting with sleep. It also calms digestive disturbance from nervous tension and is a constituent of many herbal blends for depression due to its soothing effects.

Passion flower was approved as part of the United States Pharmacopeia for treatment of anxiety until 1978 but was removed, as were almost all traditional herbs, because of lack of "clinical data" to support safety and efficacy. Nonetheless, today the National Institute of Mental Health ranks natural remedies by their likelihood of efficacy. Passion flower is deemed, by current evidence, likely to be effective for alleviating symptoms of many types of anxiety.[17]

Herbalists consider passion flower to be a sedative of moderate strength. It is safe and not habit-forming. In doses lower than those for adults, it can be used for older children with anxiety and/or sleep disturbance to calm and to promote restful sleep. Passion flower is a common remedy in homeopathy, where it is also used for insomnia, among other indications.

Spiritually, passion flower has a bit of wild energy in her that she will share with you if you ask. She awakens passions while calming fears. She offers assistance to those who do not know what they love or what they desire, because they have been ruled by fear and anxiety. If you have been too timid to shine, and anxiety has arisen to guide you back to yourself, look at her flowers and smile, or eat her ripe delicious fruit. Passion flower is a little sexy too; she can awaken libido that is seemingly dead, bringing you back to your true self. Passion flower will not give you passion for things or people you don't love. Instead she helps you feel more comfortable with who you truly are and what you really love.

Dosage: Tincture or liquid extracts are the most commonly used forms, though teas and capsules are also available. Eating the fruit confers some of the calming benefits. Tincture dose range for anxiety is 15–60 drops two to three times daily. Capsules might contain 25–100 mg of the herb, especially if there is a blend of herbs. Tea is usually made by infusing one or two teaspoons of dried herb. Spirit dose is 1–3 drops of tincture per day, in water.

Precautions: 1. Consult a medical doctor or naturopath before taking passion flower along with prescription benzodiazepine drugs for sleep, as the combination may result in excessive drowsiness. 2. Passion flower is not advised during pregnancy, as it might trigger uterine contractions.

Peach Leaf, *Prunus persica* or *Amygdylus persica* (Rosaceae)

Anxiety Uses: Soothes nervous stomach, eases panic attacks (especially those that upset digestion), calming, gentle

Other Uses: Asthma, food allergies, gastritis

Discussion: This is the leaf and twig of the common peach fruit tree, which is native to China but is now cultivated in temperate and subtropical climates worldwide. It is an excellent albeit underused remedy for nervous tension, especially nervous stomach. It calms and tones the stomach, is great for digestive disorders that are related to anxiety, and is used as well to soothe gastritis (inflammation of the stomach). It is quite safe and effective in both children and adults. It is used when there is nausea, and it generally calms vomiting. I think of peach leaf and twig as a front-line remedy for nervousness and panic attacks that have a major digestive component.

Peach is mildly mucilaginous and is generally used when there are signs of heat, like dryness or inflammation, in a body tissue. Peach is also used traditionally to alleviate food allergies, to treat asthma, and to balance digestion when there is a lot of intestinal gas.

Spiritually, there is a great deal of lore about this plant and its delicious fruit. In Chinese culture, peach is associated with longevity and immortality. It is the most sacred plant of Taoists. Its branches are used in dowsing and water witching in many areas, including Appalachia. I use this plant spiritually when there is excessive grief and clinging to the past, or when there is fear of death and loss. Peach nourishes a sense of the eternal and helps with an understanding of transformation as an essential part of life.

Dosage: Peach is best taken as a cold prepared tea or infusion. Both the fresh and dried herb are frequently used. This is a good "sun tea" herb. Use one teaspoon of fresh or dried herb steeped in one cup of water. Two or three days' worth can be made at a time, to be stored in the refrigerator. Often peach is taken as a tonic over several months. It can also be used as a tincture for ease of administration. Tincture doses are low: 1–10 drops two or three times daily.

Precautions: Safe

Red Clover, *Trifolium pratense* (Fabaceae)

Anxiety Uses: Calming, relieves insomnia, nervine, tonic to nervous system, nutritive

Other Uses: Helps alleviate menopause hot flashes, provides nutrition (especially for bones), soothes boils, carbuncles, mastitis, and skin rashes, blood thinner, aid to convalescence

Discussion: Red clover is a nutritive perennial herb, native to Asia but now found in fields and meadows throughout the world. It is beloved by ruminant animals such as cattle and buffalo, which will graze it preferentially. Its long roots draw minerals up from deep in the soil, thus it is particularly good for replenishing minerals in body tissues, especially the bones.

Red clover is a gentle herb, very nutritive, clearing, and cleansing. Its value in anxiety is two-fold. First, the rich profile of minerals calms and nourishes tissues, including those of the nervous system. Second, it is a mild, safe sedative. Herbalists call it a nervine, and it is useful when there is overwhelm or hectic energy. Red clover tea assists with a feeling of mild relaxation and well-being. Patients find it soothing, and emotionally they are more able to access feelings of inner well-being.

In Chinese medicine this herb is considered a "yin" tonic. The yin is the quieting, cooling, moistening half of a person's energy. Red clover is wonderful for slowly cooling inflammation and restoring tissues, including those of the nervous system and urinary tract that have been stressed or dried out by excessive heat and inflammation, including that caused by anxiety.

Spiritually, red clover is used for people who are not sure whether they want to live, or whether they have the strength to go on. It helps root these people, reconnecting them with the Earth and physical life, and gently restores the will, desire, and energy to persevere. It is spiritually clarifying (mirroring its physical uses), clearing people of bad energy/bad vibes, particularly ones they have unconsciously absorbed from others, centering them in their own true health and wholeness.

There is a great deal of lore about clovers, such as the four-leaved clover representing good luck. It is said that if two persons in love eat a four-leaved red clover together, their love will expand. And if seven grains of wheat are placed on a four-leaved clover, this supposedly enables fairies to become more visible. Red clover was widely used in medieval folkloric charms and potions for both finances and love.

Dosage: Tinctures and tea of the dried flowers or the flowers plus the herb tops are the most common preparations. For tea, use one tablespoon dried or fresh herb per cup. Tincture dose is 10 drops to a full teaspoon two to three times daily. For spirit doses, one or two drops of tincture are sufficient.

Precautions: 1. Red clover mildly inhibits blood clotting due to the presence of natural salicylic acid. Use with caution when utilizing other natural blood thinners such as fish oils, gingko, or nattokinase, and with low-dose aspirin. If using strong pharmaceutical blood thinners such as warfarin (Coumadin) or heparin, avoid using this herb unless under the direct supervision of a physician knowledgeable about herbal therapeutics. 2. Generally not used extensively in pregnancy because of phytoestrogens, red clover should be safe in small occasional doses, as phytoestrogens are found in many foods and botanicals including pomegranates and garbanzo beans. 3. Red clover is considered safe in lactation, again in small doses, as it can enrich the breast milk.

Rhodiola, also called golden root or Arctic root, *Rhodiola rosea* (Crassulaceae)

Anxiety Uses: Calming, restorative, helps promote restful sleep, nourishing, adaptogen, antidepressant

Other Oral Uses: Adrenal fatigue, fatigue, cardio-protective, antioxidant, improves memory and concentration[18]

Discussion: Rhodiola is an herbal treasure, a perennial plant with a thick, deep root native to cold and mountainous regions of Europe, Asia, and North America. It has been used medicinally and as a tonic in Europe for more than three thousand years.[19] The leaves, roots, flowers, and stems are all useful medicinally, though typically the root, which has an aroma of roses when dried, is most commonly selected. Rhodiola is adaptogenic, restorative, and nutritive. It balances the endocrine and nervous system via mechanisms that are mostly still unclear but include regulation of release of stress hormones. Rhodiola is the subject of much current research, with hundreds of papers written about its effects and benefits.[20] It alleviates anxiety, quells depression, and has been used successfully to soothe PTSD[21] and generalized anxiety disorder.[22] It can balance and improve many neurotransmitters and has been known to increase serotonin in the brain by as much as 30 percent.[23]

Physically, like many adaptogens, rhodiola helps decrease fatigue and build stamina. It also helps improve both cold and heat tolerance. Because it is gently strengthening, approved, and safe, rhodiola is popular with athletes.

Spiritually, rhodiola is grounding, calming, and helps people return to a sense of wholeness in themselves. It seems to bring people to an awareness of their true self, as distinct from the self of social conventions and the pressures of others. It aids the flourishing of self-expression.

Dosage: Often taken as capsules of dried herb or as a tincture. Capsules of dried rhodiola root are typically 100–150 mg, with one to three daily being a standard dose. Tincture: 10–30 drops once or twice daily. Rhodiola can be used for protracted periods of time. Small doses taken between meals, such as 1 capsule/day or 10–20 drops of tincture per day, are often effective in supporting healthy moods and improving endurance. If anxiety is extreme, for best results start with very low doses (1–2 drops of tincture or 25 mg of powdered herb) and gradually increase every few days, as tolerated.

Precautions: Avoid using with bipolar depression, unless under medical advice and guidance. Otherwise considered safe.

Skullcap, *Scutellaria laterifolia* (Labiatae)

Anxiety Uses: Anti-anxiety, sedative (mild/moderate), drug detox including benzodiazepines, insomnia (chronic)

Other Oral Uses: antispasmodic, eases menstrual cramps, headaches, hiccups

Discussion: Skullcap is a native North American plant that has been used by indigenous people for centuries to treat a number of conditions; one of these uses is as a nervous system tonic. Today skullcap tincture or tea is known as a popular, gentle, and non-addictive treatment for "bad nerves." Its action is slow and tonifying, so for anxiety, over time it might help build more of a sense of inner peace.

Skullcap is useful for insomnia when a person has difficulty falling asleep, since it can help one relax and stop worrying about the concerns of the day. Because it is a tonic, try it for a while, perhaps a month, to see if you find it beneficial. Skullcap has also been used to soothe frayed nerves when detoxing from drugs, especially benzodiazepines.

As a spirit medicine, skullcap promotes inner peace and a sense of connection with the natural world.

Dosage: Large doses are unnecessary with this tonic herb. Tincture: 5–25 drops one to three times daily, or tea 1–2 cups per day. Skullcap herb breaks down rapidly with exposure to light, so a fresh supply annually, stored in a cool, dark, dry place, is important if you buy the herb in bulk. Also, the essential-oil fraction is medicinally active, so steep covered if making a tea. Capsules are available as well.

Precaution: Avoid in pregnancy.

St. John's Wort, *Hypericum perforatum* (Hypericaceae)

Anxiety Uses: Antidepressant, anti-anxiety, supports restful sleep

Other Oral Uses: Arthritis, anti-inflammatory, antiviral, back pain (especially acute), herpes

Discussion: St. John's wort is commonly known as an herb useful for depression. It is a cheery, sunny-looking plant; just observing it puts many people in a good mood. St. John's wort is a great plant to explore with children. It has really cute leaves, perforated with tiny pores that are interesting to inspect when held up to the sun. Be aware, though, that about 5 percent of the population gets a contact dermatitis similar to poison ivy from touching the live plant. However, the dried herb is safe to touch. So play with this a little before trying a lot, just in case you are among the one in twenty who react negatively to skin contact.

In the United States and Europe, St. John's wort has been widely used for more than twenty years to alleviate mild to moderate depression. It raises the level of many neurotransmitters including serotonin. Like many herbs, the pharmacology of St. John's wort is complex. The "mechanism of action" is still being debated. Of its constituent biochemicals, both the bioflavones of St. John's wort and the antibacterial constituent hyperforin are known to be sedative in action, potentially assisting persons with anxiety.

The first significant study of this herb in regard to depression and anxiety was published in 1984 in *Arzneimittel-Forschung,* a respected German publication. Since then, hundreds of additional studies have been done and innumerable doses of this herb consumed throughout the world.[24]

Physically, St. John's wort has significant anti-inflammatory activity, so it can be of dual benefit for persons with fibromyalgia, back pain, and arthritis who also have depression or anxiety. It is effective as an antiviral, supporting reduction of activity of chronic viral conditions, including oral herpes.

Spiritually, St. John's wort offers help to those who want to improve a bleak outlook on life or who cannot seem to find their joy. There is an aspect of warmth and humor in the spirit doses and flower essence, as well as an inherent kindness and respect for the individual and their process. St. John's wort is a sunny, cheerful, happy-go-lucky friend who always notices the positives in any situation. Working with the essence or the plant in spirit doses can help people connect with the sunlight of their soul. In my experience, St. John's wort is an eager and enthusiastic helper. This plant wants to share its love and wonders, to help us discover the magic and mystery available for each of us.

Dosage: For teens and adults the standard capsule dose is 900–1050 mg per day, taken in a 300–350-mg capsule three times per day, or 450–500 mg twice per day. Tincture doses vary widely from 5 to 60 drops three times daily. To work with this as plant-spirit medicine only, use 1–3 drops of tincture per day and include a St. John's wort flower essence as well.

Precautions: 1. St. John's wort administered either topically or orally may cause increased sun sensitivity, making sunburn more likely. 2. St. John's wort is broken down by the liver, and in its metabolism it activates a certain group of enzymes known as the p450, which can affect how some pharmaceuticals, including birth control pills, are broken down. Activation of the p450 system of the liver is not unique to this herb. Many common foods including broccoli and grapefruit will also change metabolic parameters in the liver. So it is a good idea to let your doctor know if you plan to use St. John's wort, especially if you are also taking any pharmaceutical medications. 3. Like many substances, St. John's wort can cause upset stomach, rashes, and nausea in a small percentage of people. If you happen to experience uncomfortable side effects, discontinue using the herb.

Valerian, *Valeriana officinalis* (Valerianaceae)

Anxiety Uses: Anti-anxiety, moderate to strong sedative, calming, relaxing, improves sleep in several ways

Other Oral Uses: Antispasmodic, muscle spasms, anticonvulsant, muscle relaxant

Discussion: Valerian is a plant native to Europe and Asia. The root is the part used medicinally, and it has a distinctive odor that some people find alluring and others deplore. In folklore it was the herb chosen by the Pied Piper to lure both the rats and the children from the town of Hamlin. The story implies that valerian was appealing to children but offensive to adults. The fleshy roots must be dried in a cool or cold area or they can easily grow moldy. Valerian root breaks down with exposure to light.

Valerian is a good example of a plant that does not have just one active principle. In many studies, products standardized to one or more chemical constituents have all proven to be less effective than the whole herb. Some of valerian's biochemical effects are understood but not fully characterized.

Historically, prior to the advent of pharmaceutical drugs, valerian was used as an anticonvulsant for epileptics. It was also used as a sleep aid, muscle relaxant, and treatment for anxiety. In my experience, valerian is an excellent herb for insomnia. It decreases sleep latency (which means the amount of time it takes someone to fall asleep) as well as the number of awakenings that occur throughout the night. Technically, valerian is not habit-forming, but as with many effective remedies, emotional dependence upon it may develop. For soothing anxiety, low doses usually help with calming, without excessive drowsiness. Valerian is also an excellent antispasmodic and muscle relaxant, great for alleviating stress-induced muscle tension. It is often the perfect herb for anxious persons whose excessive muscle tension keeps them from falling asleep, as it calms anxiety, helps sleep, and relaxes muscular tension. Although valerian has a characteristically strong flavor and aroma, it is generally well tolerated. It rarely causes upset stomach.

Its strong, penetrating aroma hints at the spiritual properties of valerian. People who have used valerian have similarly strong feelings about it. They love it or hate it, find the smell strangely appealing or disgusting. Spiritually, valerian can be used for those who lack passion and enthusiasm—people who are wishy-washy not because they cannot make up their mind, but because there is an ennui or lack of caring. Valerian in spirit doses is an awakener, jump-starting passion, vibrancy, and the knowledge that to live is to connect with desire. Spiritually, valerian also helps people who lack a certain physical strength or vitality, which I associate with a lack of certainty about whether they really want to be embodied here in physical reality. It increases inner fortitude, helping people feel more of a sense of purpose in their lives.

Dosage: For sleep and muscle tension, a wide range of doses may be effective, from 200 to 1000 mg of dried herb at bedtime. For daytime anxiety, lower doses are preferable: 50–250 mg one to three times daily is a common range. For tincture: 5–50 drops at bedtime is a typical range, and lower amounts, 2–15 drops every 4–6 hours, are often used for daytime anxiety. For sleep, it may take a few weeks to notice optimal effects from valerian. For spirit dosing, 1–3 drops in some water is usually ideal.

Precautions: 1. Valerian lowers blood pressure modestly and should be used with caution in persons who already have low blood pressure. 2. I have seen a number of people who find that valerian is too strong in standard doses; it gives them a hung-over or drowsy feeling the next morning. Generally, a much lower dose is effective for these people. 3. It is important with valerian to be cautious with plant identification. True valerian will not give a rebound agitation, meaning it will not cause anxiety several hours after it is used, but several related plants do cause this rebound effect. If you become agitated after using valerian, the supplier may have misidentified the plant. This should ease in a few hours, but discard that product.

Vanilla, *Vanilla planifolia* (Orchidaceae)

Anxiety Uses: Calming, helps sleep, sedative (very mild), uplifting, soothes claustrophobia and other phobias, antidepressant

Other Oral Uses: Aphrodisiac, antioxidant, soothes intestinal gas and gas pains, can lower fevers, detoxification aid

Discussion: The seed pod of a tropical orchid, vanilla is widely used in foods and fragrances. It has long been valued for its anti-anxiety, soothing, and calming properties; and because it is also uplifting and restorative, it is useful for anxiety and depression. Vanilla helps sleep to be more restful and sound, especially in persons who suffer agitation, restless mind, or anxious thoughts. A still popular, old-fashioned remedy for sleep is vanilla extract in warm milk, taken at bedtime. Vanilla also soothes digestion and dispels gas.

Vanilla is used in aromatherapy for phobias, especially claustrophobia. It can be used as a food or extract for this purpose. It also helps calm restlessness, irritability, frustration, and anger.

Spiritually, vanilla is comforting and soothing, with the addition of a spicy and exotic energy. It helps people be more comfortable with stepping out of their habitual patterns, and more open to trying new things. It contributes to developing a cheery inner strength and fortitude.

Dosage: Varies widely. A usual dose of extract is 1/2–1 teaspoon in a hot beverage one to three times daily.

Precautions: Safe

Vervain or Blue Vervain, *Verbena officinalis* (Verbenaceae)

Anxiety Uses: Anti-anxiety, calming, sleep promotion, sedative (mild), calming, uplifting, mild muscle relaxant

Other Oral Uses: Gallbladder problems including biliary stasis, PMS, menopausal hot flashes

Discussion: A common perennial herb native to Europe, vervain has played an important role in European folk medicine for hundreds of years—so much so that it was called "holy herb" and "herb of grace." The ancient Egyptians referred to it as "Tears of Isis." In folklore vervain has long been associated with protection from supernatural forces. It was used in Druidic rituals.

Vervain has many benefits for relief of anxiety. It can be used for general nervousness and insomnia, but has specific indications as well. It is generally prescribed for people who are "highstrung" or "tense." These are often perfectionists who are driven to achieve, or people who are judgmental of others or themselves and suffer for their excessively high standards. They are frequently tired or exhausted and exhibit signs of adrenal stress but find it difficult to let up, especially on themselves. They may be angry at injustice, either in the world or in their personal experience. Herbalists including myself have noted that this can be a great remedy for tense people who have tight neck and shoulders. It can also be quite effective for tension headaches. Vervain is great for people who think too much or suffer endless mind chatter, where their thoughts never seem to shut off.

Vervain is a tense-looking plant, with serrated leaves and blue/white flowers at the ends of spiky branches. Energetically it is cold and very bitter. It is also an important flower essence to reduce tension, among Dr. Bach's original thirty-eight essences.

Spiritually, vervain is helpful for people who have rigid ideas about how things should be in the world, especially when reality does not conform to their desires and expectations. Often people who most benefit from spirit doses of this plant are aware that they might be happier if they could just "let go" but are unsure how to make that happen. They may be overworked or driven, with little down or personal time. Spiritually, vervain can help unhappy idealists and activists find greater ease and serenity with things as they are, and to gently discover, as Peace Pilgrim pointed out during the Cold War era, that true peace in the world begins with inner peace.

Dosage: This is a low-dosage plant, since it is very cold (cooling) and very bitter. It is generally taken as a tincture or as a tea of the leaves, though the flowers are sometimes added to salads. A typical dose is 3–10 drops of tincture one to two times daily, or 1/2 teaspoon of herb as tea in a cup of water. Spirit dose is 1 drop in water daily, or use the flower essence.

Precautions: 1. Unsafe in pregnancy, as vervain may cause miscarriage. 2. Not advised while breast-feeding.

Wood Betony, *Betonica officinalis* or *Stachys betonica* (Labiatae)

Anxiety Uses: Relief of insomnia, nervine, mild sedative, makes one
more cheerful

Other Oral Uses: Fatigue, fibromyalgia, menstrual cramps,
migraines, may slow heavy menstrual bleeding, can relieve irritable bowel, asthma relief

Discussion: Wood betony is a helpful albeit underutilized herbal
sedative. A member of the mint family, it is a gentle nervous system and digestive tract restorative tonic. It is an herb with a long
history of use that has gone in and out of favor in various eras.
In some periods, such as the ancient Greek and Roman epochs,
it was regarded as a panacea, good for almost everything, whereas
in other periods it was overlooked or abandoned.

Emotionally, wood betony is good to utilize over time for nervous exhaustion, gastrointestinal issues, and insomnia. It is particularly helpful for those experiencing agitated insomnia who are
worn out by their worries. Wood betony is especially useful when
there are longstanding emotional problems, and gentle encouragement is needed. It can be useful in people for whom too much
pushiness might overwhelm the healing process. It provides mild
but long-lasting nourishment and restoration of the nervous
system and the digestive tract. It can be useful as a restorative in
persons with irritable bowel syndrome, especially those whose
gastrointestinal issues are related to anxiety and stress.

Physically, wood betony is gentle, yet like many mints it
moves stagnant energy and is helpful in slowly improving
chronic pain syndromes and chronic tension, especially where
there is an emotional component. In Chinese medicine, it moves
stagnant liver Qi and nourishes weak stomach and gallbladder
Qi. It can be slightly laxative even in small doses. It is used in
chronic fatigue when sleep is not restorative, and for people who
are tired all the time and do not get quality sleep. It can be useful in fibromyalgia as a nervous restorative. Wood betony can be

helpful as an expectorant, and it is sometimes used in asthma, especially when there is concurrent emotional upset. It is also nutritive, helping strengthen the tone of the GI tract so that digestion is improved and nutrients more easily absorbed. It is therefore useful as a tonic in convalescence and in the elderly.

Spiritually, wood betony likes to be invited, noticed, and used with consciousness. It does not reveal itself quickly, but is very kind, loving and soft. It can help stabilize emotional swings by enhancing feelings of peacefulness and comfort. It is very helpful for people who are not in touch with their emotions, or who have trouble processing them. For people who are secretive because of fear or shame, it helps them to shine more, allowing themselves to be seen. It can be very grounding, relaxing, and stabilizing.

Dosage: Usually taken as a tea of the leaves, 1/2–1 cup per day, alone or in blends. Can also be used in tinctures, 2–20 drops one to three times daily. Wood betony is often combined with other herbs. I typically advise small doses for long periods of time (several months). For spirit doses, use 1 drop.

Precautions: 1. Uterine stimulant—do not use in pregnancy. 2. Large doses are contraindicated and may cause nausea and vomiting.

Common Herbal Preparations

Infusions: These are herbal concentrates made with water and dry or fresh herbs. A "standard infusion" is an herbalist's term, referring to a preparation made with one ounce of herb steeped in one pint of freshly boiled water. Flowers are usually steeped (meaning soaked, off the flame) at least 15 minutes, but usually not much longer. Leaves can be steeped anywhere from a minimum of thirty minutes to four hours. Roots are generally steeped at least two hours or longer. Cold infusions and sun infusions can be made by steeping plant material in room-temperature water or water placed in a jar in the sun. Generally, these take longer to extract than boiled-water infusions, but they can have a gentler effect, which is sometimes preferable.

Tinctures: For these herbal preparations the herbs are extracted into either grain alcohol or cider vinegar, concentrating those plant constituents that extract best into those media. As an alternative, there are glycerin preparations on the market in which the herbs are first extracted into alcohol; the alcohol is then removed and replaced with glycerin. Infusions and tinctures are usually used to treat physical conditions and ailments, although they can also be used for emotional and spiritual healing.

Tea: This is a common method of herbal preparation and consumption. Tea can be made from fresh or dried herbs. Typically, to make tea 1 teaspoon of leaf, 1 tablespoon of flowers, or 1/2 teaspoon of root is used per cup of water. Many herbs have volatile essential oils that will escape with steam, so it is a good idea to prepare teas covered with a lid or a saucer.

Decoctions: These herbal preparations involve boiling the fresh or dried herb. Decoctions are often made from roots, which are slower to extract into tea.

Capsules: Most capsules contain dried powdered herb, although some are made from concentrated herbal extracts. Capsules of dried herbs often have a short shelf life, as the herb begins to degrade after it is powdered. Concentrated herbal extracts and "supercritical extracts" are more expensive but are often of higher quality.

Tools for Transformation: Appreciating the Spirit Wisdom of Plants

Scientific inquiry is one of many possible routes of investigation to help us understand our world. While it is a useful method, it is relatively new on the scene of human experience. Science has its own limitations and biases. Fundamentally, science as it is currently practiced *objectifies*. It assumes a division between the examiner and the field of examination.

This means that certain types of perception, particularly ones that rely on interrelationship and subjectivity, are excluded from contemporary scientific methodologies.

There are older, venerated modes of perception for gaining insight about the nature of things. Among these are tools for direct perception, which allow for a pure communication with the natural world. The comprehension that arises from this type of inquiry is symbolic, multi-layered, and personal. Working with plants spiritually utilizes ancient methods of direct perception. It can be extremely rewarding, fostering greater self-awareness and enhanced cognizance of the interconnected nature of physical life.

My observations and advice regarding spirit-medicine tools in this exercise, and in connection with the herbs I have discussed, do not come from a particular tradition. While I have studied many areas of traditional wisdom, these observations are uniquely my own, formed in cooperation with nature, through personal experience.

Each of us hears, sees, perceives, interprets, and knows in our own unique ways. I chose to offer a "free-form" exercise for this chapter, to facilitate interested persons in their ability to communicate with plants, trees, animals, insects, and other elements of the natural world. Since this is a chapter about herbs, I frame it as communication with plants, but it can apply to diverse circumstances. With a willing heart and open mind, you can learn to communicate with any aspect of the natural world, great or small.

Exercise: Forming Therapeutic Alliances with Herbs

1. It can be of great benefit to communicate with plants that interest you, especially before embarking upon a course of treatment. This establishes a relationship that is based upon mutual trust, love, and respect. It fosters cooperation, integrity, and wholeness by acknowledging our interconnections. There are many ways to open the channels of connection, and there are also many ways to receive it.

Initially, one might check in with the herb under consideration by visiting a live plant, if it is local and in season. Reading any folklore about the plant can give you additional insight into the nuances of its personality, especially if the plant has cooperated with humanity for a long time. If it is not a plant that you can meet "in person," look at photos of it. After "meeting" the herb, allow yourself to grow quiet and receptive, perhaps by applying one of the meditation techniques discussed earlier in the book.

Next, communicate with the plant, either by speaking or in your heart/ mind, and let it know how you imagine working together. Let it know why you have chosen it, at this time. You can ask for its assistance on your journey to greater well-being, and express your appreciation for any contributions it might make to you, and for how it has helped others. You might also ask the herb if it is appropriate for you to work with it, in this way, at this time.

2. Then listen inside yourself and observe how you feel. Notice what you notice. Observe any impressions. Understand that impressions may come in many forms. They can be visual, auditory, olfactory, sensory, or emotional. Part of what you can learn by working in this manner is how you experience communication with the natural world. There is not just one right way. Each of us is unique, and spirit communicates with each of us in our own best way. Nothing is irrelevant—internal images, elusive scents, the hum of an insect, a flicker of light, a leaf fluttering, a slight breeze upon your cheek—all of this, and more, is meaningful. Notice your emotional state. Let yourself be quiet, and perceive without expectation or judgment. Follow your breath.

A feeling of well-being, love, or appreciation tells you that you are on a good track. The universe of communication opens to each of us in a meeting place of love. Feelings of unease, sadness, discomfort, or disconnection can indicate that this herb might not be a good choice at this good time. Notice if another suggestion is offered, again as an impression, that feels more whole.

If you are unsure how you are feeling, that is okay. Just share with the plant that understanding more clearly how you are feeling is another thing you want help with, and leave it at that for the time being. The natural world is very loving and willing to help. Impressions and intuition may come later, in dreams or flashes of insight.

Relying on your intellect, especially at first, is also fine if you are unsure whether you are getting any messages from the plant world. In my experience, an herb will be honored and pleased that you have connected, or made an effort to connect, to its spirit, and will be a much better ally for you, whether or not you believe there was any clear communication.

I have found that by spending just a few minutes connecting energetically in this way, prior to a course of action, many people experience a much better outcome. I have also seen many times that when working in this manner, much lower doses can be effective.

3. After you have been working with an herb for a while, periodically check in with it again and express appreciation for its contribution to you. You can do this with a formula as well. Let it know what has improved, and what you think you still need in order to feel better. Ask the herb, or herbs, if this is still the right choice. Perhaps other herbs might be good to combine with it, or possibly there is something even better for you at this new juncture. Once again, listen inside; see how you feel. Take some time with this. Many people worry when they receive impressions that they are "making them up." Do your best not to overanalyze or judge. Allow your experience to speak for itself. The experience is subjective and highly personal.

4. Remember, these tools, like any others, become easier and more fluid with practice. With these methods you can develop your skills in communicating with the spiritual aspects of plants. You will find your own style of perception and discover many things about the essence of yourself in your communication with nature. You can perceive how nature speaks with you, through you, and in you. Communion with nature is a powerful catalyst for inner peace.

CHAPTER 12

༄

Traditional Chinese Medicine, Acupuncture, and Acupressure

A cupuncture is a part of the complete healing system of Traditional Chinese Medicine and has been utilized for thousands of years. It is based upon an ancient understanding of the flow patterns and channels of vital force (Qi) throughout the body. Chinese medicine and acupuncture address patterns of imbalance that lead to physical, emotional, and spiritual diseases. Ideally in Chinese medicine, imbalances are discovered and addressed *before* physical or emotional illness manifests. Chinese medicine includes advice and therapeutics relating to diet, medications, herbs, movement and exercise, massage, and of course acupuncture. Over the years, many diverse varieties of this system evolved, each with a particular viewpoint and nuances of practice. Chinese medicine migrated to other areas of Asia and influenced traditional healing systems in many lands. For example, Kampo, the traditional healing system of Japan, traces its origins to the Chinese system; and Thai massage and traditional Thai healing, traditional Korean medicine, Tibetan medicine, and Mongolian medicine were all cross-fertilized with Chinese medicine.

Acupuncture generally involves the insertion of thin needles into specific points on the body located on channels of energy flow called meridians. Traditionally needles were gold or silver, but today they are most often stainless steel. Meridians are conduits for the flow of vital force (Qi). All meridians connect with one another, end to beginning, in a seamless whole. Most meridians are paired, connecting yin to yang, and yang to yin. There are both external (surface of the body) and internal (inside the body) flows of

Qi in each meridian, though the internal pathways cannot usually be accessed directly by points on the surface. There are approximately three hundred sixty regular acupuncture points located along the meridians of the human body. There are additional hand, ear, and scalp points with their own numbering and labeling system and their own correspondences and flow patterns that are not categorized by meridians. There is a collection of extra points as well that are not located on meridians.

Acupressure is similar to acupuncture in its use of the meridians of Qi flow as a conduit of therapeutic effects. With acupressure there are no needles; instead, a varying amount of pressure on particular points and areas is applied by fingers, elbows, knees, or occasionally various implements. Some of the points used in acupressure may differ from classical acupuncture points.

Types of Acupuncture and Acupressure

There are many contemporary varieties of acupuncture and acupressure. Each type has its advantages and adherents. Some that are most commonly useful for persons with anxiety are discussed briefly below.

Traditional Chinese Medicine (TCM)

TCM is the most widely practiced form of acupuncture. It is also called Eight Principles acupuncture. TCM Practitioners are trained in the use of Chinese herbal therapeutics, and some also train in traditional Chinese medical dietetics. This system looks at symptoms and health by examination of complementary forces: yin/yang, cold/heat, interior/exterior, and excess/deficiency. There is also an understanding of the five Elements—fire, water, earth, metal, and wood—and their relationship to balance and harmony in the body, mind, and one's overall physical health. The elements correspond to body tissues, colors, times of day, seasons, and emotions.

Diagnosis in TCM involves an extensive interview with a patient and an examination of pulse, tongue, facial color, and other physical signs and symptoms. The practitioner seeks to understand the unique patterns of disharmony and imbalance in the client. Generally, several patterns are present.

In Chinese medicine, organs and meridians are acknowledged to have emotional correlates, and there is no separation between physical and emotional symptoms when identifying patterns of imbalance. Treatment might include needles, electro-acupuncture (insertion of needles that are then stimulated via current passed through electrodes), moxibustion, cupping, and gua sha, which is a therapeutic method of scraping or vigorous rubbing.

After the Cultural Revolution of the 1950s, many of the most spiritual elements of TCM were unfortunately eliminated from the TCM academies of China. Practitioners were instead trained to focus on physical symptoms and external causes of disease, though emotional issues were still understood to be interwoven with physical ailments. Today some Western practitioners of TCM have reincorporated the more spiritual understanding. TCM, especially with a practitioner who combines elements that emphasize spiritual well-being, can be very helpful in transforming anxiety.

Five-Elements Acupuncture

Another main branch of acupuncture in the West today is Five-Elements Acupuncture. It is thought to have originated more than two thousand years ago and was influenced by observation of natural laws and their relationship with human health. In this system the balance and distribution of the five elements (earth, metal, fire, water, and wood, mentioned above in the discussion of TCM) are examined in detail in each patient. Practitioners rely upon pulse, tongue diagnosis, skin color, body odor, tenor of the voice, emotional state, and other signs to diagnose and treat imbalances. In this system, like in so many holistic systems, physical and emotional illness are thought to originate with distress at the emotional or spiritual levels. These original imbalances must be addressed for the client to heal completely, whether that is physical or emotional health. Five-elements acupuncture observes that each element corresponds to emotions, and it teaches that emotions must be balanced to support both emotional and physical health.

Five-elements acupuncture places its focus on the unity of body, mind, heart, and spirit. Because of the emphasis on the integration of spirit in the health of the whole person, this ancient form of acupuncture is not practiced today in China. Contemporary teachers of five-elements acupuncture learned its concepts and techniques from individuals who studied in China prior to the Cultural Revolution.

Treatment in five-elements acupuncture often involves fewer needles than TCM. Electro-acupuncture is not frequently used in this system, but cupping and moxibustion are commonly added. Five-elements practitioners sometimes use herbs adjunctively, but less frequently than TCM counterparts. In my experience, five-elements acupuncture is often one of the most effective Chinese-medicine tools for treatment of anxiety.

Medical Acupuncture or French Energetic Acupuncture

Generally practiced only by MDs and DOs, this type of acupuncture expands on a traditional understanding of Chinese medicine that was popular among the Jesuits who visited China in the seventeenth and eighteenth centuries. It emphasizes relationships between paired yin and yang meridians. Physician practitioners qualify for membership in the American Academy of Medical Acupuncture after about 200 hours of training.

Medical acupuncture can be helpful for treatment of anxiety, though most physicians who practice it focus more on physical problems such as pain management and musculoskeletal health problems.

Non-needle Techniques

There are a few types of acupuncture where needles are not inserted. One is Acupuncture Core therapy, also known as Shaku Jyu Chikyo. With this technique, trained acupuncturists (usually TCM-trained) use blunt silver or platinum needles *(teishin),* which are placed on the point but not inserted. Skilled practitioners can apply this gentle treatment to address blockages of energy and improve Qi circulation as well as a host of other physical and emotional imbalances. The non-insertion technique can be as deep and effective as other acupuncture modalities. Practitioners may also apply moxibustion and/or cupping during treatments.

Japanese Traditional Acupuncture: Kampo or Meridian Therapy

This type of acupuncture is similar to TCM, but needles are thinner and are not inserted as deeply. In meridian therapy, an effort is made to feel the flow of Qi in the entire meridian. This type can be very helpful for anxiety, though there are far fewer practitioners of this technique than there are TCM providers.

Auriculotherapy

Auriculotherapy is branch of acupuncture that treats specific points on the ear. As with the hand and the foot, all the points on the body are considered to be reflected in the ear. Most trained acupuncturists, especially those with TCM and Medical Acupuncture training, are familiar with this treatment. Some acupuncturists may apply adhesive-backed silver or gold pellets to specific points to extend the effects of a treatment with home care. There are several different "maps" for auriculotherapy, so practitioners may not agree on the location of points. Nonetheless, treatment of ear points can be quite useful, and there are many points that are helpful in soothing emotional distress and anxiety.

Korean Hand Acupuncture

In this traditional Korean healing system, needles are inserted only in the hands, and the needles are smaller and thinner than those used in TCM. The system developed from elements of TCM and Japanese acupuncture. In this system, points on the hands and feet are thought to mirror the entire physical body, and they have higher concentrations of Qi than most body points. Thus any physical condition can be addressed by treatment of the corresponding points on the hands. The system evaluates a patient's body type and constitution to determine an appropriate diagnosis and course of treatment. I generally see this type of treatment as addressing mostly physical ailments; however, a trained practitioner could direct you to emotional self-care points on the hand.

Overview of the Traditional Chinese Medical Understanding of Anxiety and Agitation

The diagnosis of anxiety is a modern Western one and did not exist, per se, in Traditional Chinese Medicine. Still, there were many patterns of disharmony in TCM that would correspond to our contemporary diagnosis of various anxiety disorders including generalized anxiety, panic attacks, obsessive compulsive disorder, phobias, and PTSD. Thus acupuncture and Chinese medicine can alleviate a whole host of anxiety-related symptoms such as restlessness, irritability, worry, startling easily, general tension, forgetfulness, edginess, tendency to weeping, and sleeping problems, as well as physical-emotional symptoms like heart palpitations, nausea, muscle tension, and headaches. Practitioners of Chinese medicine would tend to look at a person with anxiety in terms of their presenting physical or emotional symptoms. They would use a physical exam to check for such signs as dry eyes, mouth, hair, nails, redness of face and cheeks, and pallor, performing a careful examination of the pulses and the tongue.

A diagnosis would illuminate the pattern or patterns of disharmony that underlies the anxiety. This would be addressed with various techniques that might include needles, cupping, moxibustion, or massage. Generally there are several concurrent patterns, and treatments are customized to best support balance in the individual. Chinese medical patterns use the names of Western organs but rarely correlate with physical disease in those organs. So someone with Spleen Dampness or Heart Fire will generally not have a problem with either the spleen or the heart. There are many common patterns of disharmony that might lead to anxiety. It is interesting to note that Nobel Laureate Candace Pert, PhD, who discovered opiate receptors, also found that receptors for neurotransmitters that correspond to various emotions are concentrated not only in the brain, but on the physical organs. So the liver, spleen, heart, and other body organs all have receptors for neurotransmitters of various emotions, and these are distributed in a manner predicted by Chinese medicine. Each organ has distinctive symptoms associated with it.

Acupressure

Acupressure, or pressure on acupuncture points with fingers, hands, or implements, is another ancient system of healing with origins in Chinese medicine. It is very popular with clients and practitioners and has multiple self-care applications.

There are many forms of acupressure treatment by practitioners. These can be generally balancing to the whole body. Practitioners can identify areas of imbalance for home self-care. Some of the most well known forms of acupressure massage treatment are shiatsu (Japanese), tui na (Chinese), and Thai massage. While acupressure is not as strong as acupuncture, over time acupressure massage techniques, performed by a skilled practitioner, can achieve much of the same benefits as acupuncture.

Tools for Transformation: Self-Acupressure Massage Points for Emotional Calm

Self-acupressure is a great way to calm and center. Acupressure gently stimulates the natural healing abilities of your body, providing relief for body, mind, and spirit. It is, of course, free, and something you can do at any time. It is a safe and supportive way to help yourself shift your focus to a self-loving, self-nurturing train of thought. Even a few minutes performing self acupressure are often minutes well spent!

How to work with self-care points:

Select a point or series of points that seem appropriate to your situation. When needed, some points, like those on the arm and wrist, can be utilized in a discreet manner, even while you are engaged in other activities like public speaking or a business meeting. In these cases, it is good to know ahead of time which points tend to be most helpful for you.

Use your thumb or the pad of any finger to press the point you have selected. You do not need a lot of pressure. Even just resting your finger against a point makes a circuit that brings the body's attention to the area. If it feels comfortable, press firmly or massage the point with a gentle circular motion. Avoid pressing to the edge of discomfort. If you feel any pain, just back off to a level that feels good, or move on to another point. In many people, working with the points for a minute or two will really promote a sense of calm, but in others, five to ten seconds is sufficient. As always, listen to your body. Stimulate the points for as long as you like.

You may start to feel a gentle pulsing at a point as you work with it. This is an indication of increased circulation to the area. Acupressure self-massage works whether or not you feel a pulsing.

Most acupressure points on the body are bilateral. It is good (when convenient) to stimulate the same point on both sides of the body. For example, if you choose to work with Heart Seven (HT 7), you will find the same point on both wrists. The midline meridians of energy flow, called Conception Vessel (CV) and Governing Vessel (GV), are not paired, so there will be only one of each CV or GV point on the body. It is generally advisable to be particularly gentle when stimulating CV and GV points, especially those on the head or neck.

As a precaution, employ common sense. Never press on a point that overlies an open wound, a bruise, inflamed skin, or an area where there might be an underlying broken bone or ruptured tendon. Do not do acupressure in the area of a known tumor.

The Points

Conception Vessel Seventeen (CV 17)

CHINESE: SHAN ZHONG, "SEA OF TRANQUILITY," ALSO "PRIMORDIAL CHILD" AND "CHEST CENTER"

Location: In the center of the breastbone, between the fourth and fifth ribs, in the spot where the thumbs naturally rest against the chest when the hands are in a "prayer position." In men, this is directly between the nipples.

General Health: Nourishes the physical heart, alleviates cough, and is helpful in quieting asthma. Clears hiccups. Supports lactation. Overall strengthening of vital force (Qi) of body and spirit.

Anxiety Relief: Calming and centering, helps individuals to ground themselves in soothing heart energy. In the chakra system, this is the physical anatomical center of the heart chakra. The point balances emotions and relieves tension, depression, hysteria, nervousness, and anxiety. It is noteworthy that people who have received a shock or fright often instinctively bring their hand to this area of the chest. Alleviates sorrows. It can be especially helpful and calming to stimulate this point together with, or just before working with, the next point, GV 24.5.

Governing Vessel 24.5

Chinese: Yin Tang, "Hall of Impression" and "Hall of the Seal," also Third Eye (ajna center)

Location: In the midline of the forehead, at the spot between the top of the arches of the eyebrows. Most people will notice a small notch at this point.

General Health: Helps with frontal headaches, nasal and sinus problems including nosebleeds, also dizziness, trigeminal neuralgia, eye problems, and many head and brain issues.

Anxiety Relief: Helps activate awareness of the peaceful, calm, always supportive and loving observer in each of us. Pressing this point calms the mind and is balancing to body, mind, and spirit. It can alleviate nervousness and tension and is also great for insomnia, especially when related to stress, anxiety, or tension. Yin tang helps us to take a step back and look at the bigger picture. It decreases anxiety and stress, and supports spiritual balance while potentially providing clarity and insight. It can be especially helpful and calming to stimulate this point together with or just after working with the prior point, CV 17. The combination connects the heart to intuitive wisdom, especially when a conscious connection is made between these two spots.

Governing Vessel 20 (GV 20)

CHINESE: BAI HU, "ONE HUNDRED MEETING POINT" OR
"HUNDRED CONVERGENCES"

Location: In the hollow in the center of the crown of the head, on a line directly between the meeting points of the tips (apices) of the ears. "The point at the top of the head."

General Health: Soothes headaches and tension, and used to address all sorts of emotional issues. Used also as a main point to counter organ prolapses anywhere in the body, since this point is generally balancing and rejuvenating. Also helps diminish dizziness, visual disturbances, and memory loss and is used in treatment of seizures. Helps alertness and can be stimulated while studying or before exams for greater mental clarity. It is the GV meeting point of all six yang channels, thus it is the connector for more than one hundred points. It regulates yang, either insufficient or excessive.

Anxiety Relief: Calming, helps thoughts and senses to become clearer and more coherent. Also helps self-confidence, optimism, and overall sense of well-being. Calms the mind and the spirit. Dissipates irritability and irascibility. Supports calm clear energy, lifts the spirits, alleviates depression, and supports constructive thought patterns. Also associated with the crown chakra, this point can help us to connect with our higher wisdom, when we are ready.

Governing Vessel Sixteen (GV 16)

CHINESE: FENG FU, "WIND MANSION"

Location: On the back of the neck, in the hollow at the center of the intersection between the neck and spinal column. Be particularly gentle when massaging this point!

General Health: Head and neck problems, stiff-neck headaches, earaches, dizziness, nosebleeds; also treats ailments in feet and legs. Used for tremors and numbness.

Anxiety Relief: Calming, balancing, and centering, helps clear agitated jumpy thoughts that go from one unpleasant subject to another, as well as repetitive, stuck, and recurrent thoughts. Calms and soothes temperamental and irritable dispositions. Can be useful even in extreme anxiety and panic attacks. Can also be used to calm nervous tics and twitching. A "window-of-the-sky point," this one helps connect our body with our mind and spirit, and even our highest inner wisdom.

Stomach Thirty-Six (ST 36)

CHINESE: SU SAN LI, "LEG THREE MILES"

Location: On the outside (lateral side) of the calf, near the shin bone, about four finger-widths below the inferior (bottom) edge of the kneecap. It feels like your finger "falls into a hole" when you locate the point.

General Health: An energizing point, this alleviates fatigue, strengthens the immune system and respiratory tract, and alleviates nausea, diarrhea, and stomach and intestinal rumbling. Do not use this point to overstimulate or push yourself when you are already tired, as overuse can exacerbate burnout. One of the most commonly used acupuncture points, ST 36 is considered by some teachers to be the most important point, as it "corrects the Qi" and promotes healthy longevity. Used also for asthma, muscle pain, cough, and chest pain, as well as leg and foot problems.

Anxiety Relief: Helps decrease overall tension, and addresses a wide range of emotional disturbances including mania, depression, eruptive anger, hysterical laughter, and fright. It is especially helpful for diminishing excessive thought and rumination, as well as butterflies in the stomach. Stabilizing and grounding. Calms worried minds. Calms the spirit.

Pericardium Three (PC 3)

CHINESE: QU ZE, "MARSH AT THE BEND" OR "CROOKED MARSH"

Location: In the inner portion of the arm (ventral surface, ulnar side), at the upper tip of the crease of the elbow when the elbow is bent. Anatomically it is on the ulnar side of the biceps tendon, medial to the brachial artery.

General Health: Used to treat arm and elbow pain and problems including arthritis and tennis elbow; also settles digestion and treats nausea and diarrhea. Used for chest pain, angina, and cardiac issues. Settles tremors of the hand and is sometimes used in treatment of Parkinson's disease. Clears heat from the blood, as this is the water point on a fire meridian.

Anxiety Relief: Helps clear nervous tension related to nausea and palpitations. Also helpful in alleviating generalized sadness, especially the kind that comes in waves, or that seems to come out of nowhere.

Pericardium Six (PC 6)

CHINESE: NEI GUAN, "INNER GATE" OR "INNER PASS"

Location: On the palmar side of the wrist, about two inches or three finger-breadths from the wrist crease, in the center of the inner forearm between the two tendons.

General Health: Best known as the "seasickness relief point," PC6 helps relieve nausea and vomiting of all sorts, even from pregnancy (morning sickness), car sickness, gastroenteritis, or chemotherapy. For nausea it is best used in combination with Stomach 36. Also stimulates circulation and supports a normal heart rate and function. Nei Guan "opens the chest" and is used to treat cough, asthma, and chest pain as well as seizures and dizziness. Great for clearing hiccups, it is also known as "the hiccup point." Helps many other gastrointestinal problems including heartburn, GERD, constipation, and indigestion.

Anxiety Relief: Good for all sorts of emotional upsets, this point is calming, relaxing, and balancing. Useful for soothing fear, anxiety, heart palpitations, worry, nervous stomach and stomachache, and insomnia. Helps diminish stress-related memory loss and forgetfulness. It can be especially calming and balancing to the whole body to stimulate this point together with the next point (TW 5) by utilizing the thumb and forefinger.

Triple Warmer Five (TW 5)

CHINESE: WAI GUAN, "OUTER GATE" OR "OUTER PASS"

Location: On the dorsum (outer part) of the arm, at a natural depression between the ulna and radius bones, about three finger-widths or two inches behind the wrist.

General Health: Wrist pain, headache including migraines, chest pain, problems with forearm, elbow, hand, and fingers. Also used to address tremors (especially of the hand) and shoulder pains, as well as constipation and abdominal pains.

Anxiety Relief: Helps diminish nausea, especially from nervous tension, anxiety, heart palpitations, and insomnia. It can be especially calming and balancing to the whole body to stimulate this point together with the prior point (PC 6) by utilizing the thumb and forefinger.

Triple Warmer Fifteen (TW 15)

CHINESE: TIAN LAO, "HEAVENLY REJUVENATION" OR
"HEAVENLY CREVICE" OR "CELESTIAL BONE HOLE"

Location: On the upper shoulder, three fingers from the base of the neck, just above the angle of the scapula

General Health: Neck and shoulder and arm tension and pain (it almost always feels good to be rubbed here!), as well as neck pain and tension. Also used to treat fever, colds, and flus, to improve immune resistance to URIs (upper respiratory tract infections), and to strengthen the lungs.

Anxiety Relief: Calms nervousness, soothes emotional neck and shoulder tension.

Heart Seven (HT 7)

CHINESE: SHEN MEN, "SPIRIT DOOR" OR "SPIRIT GATE"

Location: On the edge crease of the wrist, on the side of the pinky finger, in the depression formed between the pisiform bone and the ulna. This would be the dip on the hand side of the large bump on the pinky side of the wrist.

General Health: Used mostly for emotional issues and physical heart problems including heart palpitations, chest pains, and angina. It is considered a point to tonify and steady the heart. But it can also be helpful in a wide range of physical problems including treatment of jaundice, constipation, arm and shoulder pain, and motion restriction.

Anxiety Relief: A great point for insomnia, especially when there is worry and over-thinking; also good for alleviating anxiety-related heart palpitations and agitation. Calming for people who lie down to sleep and perceive they are hearing their heartbeat in an emotionally disturbing manner, whether or not it is actually rapid. Also calming for stage fright, performance anxiety, panic attacks, worry, nausea from anxiety, nervous sweating, hysteria, shock, and PTSD. It supports mental clarity and is great for alleviating forgetfulness or cloudy and confused thinking in the presence of anxiety or stress. It is particularly useful for people with phobias, especially social phobias that have closed them off from interaction with others. It gently opens the spirit to expanded possibilities and awakens hopefulness. An overall soothing point, it can be stimulated discreetly during many activities.

Gallbladder Twenty (GB 20)

CHINESE: FENG CHI, "WIND POOL"

Location: On the nape of the neck, in the hollows on either side of the base of the skull, about 1 1/2 inches from the center of the spine. Level with GV 16.

General Health: The point is used traditionally to address headache (especially occipital, or back of the head), heartburn, high blood pressure, vertigo, as well as all manner of problems with the head including seizures, issues with sensory organs (impaired vision, taste, smell, and hearing), and neck or shoulder tension. Also helpful in upper respiratory tract problems including the common cold.

Anxiety Relief: Wonderful for alleviating tension or anxiety-related sleep issues and insomnia. Also helps fatigue and rejuvenates the mind.

Liver Three (LV 3)

CHINESE: TAI CHONG, "GREAT SURGE" OR "SUPREME SURGE" OR "GREAT RUSHING"

Location: On the top (dorsum) of the foot, in the depression between the first and second metatarsal bones. Feels like a natural stopping place or "hole" as you run your finger along the first metatarsal bone toward the ankle.

General Health: Helps alleviate headache, heartburn, high blood pressure. Strongly supports the immune system. Clears stagnation throughout the body. Also helps numerous eye disorders (including red eyes, blurry vision, and eye pain), breast problems, gastrointestinal problems including constipation and dry or painful defecation, IBS, IBD, and menstrual issues including cramps, PMS discharges, and irregular menses—all are treated though this point. It is one of the most widely used points in Chinese medicine.

Anxiety Relief: Decreases feelings of irritability, anger, and frustration. Helps people who feel stuck in the same tired patterns to get moving. Useful for people who have suppressed emotions and emotionality; it allows the emotions to flow. Also used for insomnia, excessive or repetitive thought patterns, fearfulness or acute fright, and general stress reduction.

Kidney One (Ki 1)

CHINESE: YONG QUAN, "GUSHING SPRING" OR "BUBBLING SPRING"

Location: On the sole of the foot, in the center of the crease formed when the toes are bent in plantar flexion. It is one third of the distance from the bottom of the toes to the heel. It is the only acupuncture point on the sole of the foot. In Vedic medicine it is known as the foot chakra.

General Health: Used as an emergency point when energy has collapsed, from loss of consciousness or via shock or trauma. Also used in non-emergency situations for headache and back pain, hot flashes, night sweats, tinnitus, insomnia, poor memory, heat in the soles of the feet, and heart palpitations.

Anxiety Relief: Revivifying yet wonderfully grounding, this point can be used when there is mild or severe distress, fright, or panic attack. Also when there is anger or worried feelings or fear of being out of control. Used for anxiety, especially when there is rumination. Can revitalize the body, mind, and spirit and reconnect you with your purpose in life and your link with the Earth. It is great for insomnia too. For anxiety or insomnia, try doing a foot bath, perhaps with an essential oil and/or magnesium chloride or Epsom salts, then massaging this point. To connect with the Earth, and your inner sense of purpose, it is also nice to massage this point after standing outside barefoot. It is a particularly useful point to work with when things feel like they are moving uncomfortably fast.

Kidney Six (Ki 6)

CHINESE: ZHAO HAI, "SHINING SEA"

Location: One inch distal (down toward the foot) from the medical malleolus (inner ankle bone), on the medial (inner) side of the ankle, in the space between the ankle bone and the Achilles tendon.

General Health: Constipation, eye and vision problems, fevers, sore throat, sensation of lump in throat, hoarseness and laryngitis, numerous menstrual concerns including discharges, cramps, and some forms of infertility, male sexual health issues, night sweats, hot hands and feet. Also helpful with some forms of epilepsy.

Anxiety Relief: Commonly used for sleep issues, relief of nightmares and anxiety, especially anxiety that amps up at night or before sleep. It can be especially helpful to grasp both this point and the next (UB 62) at the same time, with the thumb and forefinger. Decreases fearfulness, is grounding and soothing.

Bladder Sixty Two (UB 62)

CHINESE: SHEN MAI, "EXTENDING VESSEL"

Location: One inch below the lateral malleolus of the ankle, in the center of the lower hollow on the lateral (outer) side of the foot between the ankle bone and the Achilles tendon.

General Health: Low back pain, neck pain and stiffness, leg pain, sciatica, headaches, dizziness, some forms of epilepsy, fatigue.

Anxiety Relief: Calming and cleansing; supports detoxification of the spent neurotransmitters of anxiety. Used for clearing nervous tension, agitation, worries, and insomnia; supports restful sleep and calm mood. Also grounding. It can be especially helpful to grasp both this point and the prior one (Ki 6) at the same time, with the thumb and forefinger. The point and combination are particularly useful for relieving nervousness at night that causes insomnia.

ACU-POINTS AND THEIR USES: QUICK REFERENCE TABLE

Points	Key Anxiety Relief Indications
CV 17	Good for centering; heart soothing; alleviates sorrow and fright
GV 24.5	Quiets insomnia; calms nervousness; enhances intuition and mental clarity
GV 20	Clears muddled thoughts and senses; aids self-confidence and optimism; helps access higher wisdom
GV 16	Helps calm agitation, irritability, extreme anxiety or panic; helps release stuck unpleasant thoughts; helps access inner wisdom
ST 36	Helps with excessive thought and rumination; eases nervous tension in stomach; stabilizing, grounding
PC 3	Eases tension resulting in nausea and/or heart palpitations; helps soothe sadness
PC 6	Quiets insomnia; helps with forgetfulness, fear, worry; aids balancing, relaxing
TW 5	Quiets insomnia; calms nervous tension, nausea, anxiety, heart palpitations
TW 15	Eases neck and shoulder tension caused from stress and worry
HT 7	Quiets insomnia, worry, over-thinking, palpitations, performance anxiety, social phobias, and panic attacks; aids mental clarity
GB 20	Quiets insomnia; relieves fatigue, anxiety, tension; rejuvenates the mind
LV 3	Quiets insomnia; eases frustration, irritability, repetitive thoughts, fearfulness; releases stuck old patterns; aids in stress reduction and emotional flow
Ki 1	Quiets insomnia, anxiety, distress, panic attacks, excessive rumination; aids grounding and connecting with inner purpose
Ki 6	Relief from nightmares, insomnia, anxiety at night; aids with grounding
Bl 62	Calms nervous tension, worries, anxiety, especially nighttime anxiety

Ear, Foot, and Hand Acupressure

The ear, the hand, and the foot each have points that correspond to every area of the body. Massage or self-massage of these areas can be soothing and relaxing, an outstanding self-treatment for anxiety. Foot massage can be especially grounding and is wonderful at bedtime to help aid peaceful sleep. One ear point worth mentioning for acupressure self-massage is called *shen men* (like Heart 7). It is located in the upper portion of the ears.

CHAPTER 13

Aromatherapy

Aromatherapy is a well-established branch of healing that employs the use of essential oils extracted from flowers, leaf, bark, or roots of plants for physical and emotional health. The term *aromatherapy* was coined by the French chemist Rene Maurice Gattefosse in 1937 after he observed that topical application of dilute lavender essential oil greatly enhanced healing from burns he personally sustained, clearing a case of gangrene.[1] This was in the era of medicine prior to the widespread use of antibiotics, so it was a profound discovery.

Essential oils have been utilized since ancient times in numerous lands and cultures, including China, Egypt, India, and Southern Europe. Essential oils of cedar, myrrh, clove, cinnamon, and nutmeg were applied to the dead as part of the embalming process. Their residues have been found in tombs over two thousand years old.[2] Aromatherapy was advanced by French surgeon Jean Valnet, who read Gattefosse's book and was inspired when medications were scarce to use essential oils to treat injured soldiers during World War Two.[3]

Smell is one of our primary five senses. It triggers powerful emotional responses. We process information from our sense of smell in an area of the brain adjacent to the limbic region, our area of emotional processing and memory recall. When the scent of an essential oil is inhaled, molecules enter the nasal cavities and stimulate a firing of emotional response in the limbic system of the brain. The centrally located limbic system influences many other areas of the body and brain, including the nervous system and many hormone-producing glands such as the adrenal glands, hypothalamus, and pituitary. These in turn regulate stress or calming responses such as heart rate, breathing patterns, production of hormones, and blood pressure. Aromatherapy oils have been demonstrated to assist all these systems.

Aromatherapy is not generally employed as a sole therapy but is a wonderful adjunct, for some, in relief of anxiety and general mood support. There has been much scientific study of aromatic essential oils. For example, studies have shown that for most people, the smell of cinnamon is one of the most comforting. It reminds people of homemade cookies and cozy domestic interactions. It puts many people at ease. If you are interested in learning more about essential oils, there are some resources to get you started in the bibliography.

Essential oils can be added to baths, massage oil, compresses, inhalations, and aromatherapy diffusers. It is important to note that some essential oils can be irritating or caustic. While a few are used directly on the skin or even internally (orally), this is always done under supervision of a physician or an advanced practitioner. Generally oils applied topically are quite dilute and blended with a carrier oil like sweet almond, jojoba, coconut, olive, or avocado oil. Never ingest any essential oils or apply them undiluted to the skin without proper training or medical supervision. Here are a few of the most common and safe essential oils used for emotional support, anxiety relief, and stress reduction.

Bergamot, *Citrus bergamia*

Emotional: Bergamot has an uplifting fragrance and is used alone or in blends as support during anxiety and depression. Its uplifting, encouraging energy helps with insomnia, relaxation, and agitation.

Physical: This is the herb that gives Earl Grey tea its distinctive floral taste and aroma. It alleviates gas, helps digestion, soothes coughs, and is a good antispasmodic.

Safety: Generally safe but like all members of the citrus family bergamot is photosensitizing, meaning it can increase the risk of sunburn and rash. So do not use it topically, even in blends, within 12 hours of sun or tanning-bed exposure.

Caraway, *Carum carvi*

Emotional: Caraway, like many seeds of plants from the botanical family Umbilliferae, calms nervous stomach.

Physical: Decreases gassiness, supports good digestion and appetite, increases breast milk flow, anti-histaminic, anti-inflammatory.

Safe

Cedarwood (Eastern Red Cedar), *Juniperus virginiana*

Emotional: Used to assuage worry and repetitive thoughts. It is calming, grounding, and helps focus.

Physical: Used often in blends for bronchial concerns, like coughs and colds. Its woody aroma is a note in many men's fragrance blends.

Safe

Chamomile Roman, *Chamaemelum nobile*

Emotional: Longstanding use as a peaceful, calming scent; helps support sleep and inner harmony; decreases irritability, over-thinking, anxiety, worry; and generally soothes frayed nerves.

Physical: Alleviates muscle spasms, is a good antiviral, calms digestive upsets, menstrual cramps, and restless legs.

Safe, except some small risk of allergy, especially with persons who have allergy to ragweed.

Clary Sage, *Salvia sclarea*

Emotional: Uplifting, soothing, and slightly euphoric fragrance that enhances feelings of well-being and connection with others and with the natural world.

Physical: Helps alleviate fatigue and muscle spasms, including bronchial spasm, so it is often used in blends for asthma. Used in many women's blends for hot flashes and menstrual cramps.

Safety: Generally safe but it can increase menstrual flow, so clary sage is not a good choice with heavy menses or during pregnancy; also avoid using in estrogen-dependent breast cancer unless under medical advice.

Frankincense, *Boswellia carteri* or *Boswellia sacra*

Emotional: Calming and tranquil energy, as well as spiritually grounding. Included in many types of incense to help deepen meditation and quiet the mind.

Physical: Used often in respiratory blends for calming spasmodic cough. Moistening, and used in many cosmetic blends for aged or dry skin. Decreases gas, supports healthy immune function.

Safe

Geranium, *Pelargonium roseum* × *asperum*

Emotional: Used for alleviating anxiety and depression, restorative, with a calming and relaxing energy. Balances mood swings. Often used in combinations with citrus.

Physical: Helps vitality, is antiviral and antibacterial, decreases bloating and fluid retention, antispasmodic. Used often for PMS.

Safe

Jasmine, *Jasminum grandiflorum* or *officinale*

Emotional: Calms stress reactions, helps with optimism and self-confidence. May be utilized effectively for improvement when there is lack of motivation, indifference, fearfulness, or feelings of repression.

Physical: Beautiful fragrance much used in perfumery and skin-care products. Antispasmodic and generally strengthening.

Safety: Generally safe but can inhibit breast milk production, so avoid in nursing.

Lavender, *Lavandula angustifolia*

Emotional: This is the most common oil used for calming anxiety and is the base of many popular soothing blends. It is considered a nervous system restorative and helps with inner peace, sleep, restlessness, irritability, panic attacks, nervous stomach, and general nervous tension.

Physical: Alleviates menstrual cramps, spasmodic cough, tension headache, and skin problems and has mild antibacterial properties.

Safe

Lemon, *Citrus limon*

Emotional: Cheerful scent, encourages optimism, has an expansive happy energy that supports people who feel constrained or hemmed in.

Physical: Antibacterial, decongestant, supports the liver and the immune system; used in many household cleaners, as lemon is also a good de-greaser.

Generally safe but like all members of the citrus family, lemon is photosensitizing, meaning it can increase the risk of sunburn and rash. So do not use it topically in blends within 12 hours of sun exposure. Most commonly used in a diffusor.

Lemongrass, *Cymbopogon citratus*

Emotional: Relaxing and uplifting. Common in massage blends.

Physical: Pain-relieving, analgesic, anti-inflammatory, antifungal, antibacterial, used often when there are injuries, including to bone, muscle, or tendons. Fatigue-relieving, and generally strengthening and tonifying.

Safety: Generally safe but can be an irritant to sensitive skin. Generally not advised in topical blends for small children (under age three).

Melissa, *Melissa officinalis*

Emotional: This is the essential oil of lemon balm. Very calming, it is considered a moderately strong sedative. Use tiny amounts, 1–3 drops per ounce of base oil, in blends for sleep, panic attacks, to settle racing thoughts, and to uplift during anxiety, depression, excessive grieving. It is good that tiny amounts are used, as it tends to be among the most costly essential oils.

Physical: Antispasmodic, antiviral, calms digestion (think of lemon balm tea), eases herpes.

Safety: 1. Do not ingest this oil. 2. May cause skin sensitization if used topically.

Myrrh, *Commiphora myrrha*

Emotional: Calms, promotes inner peace and tranquility. A meditator's fragrance, as it is spiritually expansive yet grounding, and helps quiet the mind and decrease inner chatter, leading to improved focus. Like sandalwood, it is common in incense.

Physical: Oil has been used for more than four thousand years. Anti-inflammatory, anti-infective, antibacterial, antifungal, analgesic. Used for skin problems including infections, wounds, rashes, and boils, and for respiratory tract ailments including cough; clears mucus. Assists in balancing thyroid. Strengthening overall.

Safe

Orange, *Citrus sinensis*

Emotional: Good for nervous stomach including nausea. Bright, lively, and inspiring energy that supports optimism and fresh thinking.

Physical: Digestive problems of all sorts—gas, poor digestion, nausea, feeling like food just sits there, irritable bowel syndrome. Antispasmodic and antibacterial.

Safety: Generally safe but like all members of the citrus family orange is photosensitizing, meaning it can increase the risk of sunburn and rash. So do not use it topically in blends within 12 hours of sun exposure. Use only organic oils, as citrus is heavily sprayed.

Ravintsara, *Cinnamomun camphora*

Emotional: Calms nervous tension, helps with sleep and stress. Can help self-confidence and reduce fearfulness. In Madagascar it is known as "the oil that heals." Like lavender, it has a broad range of uses.

Physical: A relative of cinnamon, ravintsara is an excellent antiviral. It is used for colds, flu, and other viruses including herpes. Decongestant, used often for allergies, and over time can diminish allergic responses.

Safety: Can be sensitizing, not recommended for use topically or in steam inhalation with children under five years old. Use with caution in asthma.

Rose, *Rosa damascena*

Emotional: Very settling to the emotional heart, perhaps the second most popular essential oil after lavender for anxiety and depression. Associated with love and promotes feelings of love and spiritual connection. Nervous system restorative and tonic; helps with panic attacks, grieving, and shock.

Physical: Used often in cosmetics and perfumery. Anti-infective, anti-inflammatory, antispasmodic, excellent for dry or aging skin. Helps with hormonal balance, especially for women.

Safe

Rosemary, *Rosmarinus officinalis*

Emotional: Cheerful, resilient, expels doldrums and helps with emotional balance. Uplifting but can be stimulating, so not for use with insomnia.

Physical: Musculoskeletal concerns, respiratory tract including cough and cold, anti-inflammatory, anti-infective. Used often in shampoos and other products for healthy hair and scalp.

Safety: Avoid in pregnancy, children under 10, and seizure disorders. Some authorities also discourage use in high blood pressure, but others disagree.

Sandalwood, *Santalum album*

Emotional: Soothing, calming, promotes relaxation, another meditator's fragrance that helps with inner peace, improving focus, and quieting mental chatter.

Physical: Antiviral, antifungal, antispasmodic, decongestant; widely used in respiratory tract problems, especially sore throat.

Safety: Safe, but increasingly rare because of overharvesting, so be sure to purchase from a supplier who guarantees that it is harvested sustainably.

Vetiver, *Vetiveria zizanioides*

Emotional: Tranquil, grounding, and reassuring energy, used in trauma, helps with self-awareness and is calming and stabilizing. A nervous system tonic, it decreases jitteriness and hypersensitivity; useful in panic attacks and shock.

Physical: Antifungal, immune support, helps vitality. Widely used in perfumery and cosmetics. A powder of this root is used in Ayurveda to reduce fever.

Safe

Ylang Ylang, *Cananga odorata*

Emotional: Calming and uplifting, helps with cheerfulness, courage, and optimism, used for anxiety and depression as well as soothing fearfulness and even shock. Calms heart agitation and nervous palpitations. Moderately strong sedative, helps insomnia. Widely used in perfumery.

Physical: Antispasmodic, anti-inflammatory, lowers blood pressure, lowers rapid heartbeat.

Safety: Can be sensitizing or irritating to skin; avoid using in conditions of low blood pressure.

CHAPTER 14

⚭

Homeopathy and Emotional Support

What Is Homeopathy?

Homeopathy is a multi-faceted system of healing that differs from contemporary allopathic medicine. It has been employed for more than two hundred years, has an outstanding safety record, and has resulted in many remarkable cures. A foundational concept of homeopathy is "like cures like." The German physician Samuel Hahnemann (1755–1843) introduced the modern practice of homeopathy. He observed that substances that can cause specific symptoms in a healthy person could cure those same symptoms if given to an ill person in minute amounts. This is explained by the homeopathic understanding that development of symptoms is a result of the body's attempt to regain health. In the nineteenth century, homeopathy was the dominant form of medicine practiced in the United States.

Homeopathic remedies can be prepared from almost anything including herbs, minerals, snake venom, and milks of various animals. They can even be prepared from modern substances like pharmaceuticals, aspartame, and chemical food additives. To make a remedy, a measure of the substance is dissolved or titrated into a neutral medium (usually water, alcohol, or milk sugar) and then shaken and slapped, a process called "succussion." This blend is divided into tenths or hundredths, and one portion is diluted into a fresh portion of the neutral medium and again succussed. This process is repeated over and over.

Potency in homeopathy refers to the number of times a particular remedy has been extracted and succussed. 1× is a ratio of 1:10, and 1c is a ratio of

1:100. The fewer times succussion has been performed, the lower the potency of the remedy. Low potency does not here translate as less effective. A low-potency remedy is more likely to have physiologic effects, from presence of the actual substance. Higher-potency remedies, those above 12×, are unlikely to contain any molecules of the original substance. So common dilutions available commercially, 30c, 100c, and 200c, contain no molecules of the original substance.

What is in a homeopathic remedy, then, if there are not molecules of the original material? The neutral medium is thought to hold a vibrational imprint, an impression of the vital force of the substance. Low-potency remedies hold this imprint along with some actual physical material, while high-potency remedies contain only the vitalistic impression. References to vital force, of course, are controversial, and conventional medicine often dismisses homeopathy as "unscientific" and "quackery." It is true that some biomedical studies done on high-potency homeopathic remedies have shown no biologic activity. However, when studied through the lens of quantum physics, reproducible studies have been done several times.[1] This finding supports the homeopath's claim that the mode of action in treatment is via a vibrational imprint rather than a biochemical process.[2] The late French scientist Jacques Benveniste, who coined the term *the memory of water*, demonstrated that water can retain the impression of substances (in this case, antibodies) after the substance is removed from the water and no actual molecules of the substance remain in it; his results were published in a controversial 1988 article in *Nature* magazine.[3] Some researchers think that homeopathic remedies interact with cells at the level of the genome, though this is still speculative.

A process called "proving" demonstrates the effects of remedies. In this process, several healthy volunteers take the substance, and each catalogues every effect he or she notices. Samuel Hahnemann and his colleagues "proved" about sixty-five remedies. Today the homeopathic materia medica contains thousands of remedies. So, for example, a substance like coffee *(Coffea cruda),* which causes wakefulness in well persons, is used homeopathically for treatment of excessive wakefulness, or insomnia. Virtually all commercial remedies made today are machine-succussed, though there is some evidence that hand succussion, while more labor-intensive, may result in a remedy with greater vital force.

Homeopathy remains very popular in the public mind and is the preferred healing modality of many notable individuals, including many members of the British Royal family. There are various approaches to homeopathy. The most well known are classical homeopathy, symptomatic homeopathy, and homotoxicology. Anthroposophic Medicine is another offshoot of homeopathy that employs a spiritual scientific approach.

Classical Homeopathy

Classical homeopathy is an exacting discipline, both in its study and in its practice. Classical homeopaths begin a patient evaluation with an extensive interview of a client and all her symptoms. Even symptoms and patterns seemingly unrelated to the complaint to be treated are evaluated. Classical homeopaths then try to find the one remedy out of thousands that most exactly matches the patient and all her symptoms. This remedy is known as a "constitutional remedy." Sometimes a patient will have the same constitutional remedy for long periods of time, even decades. Constitutional remedies work very deeply, shifting long-held patterns. Classical homeopaths generally abstain from using other symptomatic remedies while a constitutional remedy is utilized, and some prefer their clients to employ no other modalities along with the remedies.

The main complaint I have heard from patients is that constitutional homeopathy is "slow." I do not discuss classical homeopathic remedies below, as they are not self-prescribed. If you feel attracted to classical homeopathy, it is best to find a practitioner with formal training. Most certification programs take three to four years and include a clinical practicum. To find a classically trained homeopath, consult the bibliography at the end of the book.

Symptomatic Homeopathy

The variety of homeopathy most commonly employed in the general population is symptomatic homeopathy, which involves treating an acute condition with an appropriate remedy that matches the predominant symptoms of a particular illness or condition. This is the type employed by most people who use home remedies or remedy kits. Symptomatic remedies are not expected to work deeply on chronic patterns. Instead they are utilized for acute situations and symptoms. Symptomatic remedies are generally used safely when symptoms match the profile of the remedy. But it is usually a good idea, when possible, to consult with an experienced homeopath, even in acute situations.

Homotoxicology

Another branch of homeopathic practice is homotoxicology, developed by Hans Reckeweg, MD, a twentieth-century German physician who also studied and was influenced by Traditional Chinese Medicine. He wanted to find ways to harmonize homeopathic practice with allopathic medicine and to extend the applications of homeopathy to work synergistically with allopathic medicines, while incorporating some of the understanding of TCM. It is therefore not surprisingly a type of homeopathy often utilized by allopathic physicians. It is increasingly popular with alternative medical practitioners such as acupuncturists, chiropractors, and naturopaths.

Reckeweg was very interested in the various physiologic functions of the extracellular matrix, a sheath that surrounds every cell to some degree. It is made up of various molecules including glycosaminoglycans. The matrix is involved in cell signaling and immune regulation, and it provides the milieu that structurally supports the cells. It stores and sequesters toxins and irritants to prevent them from entering and damaging the cell. Reckeweg observed that debris, pathogens, and toxins could encumber the extracellular matrix, especially when vitality is low or detoxification is slow. An overloaded matrix hampers cell-to-cell communication and can result in poorer immune function and greater fatigue and malaise of various sorts. Reckeweg developed a variety of remedies to support detoxification of the matrix of specific cell types and organs, thus enhancing health and vitality. Through detoxification and support of the tissue matrix, homotoxicology addresses a variety of physical and emotional symptoms. Generally this type of work is undertaken with the guidance of an appropriately trained healthcare provider.

Anthroposophy

Anthroposophic homeopathy is yet another branch of homeopathy, based upon the work of the German mystic and philosopher Rudolf Steiner. It is part of a comprehensive Anthroposophic healing system, which includes eurhythmy (a system of movement and bodywork) and dietary advice. Anthroposophic medicine builds upon scientific medicine, adding in considerations of a spiritual science and honoring the individuality of the patient. All Anthroposophic medications are chosen, among their primary focus, for their ability in any individual to trigger self-healing. The choice of remedies, and even the actions of particular remedies, may differ from the interpretation of similar substances in classical homeopathy. Specially trained medical professionals, usually physicians, practice Anthroposophic medicine. Working with an Anthroposophically trained professional can be a powerful catalyst for integration of body, mind, and spirit. I have seen Anthroposophic medicine provide tremendous relief for some of my patients, including people with deep-seated, protracted anxiety and others with post-traumatic stress disorder. It is not, however, a self-care modality, so I will not discuss specific remedies below. Consult the website www .paam.net/home.html for more information if you feel attracted to working in this spiritual and holistic manner.

Tools for Transformation: Common Homeopathic Remedies for Symptomatic Relief of Anxiety

The remedies listed below are some of the ones most commonly chosen for symptomatic relief of occasional or mild anxiety. The objective in working with single remedies in homeopathy is to find the particular remedy that most closely matches your symptoms. Every detail does not have to match, but the overall picture should fit. Try to rely on the overall feeling of the remedy, especially your emotional response to it. A response of "this feels right" is usually a good indicator that a remedy may be correct for you. You can use this overview as a jumping-off point to delve more deeply into a few appropriate-sounding remedies before choosing one, or even to get a feel about whether this way of working is appealing. Even if homeopathy is clearly attractive to you, remember that your ideal remedy may not be among the ones below, as this is just an overview of some common remedies.

When there is deep-seated or ongoing anxiety, it is a good idea to work with a trained homeopath. With prolonged or deep-seated anxiety, remedies required might shift in the course of treatment, and old symptoms might temporarily resurface, even with use of simple remedies. Hering's law, a guiding principle of homeopathic treatment, states that symptoms will physically clear with homeopathy in three ways: from inside to outside the body, from top (head) to bottom (feet), and from most recent to most distant in the past. A trained and experienced homeopath can help you navigate confidently.

Well-known, widely available over-the-counter brands are Boiron, Boericke, Tafel, Dolisos, and Hylands. Usually lower potencies are used for acute relief of mild symptomatic problems: 6× or 6c, 12× or 12c are commonly chosen, while 30c and 100c are considered medium potencies and sometimes utilized, if appropriate, once an individual has developed some confidence in working homeopathically.

If an over-the-counter remedy helps, you can keep it around in case a similar situation arises in the future. If it doesn't help or it is not clearly of benefit, do not keep using it.

Single Remedies

> *Aconite:* Panic attacks, especially if sudden onset, or severe anxiety accompanied by heart palpitations, or feelings of heat like flushing of the face, or even shortness of breath
>
> *Argentum nitricum:* Anticipatory anxiety. Used when public or social events such as a wedding, public speaking, job interview, test, or important meeting trigger anxiety, especially when there is a fear that someone will be angry, critical, or disappointed in the individual. It's not uncommon in such cases for the person to actually make an error or perform poorly as a result of the anxiety. Physical symptoms of anxiety include diarrhea, asthma,

feeling of suffocation, abdominal pain, tremors, headache, and craving for sweets which, when consumed in significant amounts, will aggravate the problem.

Arsenicum album: Useful for people who focus their worries on their health, including panic attacks centering on health anxieties. Such individuals are often very neat and organized, tending toward obsessive, so control issues can be prominent.

Calcarea carbonica: For people who constitutionally tend to be cold all the time, crave sweets, and are easily fatigued. Anxiety rises when they are tired or confused, and they may have nagging fears that "the other shoe is about to drop." Also for fear of heights and claustrophobia in people with the constitutional type.

Chamomilla: Irritability, crankiness.

Coffea cruda: For jitters and insomnia.

Gelsemium: For apprehension over upcoming events, especially stage fright, test anxiety, or fear in anticipation of doctor or dental visits. Also for fear of crowds, heights, and falling. The person might have headaches, loose stools, chills, or sweats in anticipation of an upcoming anxiety-producing event. Often physically there is trembling and fatigue. This remedy can be used when anxiety follows exposure to frightful images or violence, especially in shy or timid people. With *Gelsemium* types, anxiety may cause people to clam up or freeze.

Ignatia amara: Anxiety after a loss, or when grieving or disappointed. Sometimes the person can be defensive or moody or become anxious about criticism. Also used for the feeling of a lump in the throat caused by anxiety or stress.

Kali phosphoricum: Exhaustion from stress or overwork leading to severe anxiety, "tired and wired," jumpiness.

Lycopodium: Anxiety from feeling like one is a phony or putting up a false front to hide feelings of inadequacy. Fear of failure, self-conscious, easily intimidated, especially when the person admires someone or perceives them as powerful. Lack of confidence, though often competent or excellent when they do take on tasks.

Mercurius solubilis: Anxiety from anticipation of possible abuse. Can be helpful for people who have suffered physical, sexual, or mental abuse, including bullying and teasing, and for people who have post-traumatic stress disorder. This one is best used, when appropriate, under the guidance of a trained practitioner.

Natrum muriaticum: Weepiness, tearfulness, or an inability to cry. The person for whom this remedy is appropriate often has strong and deep emotional responses. Can be shy and self-protective as well as aloof or guarded in social situations because of shyness and strong feelings. May be a feeling of past betrayal or a loss of trust, and subsequent control issues and fear of "things getting out of control" or difficulty in opening up again. Helpful for anxiety at night that causes nightmares or insomnia, headaches including migraines, and claustrophobia. Physical signs of anxiety here include asthma, headache, insomnia, and allergies.

Nux vomica: Anxiety related to time, especially being accused of wasting time, either by self or another.

Phosphorus: For people plagued with vivid fears, imaginative and creative persons who focus on the worst outcome and generally are easily startled. They like frequent social contact and reassurance, often going out of their way for others and overextending themselves on others' behalf to the point of exhaustion.

Pulsatilla: For anxiety that manifests as insecurity, clinginess, weepiness, fear of being left alone, whininess, and a constant need for reassurance. Can also be useful for hormonally triggered anxiety as in PMS, and anxiety around life-change times like puberty and menopause.

Silicea: For generally nervous and temperamentally shy people who have acute anxiety when confronted with a change of situation or a public appearance such as a new school, a new job, an examination, or an interview. Frequently vacillation and uncertainty can trigger anxiety. Can be difficult for these people to make even minor decisions, like what color shirt to wear, and they will ask others what they think they should do. Anxiety can be severe, accompanied by a feeling of dread and/or physical symptoms such as headache, exhaustion, poor concentration, and abdominal pain.

Combination Remedies

Commonly used and frequently available over-the-counter brands of combined remedies include Bio Allers, BHI/Heel, and Dr. Reckeweg. Following are some of the most popular combination remedies for anxiety and related problems.

Calming (BHI/Heel): For relief of temporary symptoms of stress, anxiety, and insomnia. I have found that for insomnia 2–4 tablets is most effective, though one or two up to four times a day is good for mild anxiety.

Calms Forte (Hylands): Tablets for mild anxiety, restlessness, sleeplessness.

Calms Forte for Children (Hylands): As above, for kids under 12 years old.

Quietiva (Bio Allers): Liquid drops; dose is 5–10 drops under the tongue as needed for mild anxiety or nervousness.

Headache Relief (Hylands): For relief of stress-related headache.

Nerve Tonic (Hylands): For nervous tension and stress.

CHAPTER 15

⌒ᗡ

Hands-On Techniques for Health

Massage and/or various bodywork techniques can be of great assistance in the journey toward inner calm. For most people, simply experiencing touch is soothing. There are numerous modalities and styles available—something for almost everyone. In this chapter I discuss a few of my favorite techniques as well as some common varieties of bodywork that are well known and available from easy-to-find practitioners. As always, if there is a type of hands-on work that you find soothing, but it is not mentioned here, please continue to utilize it. The end of the chapter offers some resources for soothing self-massage techniques.

Hands-On Osteopathic Healthcare Modalities

Cranial Osteopathy

An understanding of wholeness and health is at the heart of the osteopathic profession. Its founder, A. T. Still, MD, stated, "To find health should be the object of the doctor; anyone can find disease." Cranial osteopathy, a branch of the larger field of osteopathy, is the study of anatomy and physiology of the cranium and its interrelationship with the rest of the body. Working with gentle techniques, physicians can improve the physical and emotional health of the whole patient, since osteopathy understands that all physiologic systems are interrelated. Cranial osteopathic work can be profoundly helpful for anxious persons, even those who have experienced significant trauma, bringing real relief as balance and harmony are restored to the nervous system and physical structure.

Developing osteopathy in the cranial field was the life work of William Garner Sutherland, DO. He explored "primary respiration" and the motion of fluids. In a cranial osteopathic understanding, fluids are not just liquids—they relate to electromagnetic forces of the body. Emotional and physical illnesses result from imbalances in these forces as well as in the physical structure. Physicians trained in cranial osteopathy can work directly with fluids, and thus the nervous system, to help restore wholeness and function.

A guiding principle of cranial osteopathy is honoring the natural forces that give form to life. Still looked toward nature for illumination of the intrinsic forces of healing within human beings. He stated, "All the remedies necessary to health exist in the human body." Both Still and Sutherland understood the primary interrelationship of body, mind, and spirit, and this understanding is interwoven in cranial osteopathic therapeutics.

Study of cranial osteopathy is limited to graduated doctors of osteopathy (DO), certified medical doctors (MD), and other physicians. To help you find a practitioner, the Cranial Academy website maintains a listing of its members at www.cranialacademy.com/index.html.

Biodynamics of Osteopathy

James Jealous, DO, developed the biodynamic understanding of osteopathy. This mode of therapy built upon the wisdom and teachings of the early osteopaths, especially Still and Sutherland, and their students Ruby Day, DO, Rollin Becker, DO, and others, as well as the discoveries of leading embryologists, especially Erich Blechschmidt, MD. In his research, Blechschmidt explores the central importance of fluid fields in embryonic development. This work revealed that it is fluid fields and fluid motion rather than biochemistry that drives the development of the embryo. From his years of study and osteopathic experience, Dr. Jealous observed that these early fluid fields persist, nourishing the individual throughout his or her life. Disruptions in them, called "lesions" (which happen to almost everyone as a part of living in the world), lead to physical and emotional health imbalances. Dr. Jealous's work and teaching explore the perceptual skills necessary for finding health in any person, harmonizing with it, and letting the health of the whole create and guide the therapeutics through the fluid fields.

In practice, the biodynamic model is a quiet, gentle, deeply therapeutic, scientific, hands-on approach whereby the physician cooperates with the higher wisdom that expresses itself through natural forces in the health of the patient. Biodynamic work can be profoundly calming for persons with anxiety, allowing patients to find ease in their body and nervous system. It is profound, restorative, and effective for soothing the nervous system and bringing balance to the treatment of the whole person. Find practitioners fully trained in the Biodynamics of Osteopathy through Dr. James Jealous's website.[1]

Osteopathy-Based Bodywork Modalities

Craniosacral/Visceral

Craniosacral and Visceral Manipulation are forms of holistic bodywork developed from osteopathic techniques and principles. The main original teacher of craniosacral therapy (or CST) is John Upledger, DO, who in the 1960s extracted and modified portions of the body of work of osteopathy in the cranial field in order to make them accessible to diverse practitioners such as massage therapists, chiropractors, acupuncturists, psychotherapists, and others who have not undertaken a complete osteopathic education. John Pierre Barral, DO, and Alain Croibier, DO, are French osteopaths who developed their own system to teach osteopathic visceral techniques to a similar population in the 1980s.

There are now multiple competing institutes and schools of thought in this burgeoning field. The advantage (and disadvantage) of these types of bodywork is their wide availability and diversity. There are hundreds of thousands of people who have taken at least one "cranial" or "visceral" course. While experienced and sensitive practitioners can be extremely effective at techniques that help the body as a whole, supporting relief of stress and tension, not all who call themselves "practitioners" are experienced or sensitive. Because there are so many styles in the marketplace, it can be a challenge for clients to find and choose a suitable modality and accomplished practitioner.

Various websites list practitioners who have studied a particular school's or certification course's techniques, and some mention the amount of training those offering services have received. Since there are so many people who offer various types of "cranial," often the best recommendation of a practitioner will be from people you know and trust.

Ortho-Bionomy

Another bodywork modality stemming from osteopathy, Ortho-Bionomy is described on the website of the Society of Ortho-Bionomy, International, as follows:

> Ortho-Bionomy is a gentle, non-invasive system of healing that reminds the body of its natural ability to restore balance. It is based on a simple and profound philosophy: allow the body to correct itself. The hallmark of Ortho-Bionomy is pain relief.
>
> The founder, British-trained osteopath Arthur Lincoln Pauls, discovered how to gently stimulate the body's reflexes for self-correction in a way that supports a person's own healing mechanisms. The body is stimulated using gentle movements, comfortable positioning, brief compression and subtle contact. The result is seemingly effortless pain and tension relief, natural re-alignment, relaxation, and a deep sense of well-being. Individuals are empowered to participate in their own recovery, and through the process they can begin to rediscover the ability to heal and restore comfort, ease, and balance back into their body.[2]

Find practitioners who have trained in Ortho-Bionomy through the website: www.ortho-bionomy.org/Default.aspx. Of the practitioners listed, registered practitioners, advanced practitioners, and instructors will have the most training and experience.

Massage

Massage has been practiced throughout recorded history. There are many styles, with numerous types that are calming and relaxing. I encourage persons with anxiety, if touch is comfortable to them, to explore massage as a supportive way of calming the nervous system and settling emotions. This is clinically supported in scientific literature: a review of twelve studies showed that massage helped reduce depression and anxiety, and lowered levels of the stress hormone cortisol.[3] When possible, a weekly or monthly massage can make a big difference in nourishing well-being.

Swedish Massage

Swedish massage and its variations are what most people think of simply as "massage." One principal purpose of Swedish massage is to relax the entire body, so this type of massage can be excellent for soothing anxious persons. The massages are usually done with several soft types of strokes, over the whole body. There may be gentle kneading, tapping, or friction, in addition to long fluid stokes. Oils are frequently used but are not absolutely required if the client does not prefer them. Sometimes gentle movement of joints is offered. Clients are generally not clothed, but parts not currently being massaged are typically covered with a sheet. It is usually very easy to find a Swedish massage practitioner, even in small communities.

Shiatsu

Shiatsu, which means "finger pressure," is a traditional Japanese massage technique that involves rhythmically using palms and fingers along the meridians of the body. These are the same meridians that are utilized in Chinese medicine. Shiatsu massage is a method for supporting the flow of Qi (vital force) throughout the body. Opening the flow of Qi helps with relaxation of tense muscles, improving vitality, aiding self-healing, and restoring emotional calm. Shiatsu is usually performed with the client lying on a mat on the floor, though it can be done on a table. Clients are generally clothed. Shiatsu is usually a gentle technique and is very popular, so it is often easy to find a trained practitioner.

Tui Na

This traditional Chinese system of body massage or physical therapy is often employed in connection with other modalities, especially acupuncture, herbs, and dietary therapies, to enhance effectiveness of treatments, particularly in musculo-skeletal conditions. Most Traditional Chinese Medicine acupuncturists receive some training in tui na, and a few take more advanced studies or choose to specialize in it.

Lomilomi

Lomilomi is a traditional Hawaiian style of massage. The word *lomi* is Hawaiian for "massage." The style is very rhythmic and soothing, and the practitioner may use hands, fingers, palms, elbows, knees, and even implements such as stones or herbs to stroke and work the body. Traditional lomilomi may be performed by one or more practitioners on a single client. There are different styles originating on various islands with different families. Traditionally trained Lomilomi practitioners may also give dietary advice and/or encourage clients to meditate, which is performed with positive intention. Both the meditation and the lomilomi practice include the offering of prayer. Massages are traditionally longer than an hour and may extend several hours. When possible, work with a traditionally trained practitioner (they are most often found in Hawaii, Japan, and the Pacific Rim). This type of massage can be of great benefit in soothing anxiety and supporting health.

Chi Nei Tsang

Chi Nei Tsang is a holistic bodywork modality that focuses upon soothing physical, emotional, and spiritual tension by working on the abdominal organs. It is based upon ancient Taoist techniques. The website of the Chi Nei Tsang Institute describes the bodywork as follows:

Chi Nei Tsang is a holistic approach to the healing touch modality of old Taoist Chinese origin. It integrates the physical, mental, emotional and spiritual aspects of our being. CNT goes to the very origin of health problems, including psychosomatic responses.

Chi Nei Tsang literally means "working the energy of the internal organs" or "internal organs chi transformation." CNT uses all the principles of Kung-Fu and Tai Chi Chuan known as Chi-Kung; therefore, CNT is a form of "applied Chi Kung."

CNT practitioners are trained in Chi-Kung and work mainly on the abdomen with deep, soft and gentle touches, to train internal organs to work more efficiently. Unprocessed emotional charges are also addressed in this manner, as well as all of the body systems: digestive, respiratory, cardiovascular, lymphatic, nervous, endocrine, urinary, reproductive, musculo-skeletal, and the acupuncture meridian system.[4]

I have found that many anxious patients benefit from this work, though others do not like the deep pressure on the abdomen that is involved. The website lists certified practitioners.[5]

Manual Lymph Drainage

Manual Lymph Drainage (MLD) can be extremely helpful for persons with anxiety. Elizabeth Olivas, BFA, a Certified Lymphatic Therapist whose work I have respected for many years, taught me most of what I know about MLD. Elizabeth runs a business called The Therapeutic Alternative in Boca Raton, Florida, and graciously shares this about her experience with Manual Lymph Drainage as a relaxation technique:

Manual Lymph Drainage is highly effective when employed as a part of a stress-management program. Manual Lymph Drainage has mostly been perceived as an edema-reducing method. This method does have the ability to help the body remove waste and extra fluids. The incredible added bonus is that this technique is also very relaxing. When applied correctly the rhythmic repetitive strokes lower the sympathetic tonus in the nervous system. The parasympathetic nervous system activates and initiates a deeply relaxed state that leaves clients rested with a sense of well-being after a session.

When the body is in the state of stress, referred to as fight or flight, the function of the lymphatic system is decreased. The goal of any lymph drainage treatment is to encourage proper function of the lymphatic structures to drain the tissues. To do this most effectively the relaxation effect must be engaged. Manual Lymph Drainage can help to teach your body what it feels like to move from high anxiety to a more relaxed calm state.[6]

Rosen Method

This gentle bodywork technique was developed by physical therapist Marion Rosen. She initially studied the potential of breath and relaxation techniques, in conjunction with psychotherapy, as a powerful tool for helping clients to relax and feel comfortable in the experience of their emotions. Eventually she developed the Rosen Method to help clients reduce stress and access the body/mind connection through gentle touch. The Rosen Method website, which includes a directory of practitioners, describes the techniques in more detail.

I have found Rosen Method bodywork to be an outstanding resource for many persons with chronic anxiety, as well as for survivors of abuse or trauma, including persons suffering from PTSD. It can gently help relax and release many physical and emotional tension patterns.

Ear Massage/Ear Reflexology

Ear reflexology and massage are related to ear acupuncture. In this system there are correspondences of points on the ear to the entire body including each organ. Every region of the body is represented on the ear. Many tables and diagrams of correspondences of body and ear points can be found with a quick Internet search.

Most people find ear massage and ear self-massage delightful. The points in the upper portion of the ear can be particularly calming. Try massaging your own ears in a moment of stress or tension, and notice if it brings you more calm. To do this, sit in a relaxing place. Use your thumb and forefinger to gently massage your ear for 1–2 minutes. You can massage both ears simultaneously by using both hands, or one at a time. I find ear rubbing to be both calming and mentally clearing. I use it often as a pause when I am writing, to find the best words.

Foot Reflexology

Most people really enjoy a good foot rub. The branch of massage that focuses on the feet is foot reflexology. Most people do not know that reflexology is an ancient science, with charts of foot and organ correspondences found on the walls of certain Egyptian pyramids. The traditional Japanese branch of reflexology is Zoku Shin Do, thought to have evolved three to five thousand years ago from Chinese acupuncture and acupressure techniques. American William F. Fitzgerald, MD, who devised Zone Therapy initially as a way to relieve pain in his patients, pioneered modern reflexology a hundred years ago. Reflexology is one of many healing modalities that seek to bring the body back into balance and harmony.[7]

Reflexology can promote detoxification. Make sure if you are having a treatment, or a series of them, to drink plenty of water and avoid alcohol the day of treatment.

There are numerous subtypes of reflexology, and not all point correspondence charts are in agreement. Some better-known ones are Ayurvedic reflexology, a synthesis of Ayurvedic healing principles and classical Hindu, Japanese, and Chinese foot reflexology treatments.

The particulars of treatments can differ substantially too. The Chinese version, for example, tends to be quite vigorous and may even be painful at times,[8] whereas an average spa foot reflexology treatment might be gentler.

There are certain contraindications to reflexology. A well-trained practitioner should be aware of any cautions and contraindications, and will likely discuss any concerns or relevant history before your treatment. He or she will be able to assess if there are signs of a detox reaction, and to advise you regarding how best to move through it.

The Metamorphic Technique

This is a wonderful modality that I believe deserves a wider audience. It is great for soothing people with all sorts of anxiety. It is very gentle and is considered safe for everyone. An English naturopathic physician, Robert St. John, developed the method in the 1960s. He believed, like his predecessor Dr. Edward Bach, the developer of Bach flower essences, that physical and emotional ailments originate from patterns of emotional stress. He discovered that the body has a psychological/emotional map that overlays the physical body. His technique involves gentle touch, without any pressure, on the spine reflex points of the hands, feet, and head, which allow the emotional body to relax. With training, virtually anyone can learn the technique. It can be performed with the client seated or lying down. Often if lying down, clients will fall asleep, and this is encouraged!

The Metamorphic Association is in Britain, where classes are offered several times a year, often at Findhorn in Scotland. But there are home-study DVDs and YouTube videos available that can assist anyone anywhere in learning the basics of this supportive holistic technique. I find it ideal for people with anxiety or any emotional disturbance.[9]

Tools for Transformation: Foot Self-Massage

Foot self-massage can be a wonderful way to unwind any time there is tension. It can be a daily practice of self-love and nurturing. I often recommend it to patients as part of a wind-down ritual to prepare for good sleep.

Foot massage can be particularly soothing after a relaxing foot bath. For the latter, I recommend either magnesium chloride salts or Epsom salts, perhaps with a few drops of a calming essential oil or relaxing herbal infusion added. After drying the feet, massage them gently with nourishing oil, again possibly with a drop or two of an essential oil added.

There are several excellent massage oils to choose from. Sesame oil is popular in Ayurvedic medicine because it is calming and grounding. Coconut oil is used for massage anywhere on the body throughout Southeast Asia and is a great emollient for dry skin. Olive oil is also fine if it is the only oil you have available—it was used traditionally as a massage oil in the Mediterranean region.

Foot self-massage is great at any time of day, and especially at bedtime. Try it after Earthing to improve your sleep.

CHAPTER 16

֍

Color and Light

Everything in the physical world and everything we experience vibrates on the electromagnetic spectrum. Everything we know has its characteristic wavelength. There are specific wavelengths for all matter, including atoms, music, x-rays, starlight, amethysts, and oak wood. Even thoughts have particular wavelengths. The brain receives these wavelengths through our various sensory organs and translates them into an understanding of physical matter. All that we experience as life in the physical world, all we hear, see, taste, smell, and feel, is merely wavelengths filtered through eyes, ears, skin, nose, and mouth and transmitted to the brain for interpretation.

For example, we consider certain frequencies audible. What does this mean? What actually happens is that sound frequencies vibrate a complex apparatus deep in our ears. This creates waveforms that our nervous system passes on as electromagnetic information to our brain. We interpret these waves as sound. Our brain does not actually hear, it just brilliantly interprets vibrational data that has been transmitted. We recognize anything in the physical world by the brain's interpretations of the wavelengths. But we are so used to interpreting the wavelengths presented as external reality that we do not think of it as vibration.

Our bones, cells, DNA, in fact all of what we think of as our physical bodies is really vibrating energy. All cellular structures, including proteins and DNA, vibrate on the electromagnetic (EM) spectrum. The wavelength of DNA, for example, is 260 nm (nanometers), while that of protein is 280 nm. The vibrational difference is how the two are distinguished in scientific inquiry. Individual atoms and even subatomic particles emit and absorb light.

Each type of atom or particle is recognized by its unique emission pattern. Atoms of hydrogen, carbon, oxygen, and neon are distinguished by their specific wavelengths. There is even a plethora of distinctive patterns within individual elements. For example, most carbon on Earth is carbon-12, meaning that it has six protons and six neutrons. But other varieties exist. Carbon-14, containing six protons and eight neutrons, is a well-known radioactive form of carbon formed in the upper atmosphere; it is often used by archaeologists to date artifacts up to fifty thousand years old.

THE ELECTROMAGNETIC SPECTRUM

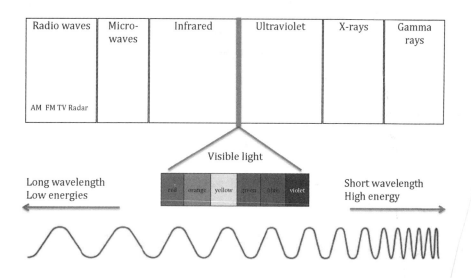

Even our thoughts, and therefore our emotions, are vibrations with measurable rates in brainwave patterns. When we are in peaceful deep meditation or contemplation, our brainwaves are slow. They are also slow when we are sleeping, unless we are in REM sleep, when they more closely resemble waking-state brainwaves. Newborn infants and babies have the brainwave patterns of adept meditators. When we are agitated or excited, our brainwaves are much faster. Both brainwaves and heart rhythms can form coherent or incoherent patterns.

Light also vibrates in the electromagnetic spectrum. The wavelength of visible light extends from 380 mn to 780 nm. "Light" is a term used generically to describe many EM emissions, even those that are not visible to us, such as ultraviolet and infrared light.

There are many commonly accepted medical uses of both ultraviolet and infrared light. Infrared light has a wavelength that is longer and lower-energy than visible light. The infrared spectrum is much larger than the visible spectrum, and infrared light is warming or heating, potentially promoting detoxification in small amounts of exposure. Many people now use infrared saunas for cellular detoxification. Interpretation of infrared light is important for thermal imaging, and far infrared light is a new technology being investigated and employed for treatment of many inflammatory conditions including arthritis, carpal tunnel syndrome, bursitis, and Raynaud's disease. Infrared LED light is also being investigated in treatment of certain cancers.

Even longer and slower wavelengths are found in the microwave and radio wave bands. Microwaves are very long and slow; they heat food by vibrating the water molecules within, which in turn heats the rest of the food. The wavelengths of AM radio are very long; one wave unit from peak to peak stretches more than the length of a soccer field.

At the other end of the visible spectrum is ultraviolet or UV light. This technically means "beyond violet" since violet light is the shortest and fastest color of light in the visible spectrum. UV light is cleansing and is used medically for instrument sterilization and certain types of phototherapy (light therapy), including psoriasis treatments. The sun produces lots of UV light, in different bands such as UVA and UVB. Many insects, including bees, can see ultraviolet light and use it to navigate. On a cloudy day bees can still see the sun from its UV light emissions and therefore will use it to find their way ͻ various flowers and back to the hive.

Although we cannot see most UV light with our eyes, our bodies are physiologically affected by it. For example, the UVB frequency, from 290 to 3ͻ nm, is essential in the chemical reaction that occurs on the skin, in which cholesterol is converted into vitamin D. Higher and faster UV frequencies can damage cells and molecules, even leading to DNA mutations. The ozone layer in the upper atmosphere absorbs most of these high-energy particles and prevents them from traveling to Earth. Oxygen and nitrogen in the atmosphere halt most of the even higher-frequency particles like the faster and shorter x-rays and gamma rays.

What we see as color is simply light that falls upon our retinas through vibratory wavelengths. It is our brains that interpret these waves as color. As is apparent from the table above, light that we perceive as visible is only a tiny part of the electromagnetic spectrum.

I became interested in the health properties of all types of light many years ago. I realized early on that it makes sense that visible light has therapeutic applications. It would seem counterintuitive, in fact, that there are medical uses for wavelengths vibrating above and below the visible spectrum, but none for light we can see. A brief review of healing modalities worldwide reveals that visible light has also been employed extensively for physical health.

Natural sunlight can be a powerful catalyst for emotional well-being and physical health. Sunlight can help wound healing and supports calm. People have associated color and positive mood throughout recorded history.

In ancient Egypt, medical solariums were designed to flood a space with sunlight and color, both of which were used for healing. The patient was placed in the room, and particular colored windows were installed to assist therapeutically. The patient or diseased part was bathed in the specific colored light.[1]

The Islamic physician Avicenna (980–1037 CE) wrote extensively in his book *The Canon of Medicine* about applications of color for treatment of various physical ailments. He noted, "Color is an observable symptom of disease." *The Canon of Medicine* was the primary medical textbook used in Europe for at least seven hundred years. In it, Avicenna frequently discussed both the diagnostic and therapeutic applications of color. Many of his findings have stood the test of time. For example, he associated liver disease with a yellow cast to the skin, an effect (called jaundice) we now understand to be caused by a build-up of bilirubin in the blood. Avicenna believed that applications of specific colors had therapeutic effects upon various organs and tissues. The color red, he thought, moved the blood and could be used to treat blood-related ailments, while white or blue subdued the energy. White light was a good color during a nosebleed but red was not, as it might increase the blood flow. Red light might be excellent, though, for someone with chilblains (cold hands or feet).[2]

Ayurvedic medicine, the traditional medicine of India, has a rich tradition of working with color as part of healing. In India colors have emotional and spiritual properties. Red, for example, is a color of protection, while green is a color of peace and happiness. Blue, the most prevalent color in nature, found in sky, rivers, lakes, and oceans, is associated with mental stability, strength of character, and the ability to overcome difficulties. Two important Hindu deities, Lord Krishna and Lord Rama, are colored blue.

The Ayurvedic system also defines the seven physical chakras—energy centers of the emotional and spiritual body that overlay and influence the physical body. Each chakra is associated with a color as well as emotional, spiritual, and physical properties. The color associations of the chakras can be used to treat the physical health of organs associated with that chakra.

Chinese medicine ascribes a color to each organ and meridian, and color in the body is observed carefully for signs of health or illness. Many of these color associations can be found in Western medicine as well. For example, a yellow hue to the skin is an indication of liver disease in either system, while overall redness can be a sign that the heart is working too hard, and white can be associated with a lack of blood (anemia). People with untreated hypertension are often noted to have a reddish cast to their skin.

The branch of healing that addresses the use of colors of visible light for therapeutic purposes is called chromo therapy or photo therapy. It is another emerging field with great opportunities for research. The understanding of chromo therapy is that the human body is an aggregation of various colors existing in a balance. A German acupuncturist named Peter Mandel used this theory to develop a system of acupuncture called color puncture, where he applies various frequencies of light to specific acupuncture points for therapeutic effects.

As a practitioner of acupuncture and a student of Ayurveda, I find that application of color makes sense. I understand that we are vibrational beings, so I believe medical application of the specific light frequencies of each visible color is probably of enormous potential benefit. Some excellent studies were done with visible light in the 1920s and 1930s. These showed benefits in a variety of areas including wound healing and organic disease. Many of these studies were done at Women's Medical College in Philadelphia (which later became Medical College of Pennsylvania, my alma mater!).

We have many traditional systems of healing on the planet that associate specific colors with the health and disease of specific organs. Building upon this wisdom would be a good place to start investigation. Applications of colored light intuitively seem to be safe, gentle, and non-toxic. Today there are many proponents of using visible light in a health-supporting setting, and more research is being undertaken. It is my hope that even mainstream physicians will soon begin to investigate the therapeutic benefits of color and light in the visible spectrum.

The importance of color for enhancing emotional well-being is already more accepted. There is widespread acknowledgment of the benefits of both full-spectrum light and sunlight in prevention and treatment of seasonal affective disorder, a form of depression related to the lack of sunlight in winter months.

The Swiss psychotherapist, Dr. Max Luscher (born 1923), has devoted his entire career to the study of how color affects emotions, and he is considered one of the founders of color psychology. He developed the Luscher color test, a psychological test widely accepted in Europe, where many colleges and corporations employ it with applicants. Even Luscher's critics acknowledge that people do have emotional response to color.

In the U.S., color is widely acknowledged to have emotional properties. Many decorators use applications of color for support of mood and harmony in the home and workplace. Pink is considered by many to be the least aggressive color and to have sedative effects. Pink is often used in prisons and mental institutions, especially in rooms used for cooling down fiery tempers. The traditional Asian practice of feng shui places great importance on both color and object placement to create balanced, peaceful, productive environments. Many U.S. individuals and some corporations hire feng shui consultants to assist in designing harmonious homes and workspaces.

Emotionally, the "cooler" colors green, blue, and violet are generally associated with calm, while the "hotter" colors red, orange, and yellow are used to lift a depressed mood. But if you want to work with color therapy, know that the experience can be subjective. If you are agitated and the "prescription" for you is blue or violet, but blue or violet seem to make you more agitated, do not use them. Since one of the objectives of this book is to teach you how to pay attention to your own inner guidance, it is good to acknowledge that no expert is more expert about you than you.

Following is a review of commonly held beliefs and associations about various colors. There are no references since this is not yet an area with much scientific data. Much of the information is investigational, drawn from a variety of sources including historical references, color therapy sites, color psychology theory, feng shui literature, and Chinese and Ayurvedic medicine. Because the chakras are associated with colors of the rainbow, in ascending order, I organize the list starting with the chakra colors, in prismatic order.

Colors Related to the Chakras

Red

Chakra: Root (first)

Chinese Medicine: Fire element (Heart and Small Intestine meridians and organs)

Discussion: Red has the longest and slowest wavelength of the colors of visible light.

Physical properties: Red is stimulating, warming, and energizing. The color of fire, red can stimulate appetite, increase heart rate, warm the body, and cause perspiration. Avicenna thought it quickened the blood and helped vitality, and he used it in treatment of blood stasis disorders such as coldness in the hands or feet.

Emotional properties: Red is associated with excitement, strong emotions, passion, love, and intensity. It is very grounding, earthy, and helps with emotional warmth, releasing passivity, and comfort. In excess it is associated with aggression, agitation, and "seeing red."

Mental properties: Red is a mental stimulant that supports assertiveness, confidence, and independence. It is a remedy for dullness and apathy.

Spiritual properties: In Ayurveda, red is considered to be protective. It is known symbolically, along with pink, as the color of love, also associated with compassion, courage, and will power.

Orange

Chakra: Sacral (second)

Chinese Medicine: Orange relates to both Fire (meridians of the Heart and Small Intestine and those corresponding organs) and Earth elements, the latter associated with Stomach and Spleen meridians (and physical organs), and to a lesser degree the pancreas (the physical organ).

Discussion: Orange is a warm, energizing color, which helps free up energy. In folklore it is associated with creativity, abundance, good luck, and procreation.

Physical properties: Orange is energizing and warming but not as much as red, stimulates appetite, aids digestion, and is helpful for lung ailments, menstrual cramps, and low energy. It may increase heart rate. Orange is esoterically associated with the adrenal glands.

Emotional properties: Associated with excitement, enthusiasm, and sociability. Wearing orange alleviates constriction and may get stuck emotions moving. It helps people have a sense that more options are available to them. Even if the color is disliked, most people feel something about orange.

Mental properties: Orange is showy and attracts attention. It is associated with dynamism and independence.

Spiritual properties: Orange helps with joy and wisdom. It eases connection and communication between people. Thus it can be helpful for social anxiety.

Yellow

Chakra: Solar Plexus (third)

Chinese Medicine: Earth element (Stomach and Spleen meridians, corresponding to the physical organs stomach, spleen, and pancreas)

Discussion: The color of sunshine, yellow is warm and highly visible. Thus it is often used for hazard signs and road work crews. It is the contemporary color of mourning in Egypt. In traditional Japanese culture, it was associated with courage. In other cultures it is associated with confidence, affirmations, cheerfulness.

Physical properties: Many color therapists believe that yellow strengthens the nervous system and the lymphatics, cleansing and purifying the body. In this, it improves digestion and helps alleviate constipation. It may be used for many digestive problems, including those of the liver, and it strengthens muscles, especially in convalescence.

Emotional properties: Yellow is cheerful, joyous, and happy. It supports will, desire, curiosity, flexibility, and achievement.

Mental properties: Yellow may improve mental clarity and confidence.

Spiritual properties: Yellow is associated with enthusiasm, *joie de vivre,* and uplifting energy.

Green

Chakra: Heart (fourth)

Chinese Medicine: Wood element (Liver and Gallbladder meridians and organs)

Discussion: One of the most prevalent colors in nature, green is associated with life and growth—trees, grass, algae, pastures, meadows, forests, and the sea. Green represents nature, springtime, grass, and good luck. As a symbol of fertility, green was the preferred color for wedding gowns in fifteenth-century Europe. Energetically green is balancing; it can aid both warming and cooling. Green is important in Irish and Islamic folklore. It is the color of four-leaf clovers. Calming and soothing, green is a color of healing.

Physical properties: Green is considered anti-inflammatory by most contemporary color therapists. It is used to treat cysts, help stomach and digestive disorders, and improve many respiratory conditions. Overall, as in nature, green is considered "health-giving." Green also may help support a calm, peaceful nervous system and reduce fatigue.

Emotional properties: Harmonizing, restful, calming, nourishing, and cheerful. This is often an excellent color for acute anxiety or chronic stress, though excess is widely associated with "jealousy" and insecurity. Balance, stability.

Spiritual properties: Associated with renewal, green is the color of life. It is grounding, balancing, and harmonizing. It can reconnect people with life and personal growth. Mystically, green is thought to have the ability to make perceptual time move more quickly.

Blue

Chakra: Throat (fifth)

Chinese Medicine: Water element (Kidney and Bladder meridians and organs)

Discussion: Blue is often considered cool and dispassionate, but with an expansive, dreamy quality of serenity. The color of the ocean and the sky, it is a popular color for bedrooms, as it is associated with sound sleep. It is also associated with activation of the pineal gland and higher spiritual wisdom.

Physical properties: Blue is felt to decrease pain, be generally physically soothing, quell all sorts of inflammation, lower blood pressure, soothe asthma, and help sleep. It could be called "antiseptic" and is useful for clearing infections. Blue light is already being used in dermatology as part of a therapy to treat some skin cancers, pre-cancerous conditions, and a variety of non-cancerous inflammatory skin conditions such as psoriasis.[3]

Emotional properties: Blue is calming and relaxing, soothing frayed nerves and supporting peaceful rest or contemplation. In excessive amounts, though, it can lead to "the blues."

Mental properties: Blue is dispassionate yet expansive, supporting healthy links between emotion and rational thought. It is associated with intelligence, strength, and clear communication.

Spiritual properties: Blue supports peace, including inner peace, hope, and mental clarity. It is a good color for meditation.

Indigo

Chakra: Brow (sixth)

Chinese Medicine: Water element (Kidney and Bladder meridians and organs). These associations are shared by blue and black.

Discussion: Indigo is the color of blueberries, twilight, and pre-dawn. In some branches of mysticism, it is the color of spiritual light, and esoterically it has been associated with St. Germaine.

Physical properties: Indigo is believed to be cooling and detoxifying. It is used to calm inflammation, inflamed skin diseases, and "hot" conditions such as infections and fevers.

Emotional properties: Indigo has potentially sedative effects in the nervous system. It is soothing, calming, and uplifting. Along with blue and green, indigo is strongly associated with calming anxiety.

Mental properties: Indigo supports the development of intuition and helps release fear.

Spiritual properties: Indigo is associated with spiritual love, the spark of intuition, awakening, and divine connection. It helps with developing inner peace and is a good color for meditation and contemplation.

Violet

Chakra: Crown (seventh)

Chinese Medicine: Violet is not usually associated with a specific meridian, though some link it with both Fire and Water elements.

Discussion: Violet has the shortest wavelength and fastest vibration of the colors of visible light. It is considered to have both warm and cool properties, but mostly cool. Found in nature in various flowers, violet is associated with royalty, romance, and the feminine. Violet windows are found in many churches, to support meditation.

Physical properties: Violet is felt to be good for supporting the nerves and nervous system. Some use it to soothe headaches, nerve pain, shingles, sciatica, and inflamed nerves. It may decrease sensitivity to pain. It is also used by many people to heal addictions.

Emotional properties: Violet is very calming and centering, an ideal color for soothing anxiety. It is even used for hysteria, as well as nervous exhaustion.

Mental properties: Violet is associated with mystery, individualism, dreams, fantasy, and nobility. It enhances imagination and memory.

Spiritual properties: Violet enhances connection with divinity and the infinite. It is a color of peace, inner stillness, mysticism, spiritual insight, transcendence, and psychic ability. It is also an overall color for spiritual healing and wholeness, and this healing may include physical transformation as well.

Magenta

Chakra: Magenta is the color of the eighth chakra, above the head, also called "the soul star."

Chinese Medicine: Fire element

Discussion: Magenta is a strong color with associations of power. Some researchers speculate that our ability to see the color magenta is a relatively new development, associated with an expansion of human consciousness.

Physical properties: Magenta is used for support of the heart and for alleviating fatigue.

Emotional properties: Magenta is associated with passion, but of a more spiritual nature than red.

Mental properties: Magenta is a color of determination, drive, and strong opinions.

Spiritual properties: Enhances alignment with one's life purpose. Associated with great spiritual power, capacity for self-realization, and completion.

Other Colors not Related to the Chakras

Pink

Chinese Medicine: Fire element (Heart, Small Intestine, Triple Burner meridians)

Discussion: Pink is warming, soothing, and comforting. While pink is now associated with children, especially girls, in Europe prior to the eighteenth century it was considered a manly color. It was too manly, in fact, for women or girls to wear. Pink is a color of the heart.

Physical properties: Pink is a color of softness and youthfulness. It can be a generally soothing color for physical health.

Emotional properties: Pink is about gentleness and nurturing. Energetically it is the least violent color. Many prisons have pink rooms into which violent inmates are placed to cool down. Pink is associated with playfulness. It also dissipates grief and helps people connect with their feelings. It reduces stress and can be a great color for clearing shock, trauma, and PTSD.

Mental properties: Mentally pink is associated with frivolity and playfulness, but also with feminine wisdom.

Spiritual properties: Associated with romantic love and also, as a heart color, pink is related to inner truth and spiritual nourishment.

Black

Chinese Medicine: Water element (Kidney and Bladder meridians and organs)

Discussion: Black absorbs all colors of the visible spectrum, so it is the absence of color. In folklore it is associated with night, silence, and coldness. Many contemporary cultures associate black with death or mourning, but in ancient Egypt black was the color of life and reincarnation.

Physical properties: Often used in clothes since black is visually slimming to appearances; it also makes a room look smaller in size.

Emotional properties: Black can be very soothing to some people, associated with deep rest, power, surety, and restoration. But others associate black with lack of power, with depression, and even menace (the color of the pirate flag).

Mental properties: Black is associated with sophistication, elegance, mystery, the unconscious, and the unknown.

Spiritual properties: Metaphysics, far journeys, freedom, the void, the black hole, no-thing-ness at the root of creation.

White

Chinese Medicine: Metal element (Lungs)

Discussion: White light is an aggregate of all colors of the visible spectrum. White light passed through a prism will yield a full rainbow of shades, so in one sense it is the perfect or complete color. In contemporary cultures white is associated with innocence, simplicity, and purity, thus is chosen by many brides, but in traditional Japanese culture white was the color of death. Most shrouds traditionally are white. In folklore it is also a color of purification, and in New Age thought, it is the color of "cosmic consciousness."

Physical properties: Physically white is both cold and warm. It is often used for healing, especially spiritual healing related to any physical malady or emotional concern.

Emotional properties: White can sometimes be associated with sterility, blandness, or "a blank canvas," but it is also a color of peace (the dove), illumination, and divine white light.

Mental properties: Cleanliness, orderliness, and simplicity are properties associated with white.

Spiritual properties: White light is a color of higher consciousness, holiness, enlightenment, unity, and oneness.

Brown

Chinese Medicine: Earth element (Spleen, Stomach, and Pancreas) as well as some association with the Wood element (Liver, Gallbladder meridians and organs)

Discussion: Brown is the ultimate "earthy, woody," grounding color. It is warming, associated with home and hearth.

Emotional properties: Brown implies comfort, nurturing, and soothing, as well as endurance and fortitude. Emotionally brown can be described as "stalwart."

Mental properties: Practicality, durability, and reliability are associated with brown.

Spiritual properties: Spiritually brown is related to groundedness and integration of experience.

Tools for Transformation:
Playing with Color and Light for Emotional Health

Color and light offer us an opportunity for playful self-awareness. You can have fun with this, because color is fun!

There are many ways you could experiment with color to alleviate symptoms of anxiety. Here are a few suggestions.

1. Make a "color diary" and take notes about how you feel with and about various colors. Note any physical or emotional reactions you have to them. Try this on various days and in different moods. See if your feelings shift or stay stable.

   Notice if you have an affinity for any colors. Which ones? Do you have them in your environment? How do these favorite colors make you feel?

2. Try deliberately wearing various colors of clothes and note your emotional state, how you react to others, and how others react to you.

3. Get some drinking glasses (made of glass) in various colors, and put water in them. Let them sit in a sunny windowsill for an hour or so. Drink the water and see how you feel.

4. Eat natural foods of various colors. The naturally occurring rainbow of pigments in fruits and vegetables indicates that these foods are loaded with antioxidants, and they may have additional emotional and physical benefits.

5. Get some natural food colorings or make them from spices and vegetables. Beets, of course make a lovely red color, and turmeric a golden yellow. Try putting some colors in a bath and see what you notice emotionally.

6. Look through colored windows. Let colored light fall upon you. Which colors calm and which stimulate you?

7. Play with a prism. Hang prisms in a window in your home and stand or lie in the rainbows.

8. Try wearing some color-filter glasses. How do they feel to you? Do they affect you emotionally?

9. Once you have identified colors that you find soothing, pleasing, and balancing, get some clothes in those shades and wear them more often. Consider painting a wall or walls in your home with calming colors. Spend time in spaces that feel emotionally supportive and restful.

10. Most of all, have fun! Let color be a supportive tool to cultivate joyousness, creativity, and wholeness.

CHAPTER 17

Essences and Other Vibrational Tools

What Are Essences?

Essences are liquids made from the energetic or vibrational impressions of a flower, leaf, gem, or other natural object or energetic force. These vitalistic impressions or signatures are stabilized in water and preserved with grape alcohol or another neutral medium such as vinegar. Since antiquity, essences have been used in healing by various cultures as spirit medicines. Dr. Edward Bach, a successful London homeopath of the early twentieth century, reintroduced essences to the modern healing repertory. In his later years, Bach had a crisis of faith in his work when he came to believe that even homeopathy did not sufficiently address the spiritual roots of illness. He found it disturbing that doctors focused on disease processes but ignored the whole person.[1] Eventually Bach left his successful practice and even discarded the scientific method, believing it was too reductionistic. He became a wanderer in the countryside, often sleeping outdoors and communing intuitively with trees and plants, and giving away his healing services for free. Through his communication with the natural world he evolved the thirty-eight Bach flower essences. These are essences of typical plants of the British countryside in the early twentieth century.

Since that time many other essences have been made from native plants of other areas, and the world of essences has expanded beyond flowers. There are falling-leaf essences, gem elixirs, planetary and starlight essences, environmental and seasonal essences, animal essences, and more. Essence practitioners understand that any part of nature can teach us about balance and harmony when we communicate with it intuitively and acknowledge its consciousness.

Essences contain no fragrance and should not be confused with essential oils. Nor are they medicinal-strength extractions of flowers or herbs, and so they should therefore not be confused with herbal tinctures or infusions. Essences are extremely dilute and generally contain few or no molecules of the original plant or flower. They have no detectable scent except that of their stabilizer: brandy, grape alcohol, shiso vinegar, or other vinegar solution.

Why Use Vibrational Tools?

Vibrational tools are not required for healing, but they can be of great benefit. They help us to focus on what we want emotionally, while simultaneously assisting us in releasing resistance to, and disbelief in, desired outcomes. I have observed that the ritual of taking a remedy or an essence is part of the healing process for many people, including myself. Working with essences allows us to focus with greater clarity on our wholeness, pointing our internal compass firmly in the direction of health.

For example, I noticed long ago that I get a wonderful "placebo effect." I can take a remedy and seconds later will often feel relief. This is much quicker than any physiologically mediated effect could be observed. I am okay with this, as I know that my positive attention is part of the healing process.

I like to utilize essences because they are safe, supportive, and gentle. I believe they work in harmony with the soul-plan of the people who use them. They do not push or force change but rather invite it, in a manner that is appropriate for the person taking it. Essences are non-toxic, without contraindications, and are appropriate for people of any age. There are no side effects from essences—they either assist or are as harmless as water and a drop or two of alcohol or vinegar. If an essence used is not correct for an individual, nothing happens. When using essence combinations, only those that are appropriate for the individual at the time they are taken will be active. They will "resonate" with the person's energetic field in a positive way or not at all.

Essences are capable of helping restore balance on mental, emotional, and spiritual levels. They connect the spirit of the plants, flowers, trees, animals, stars, gems, etc., that have willingly offered assistance with the individual or individuals experiencing imbalance. Essences are created in an intuitive manner, with the cooperation of the consciousnesses of elements of the natural world.

The natural world can assist us because it is already in harmony with the whole, and so it can teach us about our natural state of relaxation and ease. By staying in wholeness, and holding only that vibrational note, essences help us notice our limiting beliefs and patterns. They offer fresh clarity about ways to release resistance and restore harmony. Essences help especially when there are ingrained patterns, learned perhaps from family or culture, which no longer serve the growth or well-being of the person, group, or community. They are powerful tools, on the soul level, for restoring awareness of communication between one's broader non-physical self and one's personality.

How Strong Are Essences?

Essences are gentle and subtle. This does not mean they are weak or ineffective. On the contrary, I have found essences to be among the most valuable tools that I have utilized for awakening and allowing transformation. For example, in my first book, *Transforming the Nature of Health,* I shared the story of one anxious, agoraphobic patient with a history of extreme reactions to medications, herbs, and nutritional supplements. She was too sensitive to utilize any of those, so we worked, over the phone, with a succession of flower essences while she also devoted herself to a mindfulness program. Over time, she completely resolved her agoraphobia and dramatically lessened her anxiety, using only essences and her mind-body work as tools for her healing transformation.

As my patient demonstrated, the effects of essences are more noticeable as we quiet down and are able to connect with our inner selves. Tools such as journaling and meditation will help us to perceive and amplify the benefits of essences. Physical and emotional changes may ensue as patterns of disharmony dissolve and the physical self becomes more certain of its essential well-being. Sometimes essences will connect us with an understanding of the roots of disharmony that led to a physical ailment or imbalance. As we are able to reestablish balance we may gradually observe beneficial effects in the physical being.

One does not need to "believe" in essences for them to be effective. They are often used quite successfully with babies, children, animals, pets, plants, and skeptical adults, as well those who "believe" in vibrational healing. If you want to try them, then do, and see if they have anything to offer you at this time.

How Does One Work with an Essence?

Essences are used from a dosage bottle, which is prepared from a stock bottle. The entire method of preparation is quite meditative, as discussed below. Most people will begin with purchasing stock bottles of essences. Stock bottles of a plethora of brands of essences are widely available in natural pharmacies, through internet retailers, and in natural groceries. Only a few drops of stock essence are required for a dosage bottle, so the essence is quite dilute and can be very inexpensive.

Essences can be utilized in many ways. Some popular methods of administration include: oral drops in water, drops in a bath, oral drops right into the mouth or under the tongue, drops applied to a point such as an acupressure or trigger point, drops diluted in water and then applied to a body area, drops added to creams or lotions and applied to a body area, and drops added to water and spritzed in healing space or to clear the vibes in an area. If administering essences to babies, a few drops are added to bath water, or as a diluted topical application, rather than orally. The number of drops chosen is also intuitive. If you are not sure, then at first try one to five drops in any of the above formats.

Choosing and Blending Essences

Choosing essences to work with can be either a cognitive or intuitive process, or both. Cognitively, they can be chosen by reading about their spiritual properties and then selecting choices based upon which one (or ones) seems appropriate for the situation. Dowsing with a pendulum, picking flower cards, muscle testing, and running a hand past essences or names of essences are some of the intuitive ways one might select an essence. An individual can select for oneself or consult with a flower essence practitioner. A compendium or reference might be used. When reading about essences we may resonate with various ones, recognizing our own issues and desired directions of growth. Since essences are safe and without side effects, they can be easily selected by any interested person. A practitioner is not required, though working with one can be helpful.

One does not need any advanced training to study essences. Often when you read about them, certain ones will jump out at you, and you will know: "I need that one." For me, often that list is quite long and I need to prioritize, providing me with yet another avenue for self-discovery. For a program of expanding self-awareness and inner peace, you can blend several essences or choose individual ones.

Manufacturers generally have guidelines regarding how many of their essences they suggest you blend at a time. These vary a great deal from producer to producer. For example, the Bach folks generally recommend working with no more than three essences simultaneously, the Australian Bush Flower Essence teachers advise working with up to five in a combination, while Green Hope Farm gives no limit to the number of essences that may be combined. I personally have found that it is fine to combine as many essences as desired, but if you are using fewer at one time it is easier to distinguish their individual effects. I intuitively blend five to fifteen essences for patients who request them, and will mix in ones from different brands as well. But sometimes I will suggest a single essence if that seems more appropriate. There are no rules!

Many producers also make composite or blended essences with multiple constituents. These may contain up to thirty flowers and earth energies, yet they are used and blended as if they were single essences.

Types of Essences

There are many good brands available. I discuss below a few with which I am familiar and that are widely available, but there are many other excellent essences that I have not utilized. Often locally produced essences will give wonderful results, and they assist in harmonizing individuals with their bioregion.

Bach

Dr. Edward Bach was the originator of modern flower essence therapy. His original thirty-eight essences are often a good entry into exploration of this gentle healing modality. The popular "Rescue Remedy" is his most well-known essence, a combination made from five Bach remedies: Rock Rose, Cherry Plum, Clematis, Impatiens, and Star of Bethlehem. It is used for emergency situations and shock, as well as for generalized stress. Rescue Remedy can help stabilize the emotions in many situations and is an easy essence for anxious persons to start with since it is so widely available.

While any of the Bach essences might be appropriate for someone working to soothe anxiety, some of the Bach essences used most frequently for anxiety (in addition to Rescue Remedy) include:

Agrimony: For people who put on a brave face and have a forced cheerfulness but are actually experiencing inner torture. It helps people develop real cheerfulness, optimism, and a sense of the bigger picture.

Aspen: For generalized fears and free-floating anxiety that is not attached to a specific thought or experience. This essence encourages a gentle fearlessness, bolstered by faith and knowledge of the inner peace that dwells in each of us.

Cherry Plum: For deep feelings of dread, fear of losing control of thoughts or actions, or fear of going out of one's mind. Cherry Plum helps with stabilizing the feelings of calm courage and sanity, and knowledge of the deep inner truth of our wholeness.

Mimulus: For people who have specific fears, and for anxiety of a known origin. This is the Bach remedy for phobias, and for those who focus excessively on a specific disturbing topic. It helps with peace of mind, gentle humor, and equanimity.

Red Chestnut: For people who worry overly about the welfare of others. Usually this is anxiety directed toward what might happen to close friends or family members, but I have used it successfully with people who worried excessively (and in a disempowered, fearful way) about politics, animal welfare, and the environment. For worry about world circumstances, Red Chestnut is often used in combination with Vervain. It encourages feelings of security and safety, and the ability to respond to a crisis with calm strength.

Rock Rose: Used for terror and extreme fright, and for calming after shocking events. A component of Rescue Remedy, Rock Rose encourages ease with fearlessness and courage.

Vervain: For intense people who experience nervous exhaustion, stress, and strain, or perfectionism that leaves them unhappy. "Vervain types" often have heart palpitations. It is also for unhappy zealots who want everyone to believe as they do. It encourages open-mindedness, self-acceptance, unconditional love, and the deep understanding that everyone has the right to their own opinion.

White Chestnut: For looping thoughts, incessant negative mental chatter, and mental arguments. White Chestnut encourages a quiet, calm mind and greater access to inner peace. A great choice for calming people who have difficulty meditating because of excessive or intrusive-feeling thoughts.

It is easy and fulfilling to learn about essences. While beginners will often start with the Bach essences, there are many others that are simple to use and can also provide an entry point.

One of my favorite lines is the Green Hope Farm essences, based in Meriden, New Hampshire.[2] Their lovely website is chock-full of gorgeous pictures of flowers and moving descriptions of their essences. A first purchase of several essences will get you a free copy of their current book if you request it. The founder, Molly, began gardening and making essences through communication with angels before she even knew what they were!

The twenty Spirit-in-Nature essences (formerly called Master's Essences) are also simple to learn.[3] They are all made from fruits and vegetables, and were inspired by the great yogi Paramahamsa Yogananda's explanations of the spiritual qualities of some foods. There is a nice YouTube video that explains working with these essences.[4]

Other essences I personally love include: Australian Bush Flower Essences,[5] Desert Alchemy Essences,[6] Alaskan Flower Essences,[7] the Flower Essence Society Essences,[8] and Perelandra Essences.[9] Wild Earth Animal Essences are a line of animal-spirit essences that are made in ceremony with the cooperation of animal (and insect) spirits. They are great for people wanting to work with animal or insect spirits, or who have recurring dreams or visions that involve particular animals.[10]

Tools for Transformation: Creating Essences

Flower essences are infusions of flowers in water, potentized by sun, moon, or Earth vibrations, then stabilized in grape alcohol, brandy, shiso vinegar, or some other medium. This process is a spiritual one that involves intuitive connection with the spirit of the plant/flower. The resulting energetic essence can potentially stabilize the electrical system and the auric body.

Making essences is a lovely process that can, in itself, be beneficial for persons healing from anxiety. Below are instructions for making a flower essence. Read the whole method first to be sure you understand each step before proceeding:

1. Let the choice be intuitive of what flower to use for your essence. The first essence I ever made was of California Poppy. I fell in love with this plant, so much so that when I really *saw* it one day it took my breath away. I had to pull over on the side of the road to examine the glowing orange petals sitting on a showy hot-pink base and to absorb her vibes. I felt feelings of peace, excitement, and joy.

   You might ask yourself some questions such as: "What flower am I really attracted to right now? Is one showing up, all by itself, in my home or garden?" That happened to me with Nigella. I did not know what it was, but suddenly it started to volunteer prolifically in my front yard. Simultaneously my next-door neighbor, who is a photographer, had a show of her work, and the card advertising it featured a nigella blossom. Needless to say, nigella got my attention!

"Is there a flower I already feel in love with?" Personally, I have had a longstanding adoration of sunflowers. Or, "Is there something I already have growing around me that I feel an affinity toward?" I have made essences of several exuberantly blooming hybrid roses that were originally planted lovingly by the prior owners of my home.

Obviously, do not choose a flower for making an essence that is known to be toxic.

2. Once you have chosen a flower, you will need to find a stand of it, if possible, or grow it in your garden or in pots in your apartment or house. Gather a crystal bowl or clear glass bowl, some pure water (ideally in a glass container), as well as something such as food-grade alcohol or vinegar that you will use later for a stabilizer, and a jar or jug to store and transport the essence. The best water is living water, such clean spring or artesian well water, but purified water may also be used if living water is not available. If using purified water, you can energize it by immersing a clean quartz crystal in it for twelve to twenty-four hours before making the essence. A pinch of rock sea salt can also energize purified water, as can putting positive messages on its container, swirling it in a glass container, or offering a prayer or positive intention. Water that is potentizing should be in a glass container, since metal carries its own vibrations that may not necessarily harmonize with the essence.

   Usually the stabilizer is food-grade alcohol, either brandy or grape alcohol. Grape is best, as it is an energetically neutral spirit that is thought by some to augment the spirit of whatever it is added to. Bring all the collected items with you to the stand of flowers you have chosen.

3. Meditate and center yourself in or near the plant or grouping of plants you wish to utilize for an essence. Fill the bowl with pure or energized water.

4. After entering the meditative state, ask the flowers which ones wish to be made into essence medicine. Wait patiently in the meditative state, feeling your love for the flowers.

5. One or more flowers will light up in some way. They may catch your eye, or seem to twinkle a bit, or a butterfly may land on one or two, or they may stir in the breeze.

   Or you may feel their energy with your hand or whole being, if you are sensitive in this way. To do this, slowly run your hand above the flowers and notice where you pause naturally, or notice where your energy or eye is drawn. There is always some internal sense of knowing which flowers are connecting with you.

6. Once flowers are selected, they are collected and placed in the crystal or glass bowl that was filled with water. The number of flowers placed in the bowl depends on the meditative process. One is enough, but sometimes many are chosen. The number of flowers is also selected intuitively. It is even possible to ask the spirit of the flower to enter the water in a ceremony without using any physical flowers. This is only done, of course, when one feels a connection with the spirit of the flower. Or a flower can be dipped in the water while still attached to the plant. I use this method often when the plant is a rare one, and also if that is what the plant is asking for.

7. The essence is then infused (meaning left to imprint its energy in the liquid medium) near the mother plant or in a field of the plants. For example, a sunflower essence would infuse near the plant of the sunflower or sunflowers chosen, or in a patch of sunflowers. Since sunflowers express solar energy, they bloom by day, and are named after the sun, they are best prepared on a sunny day. Nocturnal blooming plants, like cereus and night-blooming jasmine, are best steeped in moonlight. This process, again, is intuitive, as is the duration of infusion. The flowers stay in the water until they are done: this may be only a few minutes, or several hours, or even a complete twenty-four-hour cycle.

8. After the infusion feels intuitively complete, the flowers are generally removed and a stabilizer added. By volume, 25 to 50 percent alcohol or 90 percent vinegar is added to the water infusion. Some flowers will ask to stay in the infusion for a while when the alcohol is added. If so, I usually take the essence home and leave them in for an additional twenty-four to forty-eight hours.

9. The resultant solution is the mother tincture, used to make stock essences. Only a few drops of mother tincture are needed for a stock essence, so each one can make hundreds or even thousands of stock essences. I generally use 3–7 drops of mother essence per half ounce of stock essence. Stock essences can be put up in shiso vinegar, cider vinegar, or a brandy, grain, or grape alcohol solution. If using alcohol, use 20 percent alcohol to 80 percent water (again, pure living water or purified and energized water) for each stock essence. These stock essences will last a few years. I also generally will hand-succuss (shake vigorously) the stock essences ten times when I add mother essence to the stock bottles.

10. Stock bottles are used for making dosage bottles. Again, I generally use 3–7 drops of stock essence per one-half to one-ounce dosage bottle. The neutral liquid in a dosage bottle can be additional diluted alcohol, or vinegar stabilizer, or purified or potentized water. Dosage bottles made with alcohol will last two to three years, and those made with vinegar about one year. Dosage bottles in water alone will retain vibrational activity only for a few weeks. This can be augmented somewhat if they are succussed (shaken and gently slapped against the palm of the hand) a few times when they are made, and again before using.

11. Because of all the dilution, there are very little if any actual chemical constituents of the flower in an essence. This makes them very safe to use, unless one is sensitive to the material employed to stabilize the essence.

12. Have fun with this, and every process!

CHAPTER 18

༚

Crystals and Minerals

Crystals, gems, and minerals have long been prized not only for their physical beauty but also for their emotional and spiritual properties. I will say at the outset that of course I understand that conventional, "evidence-based" medicine does not recognize any benefit to working with crystals. Admittedly, there is currently very little science associated with crystals, and it is probably unlikely that much more will be forthcoming in the near future. Not only are vitalistic effects difficult or impossible to prove with materialistic Western science, but contemporary studies are done at tremendous cost by vested interests that hope to earn a lot more money, and crystals are not going to be patented big earners for any pharmaceutical company.

But just because a thing has not been examined through the lens of modern science does not necessarily mean it lacks value. I do think that eventually some holistic form of study will emerge to help us understand better how to work with crystals and minerals. I am sure there is a science to them, one that includes their health-giving and emotionally supportive properties. We will discover this science in the coming eras, as we are more open-minded and open-hearted in our scientific explorations. Still, if you feel crystals are too far-out for you, please, by all means, skip this section.

Personally, I love crystals, and that is why I have included them in this book. I have lots of crystals and minerals spread around my house and office. My process in working with them is mostly intuitive. Depending on my emotional state, different crystals are likely to call to me.

There are some important clues that may point a direction for the future scientific study of crystals as tools for support of health and well-being. They form under tremendous geological forces and are geometrically precise in their structures and molecular weight. It is by these distinctive characteristics that geologists identify and classify them. Common crystals and their structures, like salt (sodium chloride), are essential in human physiology. Blood is believed to have a crystalline structure. All the common minerals in our bodies—sodium, potassium, magnesium, calcium, phosphorus, sulfur, molybdenum, copper, selenium, iron, and zinc—exist in crystalline and non-crystalline forms. These are essential in a host of biochemical processes for humans and virtually all living organisms.

We know that each crystal, gem, metal, and mineral has a distinct and unique chemical structure, and in the case of the ubiquitous quartzes, these precise structures are capable of holding and transmitting information, making them the basis of our digital communication networks. Just as a scientist can tell the composition of gasses in a distant star by analyzing the spectra of light and radiation that it emits, geologists can identify gems and minerals by chemical composition, wavelength, and molecular structure. It is conceivable that the crystalline energy of gems and minerals holds vibrational or electromagnetic information that can be of benefit for physical and emotional health.

Crystals are another type of vibrational tool. Currently there is a lot of conflicting information about the emotional and spiritual properties of crystals and minerals, none of it verified except by personal experience and heart-centered wisdom. So if you choose to work with these items, I advise you to let it be an intuitive process and not get too bogged down in what people say about the attributes of various stones. Like plants, each crystal, gem, or mineral will speak differently to people. One person might find that a crystal harmonizes their energy in certain ways, while another will feel no attraction to that crystal. The primary process of emotional well-being is always to get in touch with your own inner truth and make your decisions from a place of alignment with your greater self. Apply this principle to working with any substance, including crystals.

Working with crystals is an intuitive process, and one that can help you to open and expand your intuitive abilities as well. The simplest way to work with stones is to find ones that you are attracted to and see what you notice

278 ◄ Freedom *from* Anxiety

around them. Some people naturally pick up stones and put them in their pockets, or carry them for a while in their hand. This is the origin of the term "touchstone." To intuitively understand something or to feel benefit from it, we do not always have to translate the feelings we get into words. Sometimes a stone just feels good, right, or comfortable. This is an indication that the stone is supporting your inner harmony at that moment.

Despite a lack of Western scientific confirmation, there are many claims about the properties of specific types of crystals, and some of these are quite well known and probably have some merit. Amethyst, for example, has a long history of use as a calming stone, and one that supports sobriety. Rose quartz has a long association with the heart energy, possibly because of its lovely pink color, and is considered a gentle opener of blocked emotions. Numerous crystals, metals, and stones were mentioned in the Bible, especially the twelve associated with the ark of the covenant. Those stones are precious, but they were not the most expensive of the time. Rather, they were believed to be imbued with particular sacred properties.

Visionaries and channels like Edgar Cayce believed that crystals were important in past ages for building the pyramids and for placement of great standing stones like those at Stonehenge and Easter Island.

Choosing Stones, Crystals, and Minerals

If you feel attracted to working with stones and crystals, try being playful. Children are naturally attracted to them, picking up various stones and putting them in their pocket. I once became quite obsessed with some tumbled jasper in a rock garden display at my mom's hairdresser's salon when I was about six years old, and I had to ask the owner if I could take one home. My mom was getting a cut and curl, and I spent the whole time there trying to decide which stone was just right for me. Finally, seeing the protracted intensity of my focus and that I was down to a choice between two of the stones, the proprietress graciously allowed me to select both.

Let your intuition and feelings of well-being guide you in choosing stones. If you feel attracted to a particular crystal, mineral, or gem, you might hold it and see if you feel a sense of well-being and harmony around it. Would this be something you would like to wear on your body, or carry in your pocket, or place beside your bed? If you have no particular impression or a negative one, then that stone is not for you. But if you feel an enhanced sense of well-being or comfort, you may want to have that stone around for a time.

Cleansing Stones Energetically

When you acquire a new stone or crystal in a shop or from another person, I generally advise cleansing the stone of existing human energies or vibrations associated with it. This is especially important when working with crystals that have belonged to others, since crystals, with their lattice-like structure, can hold energy as well as encoded information. It is also a good idea to cleanse stones when you have been working with them for a while, especially if you have been dealing with thorny issues, or if the vibes around your space have been emotionally heavy, such as after an argument.

There are several methods for clearing stones energetically. One is to soak an insoluble crystal in a bath of salt water, in sunlight, for one to three days. Another is to place it on dry sea salt. This is especially important if it is a crystal of a water-soluble mineral. A crystal, metal, or gem may also merely be placed in a sunny spot for seven to ten days. That is the easiest method.

I used to be skeptical about the need for cleansing crystals, until I purchased a large collection of more than a thousand crystals and minerals at an estate auction. This was about one-fifth of the lifetime collection of a local geology professor who had recently passed away. When I brought the crystals home and put them around the house without cleansing, both my partner and I began to notice headaches, and I got fairly nauseated. It was just too much new energy. I packed up most of these, and the symptoms resolved. Then I slowly began to cleanse each of them before putting them in my house and office, and the symptoms did not recur. If you are picking up a stone in nature, the sun and Earth will have already naturally cleansed it.

Some Emotional and Spiritual/Metaphysical Properties of Selected Stones

This section explores some of the stones most often mentioned as supportive, particularly for emotional work and calming anxiety. The properties I relate here include common beliefs about particular stones as well as impressions formed from my own observations, sometimes corroborated by what others have written and what my patients report. Feel free to form your own relationships and discover what various stones and crystals have to say to you.

> Agates: There are many types of agates, each with different but overlapping properties. Agates are generally considered grounding, protective, strengthening, and gentle. Lace agates are particularly helpful for alleviating depression and despair. They do this by encouraging each person to express his or her own inner strength and beauty; they help us to let our lights shine. Botswana agates can be especially helpful for ultrasensitive persons and people with social anxiety, especially when these people need to be in public or in crowds.

> Amber: Amber is the petrified resin of an ancient tree. There may be petrified remains of ancient insects in amber, and recently scientists have begun to examine the DNA of these well-preserved insects. Amber has a steady, warming, nurturing, calming, and enduring property. It is popular in jewelry.

> Amethyst: Amethyst is the first stone I thought of when I decided to include this chapter. Amethyst is very beautiful and loves to be of service to people. The main pendulum that I use when I want to work with a pendulum is a lovely amethyst. This stone is intuitively attractive to many people. Its lovely purple shades are due to the presence of trace amounts of ferric iron.
>
> Amethyst is a variety of quartz, sometimes known as "the sobriety stone." In ancient Rome, amethyst was placed in wine cups to prevent drunkenness, perhaps by serving as a reminder

of moderation. In contemporary times, many have used it for support when attempting to curtail various addictions, including alcohol and drugs, and especially to minimize cravings. Amethyst is generally felt to have a protective, calming, and comforting energy. Persons with anxiety often use it to bolster balance, harmony, and inner peace.

It is used for many physical conditions as well, including arthritis, fatigue, fibromyalgia, and immune strengthening. Placed by the head of the bed, amethyst may support restful sleep. It can also help with developing psychic abilities, including telepathy, when one is ready. The violet color of amethyst is associated with the brow and crown chakras.

Azurite: A magnificent blue stone, azurite is sometimes called "the stone of heaven." It helps people get in touch with their intuitive guidance and thereby can improve decision-making and self-confidence. It may help decrease worry and gently awaken intuitive faculties (to the extent that people are ready for this). Azurite has been used in Native American and Mayan ceremonies to help participants connect with their spirit guides. I keep one on my bedroom window sill, appreciating the clarity I receive from its brilliance.

Barite: Barite is both grounding and energizing. A subclass of barite is a stone called the desert rose, which can be held for calming during anxiety and panic attacks.

Calcite: This common mineral is found in many forms throughout the world. Calcite is a stone with a gentle, stable energy, generally believed to help alleviate stress and fearfulness. It also helps with calming, grounding, and centering. One of my pendulums is a yellow-orange calcite, and I tend to choose it when I feel a lack of confidence.

Calcite can be a great stone for support of meditation. There are many different colors and types of calcite, associated with different chakras and supportive in various physical and emotional states. Aragonite is a type of calcite that is especially helpful for improving focus and centering. If you are new to working with minerals, consider starting with calcite.

Celestite: Another stone that comes in many colors, celestite helps decrease grumpiness and can enhance feelings of calm. The blue celestite is associated with the throat chakra and can assist with confidence in speaking one's truth. All forms of celestite are gently supportive of our spiritual growth, while calming fears and worries.

Emerald: A stone that supports hope, emerald's green color indicates a connection with the heart chakra. All types are useful, and even lower-quality, inexpensive emeralds can be very soothing for persons with anxiety. They can be used in jewelry, or carried, or placed at the bedside.

Fluorite: This is the name for a group of halide minerals that occur in a variety of colors. They are relatively soft, so are not generally suitable for jewelry, but that softness does make them amenable to stone carving.

Fluorite contains fluorine, an element that is toxic. Do not put fluorite in your mouth or wear it excessively, though it is safe to put on the body for brief periods, such as during meditation. Fluorite is calming and has long been associated with mental and emotional well-being. It has been used to soothe a troubled mind, decrease feelings of chaos and depersonalization, and enhance one's ability to focus and concentrate. I find that in the environment of a room, it has a stabilizing and calming presence. I always have one or more specimens of fluorite in my treatment room at work, and one or two in my bedroom. There is also some in the waiting room at my office. I feel it helps with serenity, fosters communication and self-confidence, and helps create a healing ambiance in the clinic. After selenite, it is the stone that patients will most often pick up and ask me what it is, or want to hold. Children especially seem drawn to fluorite and often request to hold it during visits.

Hematite: This is another mineral that can be very grounding and stabilizing. Sometimes I wear a necklace of hematite if I feel spacey or disconnected. I find it brings me back into my body. Hematite is also weakly magnetizing, perhaps supporting proper polarity in our physical systems.

Jade: Jade is valued greatly in many Asian cultures, thought to bring wealth, good fortune, and protection for health. Greener jades are most prized, so unscrupulous vendors have been known to dye specimens. I find jade calming and stabilizing.

Lapis Lazuli: Although I love lapis, it is not a stone I use to work with often. Nonetheless, when I thought about writing this chapter it was the second stone that popped into my head, and the second write-up I began. I said to lapis, "You wanted to be in there!" and felt a surge of love. Deep blue streaked with gold, lapis reminds us of the wisdom available in the depths of us. The vein of gold that shoots through it, that defines it as lapis, reminds us of the gold interwoven in each being. It is an alchemical stone. Since this write-up, I have had a lapis on my bedside table for several months, and I believe it has helped enhance my dreams and the depth of my meditations.

Malachite: Perhaps due to its rich green color, malachite is a stone commonly associated with prosperity and good fortune. It is also associated with the heart, since the main two colors often linked to heart energy are green and pink. Malachite is grounding, rooting the expansive beauty of the heart energy in the physical world. I suggest it for people who want to shift the type of person to whom they are attracted to one more suitable for their whole being, and to help people find true love, including self-love. Malachite is another stone I keep in the corner of my house and treatment room. I feel it has a friendly, generous, loving energy and promotes this in others.

Quartz, clear: There are many types of quartz, each with various properties. Several are discussed in this chapter. Quartz is used as a source of silica in manufacturing and hi-tech, so energetically it is the stone of the contemporary era.

Clear quartz crystals are a preeminent focuser of energy. Clear quartz has been used for emotional and spiritual support in many diverse traditional cultures including that of ancient Egypt, various African and Native American tribes, Celts, Scottish Highlanders, Mayans, Aztecs, Australian Aborigines, Tibetan Buddhists, and Brahman Hindus. It was thought to be used in the biblical era as one of the seven stones on the breastplate of the high priest. It is the stone that most often comes to mind when people think of "crystals."

Clear quartz deeply promotes harmony, patience, and clarity of thought and is felt by some to mediate the transfer of spiritual energies to planet Earth. Clear quartz can be supportive in any kind of emotional disturbance, providing a template of calm, heart-centered well-being. Some spiritual healers, like John of God, have crystal beds that clients lie upon after receiving treatment.

Clear quartz, despite its widely recognized power and virtues, is gentle. It is suitable for people new to working with crystals, and for children. It is not toxic, makes a nice gem elixir, and is fine to wear on the body all day long. I have dozens of clear quartz crystals around my home and office, including one right by my bed.

Rose Quartz: Rose quartz is commonly associated with the heart energy and love. I keep large rose quartz crystals in the corners of my home, especially the "love corner" as defined by the Chinese practice of feng shui. Whether this is important or not, I do have exceptionally loving relationships with my spouse, friends, and even pets.

Selenite: Selenite wands are widely believed to be repositories, like storage cells, of ancient wisdom. I keep one on my desk at work at all times. It is by far the most popular crystal in my office.

People often want to touch it or pick it up. Children are particularly unabashed and will reach for it within moments of entering the room. For persons with anxiety, selenite can help them connect with deep, ancient veins of wisdom, as well as the soul's path.

Tourmaline: Tourmalines are used frequently for all sorts of digestive disorders. For persons with anxiety, they can be soothing to nervous stomach upsets when worn or held on the body.

Turquoise: The beautiful stone known as turquoise is sacred to Native Americans, especially tribes of the Southwestern United States, who use it extensively in jewelry and ceremonial objects. It is believed to add strength and acuity in vision quests. Everywhere that turquoise naturally occurs, it has been highly regarded in local folk wisdom as a healing stone for a host of physical and emotional ills. For persons with anxiety it can be both uplifting and soothing. It can support balance, centering, relaxation, and calm deliberation and decision-making.

Gem Elixirs

Flower essences and other vibrational tools were discussed in the previous chapter. Essences of crystals are called gem elixirs. They can be made with any non-toxic mineral or crystal. There are many commercial gem elixirs available, and they are simple to make on your own too. Just be sure when making a gem or element elixir that the stone you choose is not soluble in water, and is safe for human consumption. If you are not sure if your stone is safe, look it up or consult an authority. Most hard stones that are safe in jewelry, like emeralds, quartz crystals, rose quartz, and tourmalines, are not soluble in water and are fine for gem elixirs.

Making and/or using gem elixirs can be an excellent way to connect with the emotional and spiritual aspects of a stone. If you have a favorite crystal, for example, such as clear quartz that you like to carry around, you can make an elixir with it. You can do so by modifying the instructions for making a flower essence, as you deem appropriate.

CHAPTER 19

Medical and Psychological Overview
of Anxiety

This chapter provides a synopsis of the current medical and psychiatric understanding of anxiety disorders. Conventional treatments including psychological interventions and pharmaceutical therapies for anxiety disorders are discussed here and in the next chapter. But before I dive into the details, I have a few words to offer about the concept of diagnosis and the process of deciding whether reading any particular information is right for you.

Including this chapter is logical, but it is not necessarily ideal for all readers. As a physician, I can provide a framework for a medical understanding of "anxiety disorders." But in fact I am not too fond of the idea of diagnosis, as unusual as this may seem in a medical doctor. As I alluded to in the introduction, I think that over-focus on diagnosis may lock people into unproductive beliefs about themselves. I consider a diagnosis to be "only" a momentary perception of the state of things. A diagnosis can become a problem when patients and/or practitioners become attached to it, or when it becomes a label that reduces people to a set explanatory model. Both "patients" and "practitioners" can succumb to a tendency to let the diagnosis define their perspective, and they might cease looking at the whole person in the present moment. A rigid diagnosis may lock people into old patterns, leading to a great deal of self-fulfilling prophecy and needless distress.

In my perspective, the best use of a diagnosis is as a way of classifying or discussing a temporarily existing situation. Ideally the condition is already evolving toward improvement when the "diagnosis" is determined.

A diagnosis is about what was, it is the old story, and it's not about what is becoming. The new story—which one hopes involves improved emotional and physical health—is what is emerging. Of course, in my professional work I do assign diagnoses every day in order to interface with systems that require them, such as health insurers. But I honestly do not believe in them in any fixed way, and I encourage you to let go of attachment to them as well. Each of us is a continual work in progress.

In a sense, everyone's "diagnosis" is the same. Underlying any physical or emotional "condition" there is some imbalance, disharmony, fearfulness and/ or contraction. We are all on a never-ending journey to greater joy, greater well-being, and greater wholeness. Our job in healing is to learn to let in more and more of the love. The "cure" for any distress is inevitably positive growth, joy, and consciously leaning toward greater harmony, wholeness, self-acceptance, alignment, and well-being.

While I have the above-stated misgivings about diagnosis and labeling of problems, I truly enjoy sharing information. Information is inherently neutral; it can feel empowering to some people and disempowering to others. Information, as well as interpretations and opinions about it, are abundant in our technological era. This chapter examines some of the ways that conventional medicine views anxiety and elaborates about some of the specific forms anxiety can take. It is meant for readers who might find such a discussion useful, interesting, and informative.

Before you read further in this chapter, you might continue your journey toward greater self-awareness by considering: "How does the idea of having a diagnosis feel to me?" For example, it might feel comforting to some people, like "someone finally understands me," but at the opposite pole it might feel constraining and disempowering, like a trap, pigeonhole, or dire prediction. It can feel more than one way or be neutral, like an abstract concept that has little or no emotional connection or meaning for you.

Take a moment to perceive your emotions about having a diagnosis now, before you read on. Start by taking a few calming breaths. Breathe calmly, in and out through your nose or mouth for five to ten breaths, focusing upon the flow of breath. Let go of any thoughts as they arise. Now consider for a moment the idea of anxiety disorders. Ask yourself, "How do I feel reading and learning about 'diagnoses of anxiety' and 'anxiety disorders'? How do I feel about myself or someone I love having a 'diagnosis' of an anxiety disorder?" Let yourself feel your emotion, if you notice that you have one. Whatever you feel is okay, and it is even fine if no feelings come up. Now again breathe calmly for another five to ten breaths, letting go of the emotion and returning to the ease of your breath. What did you notice? Were the thoughts pleasant, neutral, or alarming?

As we have learned, making action choices in the moment based upon what feels most comfortable is a cornerstone of finding greater wholeness and ease. Once you know and accept where you are, you can easily choose a healthier direction. Allow yourself greater ease and feel your sense of empowerment by practicing taking actions that feel comfortable to you, and avoiding those that do not. Once you recognize where you are emotionally, feel whether a thought or action takes you closer to your goal of inner peace or moves you further away.

So, if you examine the question of your personal ease with official "diagnosis" and sense any discomfort or become more anxious, then please skip this chapter and find one that feels better. Your emotions, as we learned earlier in the book, are okay. Let yourself experience them and guide you to what feels best. Avoid perusing any information that feels in any way uncomfortable to you. But if you enjoy examining all "the facts" or are happily an "information junkie," then read on.

Anxiety Disorders: A Western Medical Perspective

Anxiety disorders are extremely common in Western society, affecting almost 20 percent of people. In any given year, more than forty million American adults meet the criteria for one or more diagnosable anxiety disorders.[1] According to the National Institute of Mental Health, three-fourths of those affected by anxiety disorders have their first episode before their twenty-first birthday,[2] and anxiety disorders may render individuals more prone to other mental-health problems, especially substance abuse and depression. There is an entire book of official psychiatric diagnoses, *Diagnostic and Statistical Manual of Mental Disorders V,* referred to in short as *DSM V.* The V indicates that this manual is now in its fifth version, released in 2013. Eventually there will be a DSM VI and subsequent editions.

The *DSM V* categorizes and labels all currently accepted psychiatric diagnoses. "Accepted" indicates conditions that insurance companies, including Medicare, will pay for, and what psychologists and other emotional-healthcare providers can define as the condition they are treating when a client visits. It is good to note that the understanding of psychiatric disorders frequently changes in various editions of the DSM, reflecting various eras of history. This is unlike the agreed-upon understanding of some medical conditions like appendicitis, which remain quite stable. In recent editions of *DSM* and its predecessor volumes, some diagnoses are elaborated upon in greater detail, some are redefined, and still others are dropped completely. Amongst the currently definable mental disorders, *DSM V* includes a host of anxiety disorders.

The National Institute of Mental Health currently defines anxiety as: "Sustained feelings of fearfulness or nervousness." Anxiety disorders are different from transient moments of nervousness, as might be experienced when meeting one's boyfriend's or girlfriend's family for the first time, or when speaking in front of a large group. By definition, sustained anxiety must be present for at least six months in order to be diagnosed as a disorder.[3]

Anxiety or agitation may be accompanied by depression. Anxious persons tend to be fearful much of the time. They worry frequently about things that might occur, and may ruminate unhappily about past events. Some mentally equate possibility with probability, even for remote or unlikely events. For example, one anxious patient admitted that she worried her husband and daughter would have an auto accident every time they left the house, even though she "knew" this was unreasonable.

Obviously, none of these states feels good. Anxious persons often say that "their thoughts are thinking them" or the thoughts "just pop up, out of the blue." Disturbing thoughts can come on quickly and feel quite overwhelming. Anxious persons can exhibit a variety of behaviors, including sadness, worry, tearfulness, frustration, and fear. They may have nervous tics or perform self-destructive or addictive behaviors in a misguided effort to find relief. In some instances tearfulness may alternate with anger or even rage in seemingly random patterns.

Many physical and emotional symptoms can be attributed to anxiety; however, there is also the possibility that other physical ailments might be responsible for the symptoms. Seek the assistance and support of a qualified practitioner before assuming that physical symptoms are due solely to anxiety.

Common physical symptoms of anxiety include rapid heartbeat or feeling that the heart is pounding, excessive sweating, dry mouth, headache, dizziness, fatigue, motor (movement) disturbance including tremors and twitches, muscle aches (myalgias), shortness of breath, visual disturbances (especially blurry vision or lights flashing), gastrointestinal disturbances (including nausea, constipation, diarrhea, and abdominal pain or cramping), skin sensations (including itching, burning sensation, cold sensation, the feeling of skin crawling, pain, numbness, and tingling), frequent urination, sleep disturbances (including difficulty falling and/or staying asleep, disturbing dreams), and cognitive difficulties (including impaired concentration, feeling of the mind going blank, poor focus, and impaired judgment).

As you can see, that is quite a list, and those are just some of the most frequently observed physical symptoms caused by anxiety! Physical symptoms can be severe and may mimic other illnesses. For example, only 10 to 15 percent of emergency-room patients with acute chest pain are actually diagnosed as having a heart attack.[4] Anxiety and panic attacks, along with gastrointestinal problems, are the most common diagnosis subsequently determined to be causing the chest pain in the remaining 85 to 90 percent.

The Seven Most Common Forms of Anxiety Disorders

Generalized Anxiety

This is considered the "basic" anxiety disorder, thought to affect between 2 and 5 percent of the population. Patients affected by generalized anxiety may visit doctors frequently. They can experience a host of seemingly unrelated physical and emotional symptoms. For this reason, the diagnosis of generalized anxiety disorder may take a while to clarify.

Affected persons have chronic, persistent, and fluctuating feelings of worry and apprehensive expectation. They might exhibit any of the physical symptoms listed above, as well as numerous emotional symptoms including irrational fear, apprehension, negative anticipation of upcoming events, feeling unable to relax, expecting the worst, excessive worry, irritability, frustration, feelings of dread or impending doom, difficulty concentrating, restlessness, hypervigilance, and a heightened startle reflex.

Some researchers consider this a "personality disorder" because some patients who have it may not recall a time in their lives when they were not anxious.[5] Sufferers characterize their worries as "difficult to control." Generalized anxiety is not caused by any other specific anxiety disorder such as post-traumatic stress disorder, obsessive-compulsive disorder, or a phobia, nor is it caused by other physical health factors that may lead to anxiety such as pulmonary disease, hyperthyroid, cancer, or substance abuse.

Panic Attacks/Panic Disorder

Technically, these are considered two separate diagnoses, though they are often discussed in tandem since there is a lot of symptom overlap. Patients may have either or both of these. In the U.S., about 2.7 percent of the population experiences panic disorder or panic attacks.[6] Panic attacks are episodic and may occur at any time; however, they may happen only a few times in an affected person's life. A panic attack is defined as the sudden occurrence of symptoms such as trembling, heart palpitations, sweating, shortness of breath, or severe anxiety. Patients may feel as if they are going to die, pass out, or lose control. Panic attacks are more common in women than in men but occur in both sexes. Symptoms can last several minutes or longer and may mimic physical ailments such as heart attacks, gastroenteritis, and respiratory problems.

Panic disorder is a chronic problem characterized by repeated experience of panic attacks as well as a fear or worry of having them.[7] People may become fearful of places and experiences where their panic attacks have previously occurred, and begin to avoid any possible triggers in an effort to maintain control. Thus panic disorder can become stressful socially.

Post-Traumatic Stress Disorder

Post-traumatic stress disorder or PTSD can result from traumatic life events. This may be a single traumatic or violent episode in the distant or recent past, or a series of traumatic events. Examples of a single traumatic event that could trigger PTSD include a life-threatening accident, a rape, or witnessing a murder, especially of a friend or loved one. Examples of a series of traumatic events are a history of childhood abuse, or serving in the military in an active war zone. World War II soldiers were the first to be diagnosed with PTSD after experiencing the violent horrors of war; this condition was called "shell shock" in the old days. Symptoms might include any of those associated with generalized anxiety, with nightmares, flashbacks, hyper vigilance, and sleep disturbances being particularly common in PTSD. Patients will go out of their way to avoid any activity or experience that is emotionally linked to the stressor. There may be feelings of dissociation or disconnection.

Obsessive-Compulsive Disorder

Obsessive-compulsive disorder or OCD can be a disabling condition, characterized by persistent unwanted, repetitive, and intrusive-feeling thoughts and images. Common themes include obsessive fears of germs, bodily harm, and fear of acting upon inappropriate or upsetting thoughts—like harming a loved one. Affected persons may perform specific obsessive ritualized behaviors, called compulsions, in association with the unwelcome thoughts. Common compulsive behaviors include washing hands over and over, picking at hands or body, hair pulling, and checking behaviors such as looking many times to see that a door is locked or lights are off, and counting behaviors such as counting floor tiles or sidewalk squares while walking. People with OCD are not soothed for long when they perform these compulsive behaviors—most find only momentary relief and thus repeat the actions over and over again.

Most people who develop OCD begin to be symptomatic in their youth and are diagnosed by age nineteen. Symptoms may wax and wane, depending on other stressors.[8] Conventionally OCD is treated with psychotherapy (often Cognitive Behavioral Therapy) and medications.

Social Anxiety

Social anxiety is an unreasonable or extreme generalized fear of social interaction or social situations. This is not the same as simple shyness. Social anxiety can be especially pronounced if there are large groups or crowds. Social phobia can be quite pervasive and disabling, affecting many or most types of interaction. Affected persons will go out of their way to avoid social contacts. Ironically, they may suffer from loneliness as well.

Separation anxiety disorder, where a child dreads and resists separation from a parent or caregiver, is a subcategory of social anxiety seen in some children. Some researchers consider extreme performance anxiety, or stage fright, to be a subtype of social anxiety, whereas others classify it as a social phobia.

Phobias

Phobias are specific fears of an object or situation. They are estimated to affect about ten percent of adults.[9] Phobias of specific things are characterized under the heading of anxiety disorders, but there are hundreds of specific phobias, so this is a broad category. People with phobias will strive to avoid the object of their fear, although they usually understand that their fears are not rational. Some phobias, like social anxiety and social phobia, may be quite devastating, with profound implications for how an affected individual leads daily life. Other fears, like arachnophobia (fear of spiders), may have relatively minor consequences most of the time for affected individuals. Nonetheless, even with "minor" phobias, anxiety increases with proximity to the feared stimulus and may lead to panic.

It has been observed that alcoholics are ten times more likely to suffer from phobias than the general population. Similarly, people who suffer phobias are twice as likely to start drinking heavily as the general population.[10] If you are a phobia sufferer and a drinker, consider looking at the broader implications of how untreated alcoholism may be affecting you.

People with family members who suffer from phobias are three times more likely to develop phobias than members of the general population without a family history.[11] It seems that for any experience or object, there may be some people who have a specific phobia of it. Some of the more common phobias that patients experience include:

Acrophobia: fear of heights

Aerophobia or Pteromerhanophobia: fear of flying

Agoraphobia: a fear of going into large or open spaces, possibly extending to a fear of leaving home. This can be quite socially disabling.

Arachnophobia: fear of spiders

Amaxophobia: fear of riding in a car, with fear of driving a subcategory of this fear

Astraphobia (or Brontophobia): fear of thunder and lightning

Carcinophobia: an irrational dread of developing cancer

Chiroptophobia: fear of bats

Claustrophobia: a fear of being in enclosed spaces. Fear of being in elevators is a common subcategory of this phobia.

Cynophobia: fear of dogs

Health Anxiety/Hypochondria: fear of illness. This may include mysophobia, fear of germs, which may also be a characteristic of obsessive-compulsive disorder.

Gerontophobia: a fear of aging or old people

Glossophobia: fear of public speaking

Necrophobia: fear of death

Nosocomephobia: fear of hospitals

Nyctophobia: fear of the dark

Ophidionophobia: fear of snakes

Phasmophobia: fear of ghosts

Social Phobias: a fear and avoidance of social interaction or social situations (discussed in more detail above). Can be generalized or specific, that is, limited to one type of situation. An example of a specific social phobia is paruresis, a fear of urinating in public bathrooms.

Triskaidekaphobia: fear of the number thirteen

Trypanophobia: fear of injections or needles. Affected individuals may faint from injections.

Zoophobia: fear of animals

Phobias are often treated with psychotherapy. Common strategies include cognitive behavioral therapy as well as graduated exposure to the feared item. Desensitization is another approach employed for specific phobias. For example, a person with a fear of flying in airplanes might have a series of treatments that begin with looking at photos of airplanes, progressing to sitting in an airplane on the ground before attempting an actual flight. Sometimes medications are used as well.

Nervous Tics

Some anxious persons may exhibit nervous tics, which are repetitive, non-rhythmic motor or phonic (sound) activities. People who experience tics report a progressive build-up of tension or pressure that culminates in the performance of the tic, which temporarily relieves the tension. At times tics can be briefly suppressed by the will, but eventually the impulse to express them becomes irresistible. Because of this, they are considered un-voluntary or semi-voluntary. Not all tics are caused by anxiety; some result from an illness or medical condition such as encephalitis, head trauma, or stroke.

Some anxiety-related tics are found in association with other anxiety disorders. For example, people with obsessive-compulsive disorder will often exhibit a nervous tic such as checking or touching objects as part of their syndrome. Some of the more common tics include:

Motor Tics (when excessive and compulsive)
Examples include eye blinking, head movements, shoulder shrugging, pulling at clothes, touching people or objects, and trichotillomania (compulsive hair pulling).

Verbal Tics

Examples include throat clearing, sniffling, echolalia (repetition of what has been spoken by someone else, like an echo), palilalia (repetition of one's own words), and coprolalia (affected individuals have compulsive outbursts of foul language).

Anxiety disorders may overlap. A combination of two or more disorders is not uncommon. A person might experience panic disorders and social anxiety, and have a specific phobia about going over bridges. A common pairing is obsessive-compulsive disorder and a specific fear of germs or dirt under the nails.

Extreme anxiety may move the individual into feelings of paranoia or dissociation. These then get their own psychiatric categorizations, but at the root they can be severe reactions to persistent anxiety.

Pharmaceuticals

For some anxious persons, pharmaceutical drugs are the best choice for supporting a calm mood. They can be utilized in combination with many of the tools in this book, or alone. The choice of whether to use them is best left up to the individual and his or her physician, as well as trusted advisors. Some readers might assume that I am "against pharmaceuticals" since I have a fondness for natural remedies. While I do enjoy working with natural remedies, I make it a point to try not to cast specific types of remedies as wrong or right—largely subjective terms that differ according to culture, life experience, and individual temperament. Relief is delicious and is an improvement over tension and anxiety, regardless of how it is achieved. Most patients who consult with me on mood support do so because they prefer to work with non-drug modalities. Most, about 85 percent, are successful with this strategy. But the other 15 percent do use pharmaceutical intervention, some people for brief periods and others for extended time frames. Many patients consult me who are already on pharmaceuticals and desire to taper off them, but want to do this in a way that will be gentlest and have the greatest likelihood of success. I prescribe pharmaceuticals when they are the best choice for my patient.

Below is a brief discussion of some of the medications most commonly used in the treatment of anxiety. The medications are discussed for informational purposes only. All require prescriptions and consultation with a physician to determine if they are appropriate in any individual case.

Anxiolytics

Benzodiazepines

Benzodiazepines are medications that quickly alleviate anxiety, even when utilized at low and moderate doses. They have a significant potential for addiction and abuse, so the U.S. Drug Enforcement Agency (DEA) classifies them as schedule IV controlled substances, and they are strictly regulated. They work by binding to GABA receptors. As you may recall from chapter 10, "Nutrients and Amino Acids," GABA is a naturally occurring calming brain chemical. Benzodiazepines are used for all types of anxiety especially generalized anxiety, social anxiety, panic attacks, certain phobias like claustrophobia, and PTSD. They are also used to treat insomnia, alcohol withdrawal, muscle spasms, nausea, and some seizure disorders. At higher doses, most of these drugs are strong sedatives/hypnotics that will promote sleep. These are ideally used only briefly or intermittently as a remedy for severe anxiety. Benzodiazepines can be quite helpful together with SSRIs (discussed below) when the latter are first utilized and there is a higher risk of increased anxiety during the new drug's latent period.

Buspar

Buspar is an anxiolytic azapirone drug. Azapirones are medications that enhance effects on 5-HT1a receptors, modifying the way the brain uses serotonin. There may be further activities of buspar that are not yet characterized. Buspar is approved for treatment of generalized anxiety disorder and may improve depression as well. It is usually not helpful for panic disorder, severe anxiety, or OCD.

Beta Blockers

Members of this group of drugs block beta adrenergic activity in a variety of muscles and tissues. Beta adrenergic receptors are an element of the sympathetic ("fight or flight") part of the nervous system. They receive stimulation from the alarm hormone epinephrine. Blocking some of these receptors allows parasympathetic (or calming) tone to emerge and predominate in the nervous system. Beta blockers slow the heart rate, decrease intraocular pressure, and relax arterial blood vessels. They are best known as drugs to treat hypertension, chest pain (angina), migraines, and glaucoma but are commonly prescribed by physicians for treatment and prevention of symptoms of generalized anxiety, social anxiety, and panic attacks.[12] They are also, at times, used preventively in common situations that might lead to panic, such as "stage fright," to control physical symptoms of pounding or racing heart, dizziness, and excessive sweating. They are widely used by musicians in orchestras. The International Olympic Committee bans them for use in athletes.

Antidepressants

SSRIs

Many patients who suffer from anxiety have some amount of accompanying depression. Because antidepressants also give relief from anxiety, in some cases antidepressants may be a good choice to combat anxiety since they can work for primarily anxious as well as primarily depressed people. Selective serotonin reuptake inhibitors or SSRIs are the most commonly used type of pharmaceutical antidepressant. They are used in higher doses for treating anxiety, though paradoxically they may increase anxiety. SSRIs, when they are effective, are first-line prescriptions and in most cases can stand alone as the sole medication utilized. Since increased anxiety is a known side effect of SSRIs in the initial stages, physicians often prescribe these along with a benzodiazepine for the first few weeks, called the latent period. Among patients diagnosed with anxiety, SSRIs are most frequently used in treatment of OCD, but they can be used with caution with any type of anxiety. Sometimes if anxiety is amplified, this will only be temporary, and experienced physicians may have tools, including benzodiazepines or other medications, to help during the initial or latent period.

Wellbutrin (Bupropion)

This norepinephrine-dopamine reuptake inhibitor (NDRI) is another anti-depressant sometimes used for anxiety. It is the same medication that, at lower doses, is used for smoking cessation, and the trade name for that use is Zyban. Like the SSRIs, Bupropion can be effective in treatment of some forms of anxiety including PTSD and social anxiety, especially at lower doses or in combination with a SSRI. It is not considered effective for panic disorders or phobias. It may aggravate tics in Tourette's syndrome.[13]

Tricyclics

The tricyclics are an older class of antidepressants that block the reuptake of serotonin and norepinephrine in the brain. Low doses of these are often used to aid sleep, as they make most people drowsy. They have also been used effectively for treatment of some anxiety disorders including PTSD, generalized anxiety, and panic disorder, and at low doses as a sleep aid in anxious persons.

Other Medications

Hydroxyzine (Atarax)

Hydroxyzine is an antihistamine medication that has been used for more than fifty years. It is also used for calming anxiety and is approved by the FDA for treatment of anxiety. Calming and sedative, it is sometimes selected for individuals potentially needing help with anesthesia induction. It is low in side effects, but it is considered less effective than benzodiazepines for generalized anxiety disorder.

Pregbalin (Lyrica)

This relatively new drug is used off-label (meaning it is not officially approved yet for this indication) in the U.S. for treatment of generalized anxiety disorder. It is best known for its use in seizure disorders, fibromyalgia, diabetic neuropathy, and for post-herpetic neuralgia. It was approved for treatment of generalized anxiety disorder in the European Union (but not yet in the U.S.) in 2007. It decreases release of excitatory neurochemicals such as glutamate, norepinephrine, and substance P. Unlike the benzodiazepines, it has no effect on GABA or GABA receptors.

Lithium

Pharmacologic doses of lithium are rarely used for anxiety alone. They are more commonly selected as a treatment for bipolar disorder that includes depression and anxiety. The use of lithium in non-pharmacologic doses is discussed in chapter 10 (section on Minerals).

One current theme in psychopharmacology is to give small doses of several medications rather than large doses of one or two. This strategy can, in the hands of a skilled practitioner, have a lot of benefits. Herbalists often employ the same concept. The chance of side effects is minimized, as there is less of any one drug being given, and a number of different medications that each address some unique aspect of the patient's situation can be combined for the best overall results. Whatever the strategy, if you believe you might benefit from pharmaceuticals as a part of your program of anxiety relief, a visit to your physician or psychiatrist is in order.

CHAPTER 20

❧

Psychotherapy

Working with a therapist can be enormously helpful in reducing and resolving anxiety. There are many advantages to choosing some sort of talk therapy, especially if there is deep-seated or chronic anxiety. The mere presence of another caring person as a listener or in dialogue can catalyze a transformation. Psychotherapists may offer even more, since they are skilled professionals who can help clients illuminate and resolve buried thoughts, feelings, motivations, and behaviors that contribute to suffering. A skilled therapist can make a tremendous difference in an individual's healing journey.

Many studies comparing medications and psychotherapy have shown that therapy is as effective or even more effective than medications alone, and studies that examine the combination of the two find that this dual approach is often the most effective. Relief achieved from psychotherapy tends to be lasting, even after therapy is no longer needed, while gains from medications alone can deteriorate after medication is withdrawn.

The choice of a style of therapy is a personal matter. There is a wide array of choices in the marketplace. Anxious clients who might potentially benefit from some form of treatment can feel overwhelmed by the process of selecting a type of therapy, or choosing a practitioner. While there can be benefits to many types of therapy, there are some styles that I have found most useful for people suffering from anxiety. Some effective forms are very deep but take years to note changes, while others can improve disposition in a matter of weeks or months. A selection of common choices of psychotherapy is discussed here to help individuals choose what is best for them right now.

Cognitive Behavioral Therapy

Cognitive Behavioral Therapy, or CBT, is currently the most prominent type of therapy used in working with the full spectrum of anxiety disorders. It is a synthesis of several varieties of psychotherapy, including behavioral therapy and cognitive therapy. One emphasis of CBT is to assist the client in learning to focus on the present moment. As the spiritual teacher Thich Nhat Hanh aptly stated: "Anxiety, the illness of our time, comes primarily from our inability to dwell in the present moment."[1] Another emphasis of CBT is teaching new habits of thought, ones that serve the person better in the here and now, along with accessible tools to reinforce these new thought patterns. An advantage of Cognitive Behavioral Therapy is that it usually is not required long term unless there are many issues. Generally a CBT therapist can help clients to greater ease rather quickly, as compared with more psychodynamic methods. A typical course of treatment lasts several months rather than several years.

Many of the approaches I outline in this book are similar to concepts of CBT. Though I am trained as a family physician rather than as a psychotherapist, I discovered many tools similar to those used in CBT during my own journey toward wellness. In fact, it was only a few years ago that I even heard of this delightful and effective modality.

CBT acknowledges the vital links among thoughts, feelings, and actions. As was discussed earlier in the book, the focus of one's thoughts creates emotions, and these emotions can result in action. Most people have patterns of thought that have become habitual but no longer serve them. The effort in CBT is directed toward helping clients change their present thoughts. When they do so, new feelings and improved life circumstances frequently result. Exposing old habits of thought that are no longer productive and shifting to more concordant thoughts brings the client relief. Old dysfunctional thoughts are displaced, not by revisiting the past scenarios, but by repetition of the new, more harmonious concepts. These repetitions inform the subconscious mind of the improved, more positive habit(s) of thought. Research indicates that it takes between three and six weeks for new habits of thought and action to form, so this can be a quick process. The brain actually rewires itself, much like diverted water will begin to flow through a new rivulet. As more water flows down the new pathway, the channel becomes stronger and deeper. Similarly with the mind, as new, more productive thought pathways are followed, they become the dominant modes of thought.

CBT has been shown to be quite effective, perhaps more than medications, for a number of anxiety disorders including generalized anxiety disorder,[2] panic attacks, stuttering, social phobias, eating disorders, obsessive-compulsive disorders, and post-traumatic stress disorder. It is used as well for associated disturbances including insomnia and many forms of depression.[3] Positive results can be permanent, since in the best outcomes, the brain and its pathways have been rewired. With many of these disorders, a year after CBT treatment is completed, former patients no longer meet diagnostic criteria for the disorder. The method has been studied with children and adolescents and has been found to be effective with them as well.[4]

There is a great deal of experimental evidence demonstrating benefit and efficacy of CBT and similar approaches, especially for relief of specific symptoms including anxiety. In the United Kingdom, The National Institute for Health and Clinical Excellence (NICE) recommends CBT as the treatment of choice for several specific anxiety-related emotional-health issues including generalized anxiety disorder, panic attacks, PTSD, obsessive-compulsive disorder, and depression. NICE has run a number of randomized controlled trials, and this method has been shown to have outstanding clinical efficacy. Since 2006, NICE has recommended a trial of CBT for mild to moderately depressed individuals before instituting medications.

Exposure Response Prevention

Exposure Response Prevention is often combined with CBT for effective treatment of OCD and phobias. In this form of therapy, the client is gradually exposed to a feared stimulus over a series of treatments. For example, a person with a severe phobia of bridges might first say the word *bridge* in a treatment, and at the next session look at a picture of a bridge. Meanwhile the therapist and client would use CBT techniques for rewiring the client's thoughts about bridges. Eventually, over several sessions, the treatment would include visiting a bridge, stepping upon a bridge, and finally, when the client is ready, crossing a bridge. This type of therapy can be extremely helpful when phobias interfere with a person's ability to carry out normal life.

Somatic Psychotherapy

There are many types of somatic psychotherapy. The word "somatic" comes from the Greek root *soma* and means "body." These types of therapy address the interaction between the psyche-mind and the soma-body. In somatic therapies, there is no mind/body duality. Instead, the body reflects the mind and emotions.

Hakomi

Hakomi is a body-centered form of psychotherapy developed by Ron Kurtz in the 1970s. He founded the Hakomi Institute in Boulder, Colorado, in 1981 to teach and disseminate his methods. Hakomi joins Eastern techniques of meditation, the practice of nonviolence, and a sense of mindfulness with Western psychotherapeutic tools.

The website for the Hakomi Institute explains:

> Integrating scientific, psychological, and spiritual sources, Hakomi has evolved into a complex and elegant form of psychotherapy that is highly effective with a wide range of populations. The method draws from general systems theory and modern body-centered therapies including Gestalt, Psychomotor, Feldenkrais, Focusing, Ericksonian Hypnosis, Neurolinguistic Programming, and the work of Wilhelm Reich and Alexander Lowen. Core concepts of gentleness, nonviolence, compassion, and mindfulness evolved from Buddhism and Taoism.[5]

Hakomi is a loving and supportive type of somatic psychotherapy. A pronounced focus on the body as a reservoir of stored experience means that physical symptoms and physiologic experience are seen as a gateway to illuminating, understanding, and shifting predominant but perhaps unconscious or subconscious emotional patterns and beliefs. These subconscious and unconscious themes are referred to as "core material." Core material may encompass habits, attitudes, beliefs, and behaviors. Hakomi helps individuals discover their underlying core material to learn what parts of it are still serving them well, and which parts are no longer functional or harmonious with their current self and goals. When old, unhelpful patterns and beliefs are discovered, they are re-evaluated with new tools. There are Hakomi practitioners throughout the world. It has proven to be of great benefit for many of my patients with anxiety. A directory of trained therapists is found on the Hakomi Institute website.

Somatic Experiencing (SE)

SE is a form of talk psychotherapy that incorporates gentle touch. It is useful for resolving emotional issues related to extreme stress and trauma. It was introduced to the world by psychotherapist Peter Levine in his 1997 book *Waking the Tiger*. Through his work, Levine became fascinated with the ways that animals in the wild handle stressful and traumatic experiences. For example, a grazing gazelle that spots a distant lion will freeze or flee, while other animals might fight. When the threat of the lion has passed, the gazelle will tremble and shake before going on with her other activities. Levine found that humans who were taught to incorporate the instinctive tools of animals more easily and thoroughly released trauma and memory of trauma from their body and mind. He attributed prolonged affects of trauma in humans to a maladaption/dysregulation in the response of the autonomic nervous system (ANS) resulting from the trauma. In acute or chronic trauma, the dominant response states—fight, flight, or freeze—may be locked into the nervous system and emotional fluidity is lost. But Levine believes that humans, like animals, have innate abilities to heal from trauma, and these can be awakened and stimulated, resulting in profound and permanent shifts. These shifts allow the sufferer an improved sense of calm, wholeness, and ease.

Some but not all Somatic Experiencing practitioners are psychotherapists. The techniques are often taught to bodyworkers, parents/caregivers, and emergency response personnel. Somatic Experiencing may be particularly useful for anxiety resulting from PTSD and for developmental trauma that results from childhood neglect, abuse, traumatic birth, or difficulties with attachment. Training certification is a three-year process. Certified practitioners, and more detailed information on this helpful approach, can be located through the Somatic Experiencing Trauma Institute website.[6]

Other Somatic Therapies

There are several other types of somatic psychotherapy that can assist and soothe anxious persons. Some of these include Psychomotor Therapy, Somatic Psychotherapy, Somatic-Psychoeduction, Body Psychotherapy, Analytic Somatic Therapy, and Multimodal Therapy, the latter a synergy of CBT and Somatic Therapy. If you are attracted to somatic therapies, considering reading more about the different styles to find one that resonates with you, especially if a variety of modes is available in your area.

A number of ancillary movement and touch therapies can be performed by bodyworkers and other practitioners (not strictly psychotherapists) that include elements of somatic therapy. Some of these include Trager bodywork, Dance Therapy, Continuum Movement, Expressive Arts Therapy, Body Mind Centering, and Drama Therapy. Any of these can be of assistance for persons with anxiety.

Additional Useful Tools

Eye Movement Desensitization and Reprocessing (EMDR)

EMDR is colloquially known as "rapid eye movement." It is a widely used psychotherapy tool that engages bilateral communication between brain hemispheres. EMDR allows rapid healing of the stress response. Some patients have fully resolved PTSD from a single trauma in as little as three fifty-minute sessions, and have healed from repeated traumas in as few as twelve sessions. EMDR is widely acknowledged to work better than Exposure Response Therapy for PTSD, and for phobias that are a result of PTSD or trauma.[7]

EMDR originated with Dr. Francine Shapiro, who introduced the technique in 1990. She believed that, like the body, the mind and emotions have a natural ability to heal. Efficacy of the methodology for relief of trauma has been verified in twenty-four randomized clinical trials.[8] The American Psychiatric Institute approves EMDR as an adjunctive therapy for acute stress disorder and post-traumatic stress disorder. In 2004, it was "strongly recommended" as a treatment for PTSD by the Department of Veteran Affairs in Washington, DC. In addition to its great proven benefits with trauma and PTSD sufferers, I have found EMDR very useful for some of my patients with other anxiety disorders, including generalized anxiety disorder, panic attacks, and OCD.

Hypnotherapy

Hypnotherapy is another tool offered by many psychotherapists. It can aid a patient in rapidly resetting old, dysfunctional thought patterns and replacing them with new, supportive ones. In hypnotherapy, the patient is hypnotically inducted into a relaxed, receptive state. While in this state, new thought patterns and positive images are provided. This allows clients to more swiftly shift their inner associations. Hypnotherapy is often combined with some sort of guided imagery technique or guided visualization, and is effective along with other psychotherapeutic techniques.

Psychodynamic Therapy

"Psychodynamics" is an umbrella term for many common insight-oriented approaches to therapy that examine the psychological forces that motivate human behaviors. It is what most people think of when they hear the word "psychotherapy," though few therapists today practice only pure psychodynamic therapy. Psychodynamics seeks to illuminate the conscious, subconscious, and unconscious underpinnings of human thought and behavior. The techniques originated with Sigmund Freud. Other branches of thought include Jungian therapy, object relations, self-psychology, Ericsonian therapy, and transactional analysis.

Psychodynamic therapy, in its various forms, can be profound in its ability to help people understand and thus shift old, unhelpful patterns. It is a deep, slow type of therapy; treatment often extends over many years, and sessions may happen one or more times per week. While it can offer clients permanent improvement and deep self-awareness over time, I generally advise clients who have a great deal of anxiety to avoid classical psychodynamic therapy until the anxiety is significantly reduced.

The emphasis in psychodynamics is exploration of the past, to discover subconscious and unconscious triggers. While this may eventually be quite helpful, for persons with severe anxiety disorders, including PTSD, severe generalized anxiety disorder, and OCD, recalling past traumatic events can trigger worsening symptoms.

Over the years, I have observed this unfortunate effect in many patients, usually silently, since I did not want to undermine the therapeutic relationships or the patients' self-confidence. I have observed a few patients suffering from PTSD who were engaged in psychodynamic therapy to worsen substantially and alarmingly. Their deterioration sometimes included worsening physical symptomatology as well. Most, fortunately, came to the conclusion, on their own, that their therapy did not seem to be helping, and let go of it. Some later chose to pursue a deeper understanding when their anxiety was less troubling, and these efforts generally had good success. Over time, psychodynamic therapy may be the perfect choice for long-term healing. But I generally advise it in anxiety only for mildly anxious persons who want to go deeper, or after a successful course of CBT or a somatic therapy (or both) has substantially lessened potentially debilitating anxiety.

CHAPTER 21

⌒

Putting It All Together

Finding your personal path to freedom from anxiety can provide a spiritual journey of greater self-love, self-acceptance, and self-awareness. A variety of effective emotional, body/mind/spirit, and natural approaches to treatment of anxiety have been offered throughout this book. This chapter recaps several techniques and offers some programmatic suggestions for soothing the most common types of anxiety.

Even amongst the good choices offered here, someone seeking to alleviate anxiety should select only the items that resonate best with him or her. Over the years of my integrative medical practice, I have repeatedly noticed that many people try to do *too much* rather than too little. It is wonderful to have a strong desire for well-being, but this does not mean that you need to move in too many directions at once. Applying a few well-chosen tools, consistently, can give outstanding results.

How to choose? Look within, and find those that resonate best with you. While it is great to have trusted advisers, friends, loved ones, and a physician or holistic practitioner whom you respect, learning to connect with your own inner guidance and following it can help you forge a path that is ideal for you, amongst the chorus of suggestions offered by well-meaning others, including me. This book features many techniques to help you get in touch with your own inner guidance. Use them as you are selecting the techniques that you will apply.

Practice observing yourself and your emotions. This act of observing yourself while simultaneously noticing and accepting your emotions and the information they give you is a powerful stepping-stone toward helping you develop greater emotional flow, ease, and inner peace. Much of the book really is about learning to listen inside yourself with kind awareness. Gentleness, ease, humor, and compassion for oneself, while finding one's own individual internal compass, are the backbone of this program of self-healing of anxiety. Try to start with these concepts, and return to them over and over again.

Including one or more types of meditation or mindfulness can enhance every program of freedom from anxiety. Breathing exercises, meditation practice, meditative movement, and mindful exercise are all of benefit. Which techniques appeal to you? Practice some form of meditation or mindfulness one or more times daily. Many techniques, such as breathing exercises, can be performed briefly throughout the day. During my most anxious days, to find relief I sometimes did mini-meditations or breathing exercises several times an hour. You can do them over and over again, to continually clear a path to well-being.

Every plan can also be improved by including a program of shifting thoughts and focus. Here is a template:

1. Notice how you feel at many times throughout your day. If you find you are not sure how you feel, learn more about how to get in touch with your emotions through one of the many tools offered in the book, including checking in, heart-centered breathing, and psychotherapy.

2. Acknowledge how you feel and let yourself experience your emotions. Notice if you experience emotions physically as well as emotionally.

3. Let go of your story about why you feel the way you do. Simply feel your emotions.

4. Acknowledge that you want to feel better.

5. Find a thought that emotionally feels slightly better and focus upon it. Choose something that is not too distant from your current object of focus. You may look at the emotional scale to make your choice, or just feel around for a sense of relief.

   Alternately, you can simply change the topic. Intentionally distract yourself with something neutral or soothing music, your breath, a pet, or a joke. It is often helpful to focus on nature—a sunrise or sunset, birds chirping, cloud formations.

6. Acknowledge the relief you feel in moving away from distress, toward greater ease. Let the relief course through you.

7. Rest, and repeat as desired.

Pay attention to nutrition and nourish your body with what it is asking for. Nourishing your body is another form of self-love. Try to eat with intention, actively including your body and mind in the discussion about what is needed for finding wholeness. Consider that the nervous system may want more healthy fats, including animal fats like butter, more cholesterol, more protein, or more cooked veggies, and fewer sweets, processed foods, and stimulating foods.

Finally, consider the wide range of modalities that might be of benefit to you. Select those that are most appealing to you, given your particular situation. Even if a tool like crystals or flower essences seems "far out," notice whether you are attracted to it. Shifting yourself to decrease anxiety allows more of you to express itself. You are letting go of limiting beliefs and finding what is really right for you.

Here is a summary of the essence of this program of finding Freedom from Anxiety:

Step One: Be nice to yourself. Interrupt self-critical thoughts with kindness and compassion.

Step Two: Quiet the internal chatter through meditation, breath work, movement, or mindfulness.

Step Three: Learn to listen to your inner guidance. It will be what makes you happy, without reservations. Know that you have a quiet inner observer that never judges you. You can find solace in its perspective.

Step Four: Smile, laugh, and connect with the Earth. Reach out to others.

Step Five: Move your body in ways that are pleasurable to you.

Step Six: Nourish yourself with food and thought.

Step Seven: Select the techniques and tools that appeal to you—breathing techniques, nutritional supplements, herbs, homeopathy, crystals, color, music. Decide amongst the many possible choices by noticing which ones light up for you. Which concepts made you eager to read the chapter, and which awakened your skepticism?

Step Eight: Consider whether medication or some psychotherapy is right for you. If so, consult an appropriate professional. Be kind to yourself, whatever you choose. There is no shame in this, or any choice.

Step Nine: Enjoy the journey!

Freedom from Anxiety is built upon the recognition that life is meaningful, and that even when we struggle, we grow. Emotional well-being is the birthright of each of us—it is at the core of our being. By practicing methods that help us to be true to ourselves, we enhance self-awareness and self-esteem. True thriving can flow from our conscious understanding of the unity of our body, mind, and spirit. Even in the face of apparent difficulties, we can choose to live and express the love that is at our core, and in this way we can find ease and peace.

Freedom from Anxiety is a practice with many tools. It is like any other practice in that it becomes easier over time, as we release our uncomfortable preconceived and limiting notions of who we are and expand into understandings that give greater ease, peace, and freedom. It is my sincere hope that through the many tools offered in this book, you and your loved ones find the right combination of techniques to support and nourish you, and help you let go of excess anxiety for a freer, less stressful, more peaceful life.

Notes

ᥰᎧ

Introduction

1. The phrase "still small voice" is a commonly used phrase, found originally in the Old Testament (1 Kings 18:20–40). In that text God was communicating with the prophet Elijah after a great battle. First God sent an earthquake and then a fire, but God's voice was not in those; it was in a gentle inner whispering that Elijah heard. Many contemporary scholars and theologians believe the "still small voice" reference is an indication that God, or the wisdom of God, may speak to individuals, as happened with the prophet Elijah, in quiet moments of inner knowing and in the peaceful recesses of the heart.

2. R. C. Kessler, W. T. Chiu, O. Demler, and E. E. Walters, E. E. (June 2005), "Prevalence, severity, and comorbidity of twelve-month DSM-IV disorders in the National Comorbidity Survey Replication (NCS-R)," *Archives of General Psychiatry* 62 (6): pp. 617–27.

Chapter 1: Emotional Well-Being and Physical Health

1. The Free Online Dictionary: www.thefreedictionary.com/optimism.

2. www.thefreedictionary.com/pessimism.

3. S. C. Segerstrom and S. E. Sephton (2010), "Optimistic expectancies and cell-mediated immunity: The role of positive affect," *Psychological Science* 21: pp. 448–55; and http://pss.sagepub.com/content/early/2010/02/22/09567976 10362061.abstract.

4. "Yet Another Worry for Those Who Believe the Glass is Half-Empty," *New York Times* online: www.nytimes.com/2007/01/09/health/psychology/09essa.html.

5. Eric Giltay et al. (November 2004), *Archives of General Psychiatry* 61: pp. 1126–35, as quoted in the article "Optimism Associated with Lowered Risk of Dying from Heart Disease," www.eurekalert.org/pub_releases/2004–11/jaaj-oaw102804.php.

6. Eric J. Giltay et al. (Feb 27, 2006), "Dispositional Optimism and the Risk of Cardiovascular Death," *Archives of Internal Medicine* 166: pp. 431–36.

7. J. E. Blalock (1984), "The Immune System as a Sensory Organ," *Journal of Immunology* 132: pp. 1067–70.

8. K. W. Kelley (1988), "Cross Talk between the Immune and Endocrine System," *Journal of Animal Science* 66: pp. 2095–2108; and K. W. Kelley (2004), "From Hormones to Immunity: The Physiology of Immunology," *Brain, Behavior and Immunity* 18: pp. 95–113.

9. Robert H. Schnewider, MD, et al. (May 1, 2005), "Long-Term Effects of Stress Reduction on Mortality in Persons ≥55 Years of Age with Systemic Hypertension," *American Journal of Cardiology* 95(9): pp. 1060–64.

10. Norman Doidge, MD, *The Brain That Changes Itself* (New York: Penguin Books, 2007).

Chapter 2: Neurobiology: Anxiety and Calm

1. Candace Pert, PhD, *Molecules of Emotion* (New York: Scribner, 1997), pp. 144–45.

2. The Economics of Happiness: www.theeconomicsofhappiness.org.

Chapter 3: The Wellsprings of Inner Peace and Letting Go

1. Abraham, interpreted by Esther Hicks, is a popular inspirational/self-help teacher. Esther Hicks describes Abraham as a group of non-physical teachers. Abraham-Hicks popularized the concept known as the Law of Attraction, and they offer many tools to help individuals connect with their inner being and their own non-physical aspects of self. Abraham-Hicks is a *New York Times* bestselling author, having published many books, CDs, and DVDs.

2. Rich evidence of the truth of this statement can be found in the near-death experience (NDE) literature. So many people who have experienced NDEs report the same things as I observed during a transformative awakening experience I had at age 18 (discussed in detail in my first book, *Transforming the Nature of Health*). For a great read on a NDE and the underlying love of the universe, read Anita Moorjani's *Dying to Be Me*.

3. For an artistic rendition of this concept, consider the beautiful poem "Ithaka" by CP Cavafy, www.cavafy.com/poems/content.asp?cat=1&id=74.1

4. Thich Nhat Hanh, *The Heart of the Buddha's Teaching: Transforming Suffering into Peace, Joy, and Liberation* (New York: Broadway Books, 1999).

Chapter 5: Meditation

1. www.marceyshapiromd.com.

2. *Yantra* is a Sanskrit word with a variety of meanings that include machine, tool, instrument, or symbol. In the context of meditation, a yantra is a symbolic geometric figure used as a visual tool for contemplation. It helps with centering the mind and balancing the emotions. The Sri Yantra is a well-known example of a commonly used meditation yantra. Many images of meditative yantras are available online.

Chapter 6: Movement and Exercise

1. www.dartmouth.edu/~eap/library/spring2011.pdf and www.helpguide.org/mental/depression_tips.htm.

2. www.livestrong.com/article/478780-a-list-of-foods-with-the-highest-gaba/?utm_source=dontgo2&utm_medium=a2.

3. www.feldenkrais.com/method/the_feldenkrais_method_of_somatic_education/.

4. Ibid.

5. As quoted on the Continuum website: www.continuummovement.com/overview.php.

6. Ibid.

7. I learned this technique long ago, I am not sure where—I think it was at a Jean Houston workshop. But when writing it up, I found I was foggy on some details, so I consulted this webpage: www.chinese-holistic-health-exercises.com/abdominal-stretching.html. The page also includes some handy photos.

Chapter 7: More Useful Tools

1. "Laughter Remains Good Medicine," www.sciencedaily.com/releases/2009/04/090417084115.htm.

2. Ibid.

3. Robert Provine, PhD, *Laughter: A Scientific Investigation* (New York: Penguin Books, 2001).

4. Human Can Increase Hope: www.sciencedaily.com/releases/2005/02/050211095658.htm.

5. www.laughing-yoga.org/benefits-of-laughter-yoga/62-psychological-health-benefits.html.

6. Ibid.

7. Public Broadcasting Service (PBS), "A Sustainable Future," www.pbs.org/ktca/farmhouses/sustainable_future.html.

8. These can be purchased online through a variety of sites including through the Monroe Institute: www.monroeinstitute.org/catalog/hemi-sync-titles.

9. Arthur Gladman, MD, Emergency Series Research Progresses, www.monroeinstitute.org/research/cat/surgery/emergency-series-research-progresses.

10. Nicola Gilbert and Bob Roalfe, Hemi-Sync® and Surgery, www.monroeinstitute.org/research/cat/surgery/hemi-sync-and-surgery.

11. www.soundhealingcenter.com/explore.html#whatis.

Chapter 8: Breathing and Pranayama

1. www.abc-of-yoga.com/pranayama/basic/viloma.asp.

2. This is a phrase from an Orin meditation.

3. Thanks to author Susan Gorell for this contribution! She reports that she has had incredible spiritual insights with this technique. I tried it upon her suggestion, and agree that it is a lovely, powerful meditation.

Chapter 9: Nutrition and Emotional Health

1. http://wiki.answers.com/Q/Is_the_Dalai_Lama_a_vegetarian.

2. The following three books are good examples of researchers addressing the old questions anew: Uffe Ravnskov, MD, *Fat and Cholesterol Are Good for You* (Sweden: GB Publishing, 2009).

Mary Enig, *Know Your Fats: The Complete Primer for Understanding the Nutrition of Fats, Oils and Cholesterol* (Silver Springs, MD: Bethesda Press, 2000).

Sally Fallon and Mary Enig, *Nourishing Traditions: The Cookbook that Challenges Politically Correct Nutrition and the Diet Dictocrats,* revised second edition (Washington, DC: New Trends Publishing, 1999).

3. www.utne.com/mind-body/effects-of-fatty-foods-zm0z12mazsie.aspx#ixzz2Bxb2EHRD

4. Palm oil, however, is controversial. While it is a traditional fat and can be produced in an ecologically sustainable manner, in fact most palm oil today is a product of rainforest-destroying agribusinesses. It is used as a cheap ingredient in commercial pies, cakes, and starchy foods. Many of these products in the U.S. are also laden with GMO ingredients such as high-fructose corn syrup. So, it is generally best to avoid palm oil as an ingredient in commercial products. If you want to purchase palm oil for home use, select a brand that is rainforest-safe.

5. www.westonaprice.org.

6. http://atvb.ahajournals.org/content/24/5/806.full.

7. William Castelli (July 1992), "Concerning the Possibility of a Nut...," *Archives of Internal Medicine* 152 (7): pp. 1371–72.

8. www.cholesterol-and-health.com/Vegetarianism.html.

9. H. Peter, I. Hand, F. Hohagen, A. Koenig, O. Mindermann, F. Oeder, and M. Wittich, "Serum cholesterol level comparison: control subjects, anxiety disorder patients, and obsessive-compulsive disorder patients," www.ncbi.nlm.nih.gov/pubmed/12211884.

10. www.livestrong.com/article/501418-lactobacillus-acidophilus-and-stress-response/.

11. "Could eating yoghurt help treat depression? Study finds probiotics affect areas of the brain related to emotions and reasoning," www.dailymail.co.uk/health/article-2332772/Could-eating-yoghurt-help-treat-depression-Study-finds-probiotics-affect-areas-brain-related-emotions-reasoning.html.

12. www.sciencedaily.com/releases/2011/08/110829164601.htm.

13. www.psychologytoday.com/articles/201110/your-backup-brain.

14. Nora T. Gedgaudas, CNS, CNT, *Primal Body, Primal Mind* (Portland, OR: Primal Body-Primal Mind Publishing, 2009), p. 29.

15. www.thedailygreen.com/healthy-eating/eat-safe/dirty-dozen-foods.
16. www.ewg.org/foodnews/.

Chapter 10: Nutrients and Amino Acids

1. www.livestrong.com/article/491201-glutamic-acid-ocd/.
2. Jonathan E. Prousky, ND (2004), "FRSH1 Niacinamide's Potent Role in Alleviating Anxiety with its Benzodiazepine-like Properties: A Case Report," *Journal of Orthomolecular Medicine* 19 (2): p. 104, http://orthomolecular.org/library/jom/2004/pdf/2004-v19n02-p104.pdf.
3. www.hospitalnews.com/nutritional-treatments-to-combat-anxiety-disorders/.
4. www.webmd.com/heart/news/20120619/low-vitamin-b6-linked-to-inflammation.
5. http://biogaba.com/images/nutrients_botanicals_stress.pdf.
6. http://ods.od.nih.gov/factsheets/VitaminB6-HealthProfessional/.
7. S. Hashimoto, M. Kohsaka, N. Morita et al. (1996), "Vitamin B12 enhances the phase-response of circadian melatonin rhythm to a single bright light exposure in humans," Neuroscience Letter 220: pp. 129–32.
8. T. Ohta, T. Iwata, Y. Kayukawa, T. Okada (1992), "Daily activity and persistent sleep-wake schedule disorders," *Progress in Neuro-Psychopharmacology & Biological Psychiatry* 16: pp. 529–37, http://biogaba.com/images/nutrients_botanicals_stress.pdf.
9. www.nlm.nih.gov/medlineplus/ency/article/003705.htm.
10. M. Fux, J. Levine, A. Aviv, and R. H. Belmaker (1996), "Inositol treatment of obsessive-compulsive disorder," *American Journal of Psychiatry* 153(9): pp. 1219–21.
11. J. Benjamin, G. Agam, J. Levine et al. (1995), "Inositol treatment in psychiatry," *Psychopharmacology Bulletin* 31: pp. 167–75.
12. G. Gregersen, B. Bertelsen, H. Harbo et al. (1983), "Oral supplementation of myoinositol: effects on peripheral nerve function in human diabetics and on the concentration in plasma, erythrocytes, urine and muscle tissue in human diabetics and normal," *Acta Neurologica Scandinavica* 67: pp. 164–72.
13. M. Fux et al. (see note 10).

14. A. Palatnik, K. Frolov, M. Fux, J. Benjamin (2001), "Double-blind, controlled, crossover trial of inositol versus fluvoxamine for the treatment of panic disorder," *Journal of Clinical Psychopharmacology* 21 (3): 335–39. Also: J. Benjamin, J. Levine, M. Fux et al. (1995), "Double-blind, placebo-controlled, crossover trial of inositol treatment for panic disorder," *American Journal of Psychiatry* 152: pp. 1084–86.

15. http://ods.od.nih.gov/factsheets/VitaminC-HealthProfessional/.

16. www.ehow.com/about_6582987_lithium-aspartate-vs_-lithium-orotate.html.

17. http://tahomaclinicblog.com/lithium-the-misunderstood-mineral-part-1/

18. www.webmd.com/vitamins-supplements/ingredientmono-1065-LITHIUM. aspx?activeIngredientId=1065&activeIngredientName=LITHIUM.

19. www.clinicaltrials.gov/ct2/show/NCT00405535.

20. www.hospitalnews.com/nutritional-treatments-to-combat-anxiety-disorders/.

21. "Glycine Could Be Key to REM Sleep Behavior Disorder, Study Shows," www. sciencedaily.com/releases/2008/03/080327172155.htm.

22. M. Bannai and N. Kawai (2012), "New therapeutic strategy for amino acid medicine: glycine improves the quality of sleep," *The Journal of Pharmacological Sciences* 118 (2): pp. 145–48.

23. L. G. Kirby, F. D. Zeeb, C. A. Winstanley (Sept 2011), "Contributions of serotonin in addiction vulnerability," *Neuropharmacology* 61 (3): pp. 421–32.

24. Brain chemistry link to anorexia, http://news.bbc.co.uk/2/hi/health/4215298. stm.

25. H. E. J. Miller, J. F. W. Deakin, and I. M. Anderson (2000), "Effect of acute tryptophan depletion on CO_2-induced anxiety in patients with panic disorder and normal volunteers," *The British Journal of Psychiatry* 176: pp. 182–88. Also: K. Schruers, R. van Diest, T. Overbeek, E. Griez (2002), "Acute L-5-hydroxytryptophan administration inhibits carbon dioxide-induced panic in panic disorder patients," *Psychiatry Research* 113: pp. 237–43.

26. S. Laidlaw, T. Shultz, J. Cecchino, and J. Kopple (1988), "Plasma and urine taurine levels in vegans," *American Journal of Clinical Nutrition* 47 (4): pp. 660–63.

27. R. J. Huxtable (1992), "Physiological actions of taurine," *Physiological Reviews* 72 (1): 101–63.

28. C. G. Zhang and S. J. Kim (2007), "Taurine induces anti-anxiety by activation of strychnine-sensitive glycine receptor in vivo," *Annals of Nutrition and Metabolism* 51: pp. 379–86.

29. W. Kong, S. Chen et al. (Feb 2006), "Effects of Taurine on Rat Behaviors in Three Anxiety Models," *Pharmacology, Biochemistry, and Behavior* 83(2): pp. 271–76. Also: J. Azuma, S. W. Schaffer, W. Stephen, and T. Ito (Eds.), "Taurine 7," *Advances in Experimental Medicine and Biology,* Vol. 643 (New York: Springer 2009).

30. "EFSA adopts opinion on two ingredients commonly used in some energy drinks," www.efsa.europa.eu/en/press/news/ans090212.htm.

31. www.webmd.com/vitamins-supplements/ingredientmono-1024-TAURINE. aspx?activeIngredientId=1024&activeIngredientName=TAURINE.

32. Ibid.

33. NIMH Medline Plus: www.nlm.nih.gov/medlineplus/druginfo/natural/993. html.

34. G. C. Burdge and P. C. Calder (2005), "Conversion of alpha-linolenic acid to longer-chain polyunsaturated fatty acids in human adults," *Reproduction, Nutrition, Development* 45 (5): pp. 581–97. Also: Thomas A. B. Sanders (Aug–Sept 2009), "DHA status of vegetarians," *Prostaglandins, Leukotrienes, and Essential Fatty Acids* (International Society for the Study of Fatty Acids and Lipids) 81 (2–3): pp. 137–41; and S. Yehuda, S. Rabinovitz, and D. I. Mostofsky (2005), "Mixture of essential fatty acids lowers test anxiety," *Nutritional Neuroscience* 8 (4): pp. 265–67.

35. A. Higashiyama et al. (2011), "Effects of L-theanine on attention and reaction time response," *Journal of Functional Foods* 3 (3): pp. 171–78.

36. www.sciencedirect.com/science/article/pii/S0308814610011416.

37. J. H. Kim, D. Desor, et al. (2006), "Efficacy of as1-casein hydrolysate on stress-related symptoms in women," *European Journal of Clinical Nutrition* 61: pp. 536–42.

38. Z. de Saint Hilaire, M. Messaoudi, D. Desor, and T. Kobayashi (2009), "Effects of a bovine alpha S1-casein tryptic hydrolysate (CTH) on sleep disorder in Japanese general population," *Open Sleep Journal* 2: pp. 26–32.

39. www.lactiumusa.com/research-study-reports.html. Also: Laurent Miclo, Emmanuel Perrin, et al. (2001), "Characterization of α-casozepine, a tryptic

peptide from bovine αs1-casein with benzodiazepine-like activity," *FASEB Journal* (online), www.lactiumusa.com/pdf/restudy/characterization-of-alpha.pdf.

40. D. Lanoir, F. Canini, M. Messaoudi, C. Lefranc, B. Demagny, S. Martin, and L. Bourdon (2002), "Long-term effects of a bovine milk alpha-S1 casein hydrolysate on healthy low and high stress responders," *Stress* 5 (suppl.): p. 124.

Chapter 11: Herbs for Natural Well-Being

1. P. U. Devi et al. as quoted in Kerry Bone, *Clinical Applications of Ayurvedic and Chinese Herbs* (Warwick, Queensland: Phytotherapy Press, 1996).

2. A. Grandhi et al. (1944), Ashwagandha. *Journal of Ethnopharmacology* 44: p. 131.

3. http://clinicaltrials.gov/show/NCT00761761. Also: www.prweb.com/releases/ Sensoril_Natreon/Withania_Somnifera/prweb862204.htm.

4. R. H. Singh and L. Singh (1980), "Studies on the anti-anxiety effect of the Medyha Rasayana drug, Brahmi *(Bacopa monniera)*–Part 1, *Journal of Research in Ayurveda and Siddha* 1: pp. 133–48.

5. C. Calabrese, W. L. Gregory, D. Kraemer, K. Bone, and B. Oken (July 2008), "Effects of a standardized Bacopa monnieri extract on cognitive performance, anxiety, and depression in the elderly: a randomized, double-blind, placebo-controlled trial," *Journal of Alternative and Complementary Medicine,* 14: pp. 707–13, Helfgott Research Institute, National College of Natural Medicine, Portland, Oregon.

6. Steven Roodenrys, PhD, Dianne Booth, MSc, Sonia Bulzomi, G.Dip.App. Psyc, Andrew Phipps, G.Dip.App.Psyc, Caroline Micallef, G.Dip.App.Psyc, and Jaclyn Smoker, G.Dip.App.Psyc. (2002), "Chronic Effects of Brahmi (Bacopa monnieri) on Human Memory," *Neuropsychopharmacology* 27: pp. 279–81. See also K. S. Negi, Y. D. Singh, K. P. Kushwaha et al. (2000), "Clinical evaluation of memory-enhancing properties of Memory Plus in children with attention deficit hyperactivity disorder," *Indian Journal of Psychiatry* 42, Supplement [Abstract].

7. R. Sharma, C. Chaturvedi, P. V. Tewari (1987), "Efficacy of *Bacopa monnieri* in revitalizing intellectual functions in children," *The Journal of Research and*

Education in Indian Medicine (Jan-June): pp. 1–12. As referenced in an NCBI article: "Randomized controlled trial of standardized *Bacopa monniera* extract in age-associated memory impairment," www.ncbi.nlm.nih.gov/pmc/articles/ PMC2915594/.

8. K. Venkateshwarlu, V. S. Saxena, and A. Amit (2007). "Safety evaluation of BacoMind in healthy volunteers: a phase I study," *Phytomedicine* 14 (5): pp. 301–08.

9. University of California Center for Medical Cannabis Research: www.cmcr.ucsd. edu.

10. www.washingtonpost.com/wp-dyn/content/article/2009/10/26/ AR2009102602407.html.

11. Gregory T. Carter, MD, *Marijuana Medical Handbook: Practical Guide to Therapeutic Uses of Marijuana,* revised edition (Oakland, CA: Quick American Press, 2008).

12. Ibid.

13. K. Sembulingam, P. Sembulingam, and A. Namasivayam (Jan 15, 2005), "Effect of Ocimum sanctum Linn on the changes in central cholinergic system induced by acute noise stress," *Journal of Ethnopharmacology* 96 (3): pp. 477–78. Also: A. Bhattacharya, A. V. Muruganandam, V. Kumar, and S. K. Bhattacharya (Oct 2002), "Effect of poly herbal formulation, EuMil, on neurochemical perturbations induced by chronic stress," *Indian Journal of Experimental Biology* 40 (10): pp. 1161–63.

14. M. H. Pittler and E. Ernst (2003), "Kava extract for treating anxiety," *Cochrane database of systematic reviews* (Online), www.ncbi.nlm.nih.gov/ pubmed/12535473.

15. M. Baba and S. Shigeta (1987), "Antiviral activity of glycyrrhizin against varicella-zoster in vitro," *Antiviral Research* 7: pp. 99–107.

16. W. Tang and G. Eisenbrand, *Chinese Drugs of Plant Origin* (Heidelberg, Germany: Springer-Verlag, 1992).

17. Medline Plus: Passion Flower www.nlm.nih.gov/medlineplus/druginfo/natural/871.html.

18. *Herbalgram* (magazine published by the American Botanical Council), "Rhodiola rosea: A Phytomedicinal Overview," Richard P. Brown, MD, Patricia L. Gerbarg, MD, and Zakir Ramazanov, PhD, DS, Fall 2002.

19. Plants for a Future, www.pfaf.org/user/Plant.aspx?LatinName=Rhodiola+rosea.

20. *Herbalgram,* "Rhodiola rosea: A Phytomedicinal Overview" (see note 18).

21. www.foxnews.com/health/2012/03/07/rhodiola-rosea-natures-antidepressant/.

22. Alexander Bystritsky, Lauren Kerwin, and Jamie D. Feusner (March 2008), "A Pilot Study of Rhodiola rosea (Rhodax®) for Generalized Anxiety Disorder (GAD)," *The Journal of Alternative and Complementary Medicine* 14 (2): pp. 175–80.

23. *HerbalGram,* "Rhodiola rosea: A Phytomedicinal Overview."

24. Arzneimittel-Forschung 34 (1984): pp. 716–21, as found in the World Health Organization monograph "Folium Gingko," http://apps.who.int/medicinedocs/en/d/Js2200e/18.html.

Chapter 13: Aromatherapy

1. www.oilsandplants.com/gattefosse.htm.

2. www.aromaweb.com/articles/history.asp.

3. www.aromatherapynaturalhealing.com/history.html.

Chapter 14: Homeopathy and Emotional Support

1. L. R. Milgrom (2006), "Toward a New Model of the Homeopathic Process Based on Quantum Field Theory," *Forsch Komplementärmed* 13: pp. 174–83, www.karger.com/Article/Abstract/93662; and "Physicists Demonstrate a Four-Fold Quantum Memory," www.homeopathyworldcommunity.com/profiles/blogs/physicists-demonstrate-a.

2. www.naturalnews.com/001951_homeopathy_homeopathic_remedies.html.

3. E. Dayenas, J. Benveniste et al. (30 June 1988), "Human basophil degranulation triggered by very dilute antiserum against IgE" (PDF). *Nature* 333 (6176): pp. 816–18.

Chapter 15: Hands-On Techniques for Health

1. http://jamesjealous.com.

2. www.ortho-bionomy.org.

3. www.webmd.com/balance/massage-therapy-styles-and-health-benefits?page=3.

4. www.chineitsang.com/what-is-chi-nei-tsang/.

5. www.chineitsang.com/directory/.
6. To find a Certified Manual Lymph Drainage Therapist, go to www.vodder.org.
7. http://theraggededge.hubpages.com/hub/Foot-Reflexology-Techniques#.
8. www.chinese-holistic-health-exercises.com/support-files/reflexologyfootchart.pdf.
9. www.metamorphictechnique.org.

Chapter 16: Color and Light

1. A. Coclivo (1999), "Coloured light therapy: overview of its history, theory, recent developments and clinical applications combined with acupuncture," *American Journal of Acupuncture* 27: pp. 71–83.
2. Faber Birren, *Color Psychology and Color Therapy* (New Hyde Park, NY: University Books, 1961).
3. "Photodyanamic therapy (PDT or Blue Light Therapy)," www.medicinenet.com/photodynamic_therapy/article.htm.

Chapter 17: Essences and Other Vibrational Tools

1. http://www.bachcentre.com/centre/drbach.htm.
2. http://www.greenhopeessences.com/index.html.
3. http://spirit-in-nature.com.
4. http://www.youtube.com/watch?v=oz1rzbvfHH8.
5 http://ausflowers.com.au.
6. http://www.desert-alchemy.com.
7. http://www.alaskanessences.com.
8. http://www.flowersociety.org.
9. http://www.perelandra-ltd.com/Perelandra-Essences-C745.aspx.
10. http://www.animalessence.com.

Chapter 19: Medical and Psychological Overview of Anxiety

1. www.apa.org/helpcenter/data-behavioral-health.aspx.
2. Ibid.
3. www.nimh.nih.gov/health/publications/anxiety-disorders/introduction.shtml.

4. B. D. McCarthy, J. R. Beshansky, R. B. D'Agostino et al. (1993), "Missed diagnosis of acute myocardial infarction in the emergency department: results from a multi center study," *Ann Emerg Med* 22: pp. 579–82.

5. David H. Barlow, editor, *Clinical Handbook of Psychological Disorders, Third Edition: A Step-by-Step Treatment Manual* (New York: Guilford Publications, 2001), p. 154 (Chapter 4, Generalized Anxiety Disorder).

6. The Mayo Clinic, "Panic Attacks and Panic Disorder," www.mayoclinic.com/health/panic-attacks/DS00338.

7. www.helpguide.org/mental/anxiety_types_symptoms_treatment.htm.

8. http://www.nimh.nih.gov/health/publications/obsessive-compulsive-disorder-when-unwanted-thoughts-take-over/index.shtml.

9 http://psychology.about.com/od/phobias/p/commonphobias.htm.

10. www.webmd.com/anxiety-panic/ss/slideshow-phobias.

11. Ibid.

12. Peter Tryer (January 1992), "Anxiolytics not acting at the benzodiazepine receptor: Beta blockers," *Progress in Neuro-Psychopharmacology and Biological Psychiatry* 16 (1): pp. 17–26, as quoted in Wikipedia; http://en.wikipedia.org/wiki/Beta_blocker.

13. T. Spencer, J. Biederman, R. Steingard, and T. Wilens (1993), "Bupropion exacerbates tics in children with attention-deficit hyperactivity disorder and Tourette's syndrome," *Journal of the American Academy of Child and Adolescent Psychiatry* 32 (1): pp. 211–24.

Chapter 20: Psychotherapy

1. Thich Nhat Hanh, *The Heart of the Buddha's Teaching: Transforming Suffering into Peace, Joy, and Liberation* (New York: Broadway Books, 1999).

2. R. A. Gould, M. Otto, M. Pollack, and L. Yap (1997), "Cognitive behavioral and pharmacological treatment of generalized anxiety disorder: A preliminary meta-analysis." *Behavior Therapy* 28 (2): pp. 285–305.

3. http://psychcentral.com/lib/2005/psychotherapy-for-anxiety-disorders/.

4. Mark A. Reinecke, Frank M. Dattilio, and A. Freeman, editors, *Cognitive Therapy with Children and Adolescents: A Casebook for Clinical Practice,* second edition. (New York: The Guilford Press, 2006). Also Philip C. Kendall, PhD,

editor, *Child and Adolescent Therapy: Cognitive-Behavioral Procedures,* third edition (New York: The Guilford Press, 2005).

5. www.hakomiinstitute.com.

6. www.traumahealing.com.

7. Scott O. Lilienfeld and Hal Arkowitz, "EMDR: Taking a Closer Look," *Scientific American,* January 3, 2008. http://www.scientificamerican.com/article.cfm?id=emdr-taking-a-closer-look.

8. www.emdr.com.

Bibliography

Bach, Edward. *Bach Flower Essences for the Family.* London: Wigmore Publications, 1996.

Baker, Dan, and Cameron Stauth. *What Happy People Know: How the New Science of Happiness Can Change Your Life for the Better.* New York: Rodale, Inc., 2003.

Barlow, David H., editor. *Clinical Handbook of Psychological Disorders, Fourth Edition: A Step-by-Step Treatment Manual.* New York: The Guilford Press, 2007.

Bateson, Gregory. *Mind and Nature: A Necessary Unity.* New York: E. P. Dutton, 1979.

Birren, Faber. *Color Psychology and Color Therapy.* New Hyde Park, NY: University Books, 1961.

Bois, Danis, PhD. *Wild Region of Lived Experience: Using Somatic-Psychoeducation.* Berkeley, CA: North Atlantic Books, 2009.

Bone, Kerry. *Clinical Applications of Ayurvedic and Chinese Herbs.* Warwick, Queensland: Phytotherapy Press, 1996.

Boone, J. Allen. *Kinship with All Life.* San Francisco: HarperCollins, 1954.

Brooks, Rachel E., MD, editor. *The Stillness of Life: The Osteopathic Philosophy of Rollin E. Becker, D.O.* Portland, OR: Stillness Press, 2000.

Buchanan, Jim. *Labyrinths for the Spirit.* London: Gaia Books, 2007.

Buhner, Stephen Harrod. *The Lost Language of Plants: The Ecological Importance of Plant Medicines for Life on Earth.* White River Junction, VT: Chelsea Green, 2002.

———. *The Secret Teachings of Plants: In the Direct Perception of Nature.* Rochester, VT: Bear and Company, 2004.

Carter, Gregory T., MD. *Marijuana Medical Handbook: Practical Guide to Therapeutic Uses of Marijuana,* revised edition. Oakland, CA: Quick American Press, 2008.

Chancellor, Phillip M. *Illustrated Handbook of the Bach Flower Remedies.* Saffron Walden, Essex, England: The C. W. Daniel Company, Ltd, 1971.

Childre, Doc, and Howard Martin. *The HeartMath Solution.* San Francisco: HarperSan Francisco, 1999.

Childre, Doc, and Deborah Rozman, PhD. *Transforming Anxiety: The HeartMath Solution for Overcoming Fear and Worry.* Oakland, CA: New Harbinger Publications, 2006.

Conrad, Emilie. *Life on Land: The Story of Continuum, the World-Renowned Self-Discovery and Movement Method.* Berkeley, CA: North Atlantic Books, 2007.

Cooksley, Valerie Gennari: *Aromatherapy: A Lifetime Guide to Healing with Essential Oils.* Parnassus, NJ: Prentice Hall, 1996.

Cousto, Hans. *The Cosmic Octave: Origin of Harmony.* Mendocino, CA: LifeRhythm Books, 2000.

Davis, Patricia. *Aromatherapy, an A-Z.* Saffron Waldon, Essex, England: C. W. Daniel Company, 1995.

Davis, William, MD. *Wheat Belly.* New York: Rodale, 2011.

Doidge, Norman, MD. *The Brain That Changes Itself.* New York: Penguin Books, 2007.

Dooley, Timothy R. *Homeopathy: Beyond Flat Earth Medicine,* second edition. San Diego, CA: Timing Publications, 2002.

Eckberg, Maryanna. *Victims of Cruelty: Somatic Psychotherapy in the Treatment of Posttraumatic Stress Disorder.* Berkeley, CA: North Atlantic Books, 2000.

Eisenstein, Charles. *The Yoga of Eating.* Washington, DC: New Trends Publishing, 2003.

Ellis, Andrew, Nigel Wiseman, and Ken Boss. *Fundamentals of Chinese Acupuncture,* revised edition. Brookline, MA: Paradigm Publications, 1991.

Emery, Marcia, PhD. *The Intuitive Healer: Accessing Your Inner Physician.* New York: St. Martin's Press, 1999.

Enig, Mary, PhD. *Know Your Fats: The Complete Primer for Understanding the Nutrition of Fats, Oils and Cholesterol.* Silver Springs, MD: Bethesda Press, 2000.

Fallon, Sally. *Nourishing Traditions: The Cookbook that Challenges Politically Correct Nutrition and the Diet Dictocrats,* revised second edition. Washington, DC: New Trends Publishing, 1999.

Felter, Harvey Wickes, MD. *The Eclectic Materia Medica, Pharmacology and Therapeutics.* Sandy, OR: Eclectic Medical Publications, 1994.

Felter, Harvey Wickes, MD, and John Uri Lloyd, PhrM., PhD. *King's American Dispensatory, Volumes 1 and 2.* Sandy, OR: Eclectic Medical Publications, 1983.

Foster, Rick, and Greg Hicks, *How We Choose to Be Happy*. New York: Berkley Publishing Group, 1999.

———. *Happiness & Health: 9 Choices That Unlock the Powerful Connection Between the Two Things We Want the Most*. New York: Penguin, 2008.

Gedgaudas, Nora T., CNS, CNT. *Primal Body, Primal Mind: Empower Your Total Health the Way Evolution Intended (…and Didn't)*. Portland, OR: Primal Body–Primal Mind Publishing, 2009.

Gerber, Richard. *Vibrational Medicine: The #1 Handbook of Subtle-Energy Therapies*, third edition. Rochester, VT: Bear & Company, 2001.

———. *A Practical Guide to Vibrational Medicine: Energy Healing and Spiritual Transformation*. New York: Quill/Harper Collins, 2000.

Gintis, Bonnie, DO. *Engaging the Movement of Life: Exploring Health and Embodiment Through Osteopathy and Continuum*. Berkeley, CA: North Atlantic Books, 2007.

Gittleman, Ann Louise, PhD. *Why Am I Always So Tired?* San Francisco: Harper, 1998.

Goleman, Daniel. *Emotional Intelligence: Why It Can Matter More Than IQ*, Tenth Anniversary Edition. New York: Bantam Books, 2006.

Green Hope Farm. *A Guide to Green Hope Farm Essences*. Meriden, NH: Green Hope Farm, 2009.

Hay, Louise. *You Can Heal Your Life*. Carlsbad, CA: Hay House, 1999.

Hendricks, Gay, PhD, and Kathlyn Hendricks, PhD. *At the Speed of Life: A New Approach to Personal Change Through Body-Centered Therapy*. New York: Bantam Books, 1994.

Hicks, Esther and Jerry. *Ask and It Is Given: Learning to Manifest Your Desires*. Carlsbad, CA: Hay House, 2004.

———. *The Law of Attraction: The Basics of the Teachings of Abraham*. Carlsbad, CA: Hay House, 2006.

———. *The Vortex: Where the Law of Attraction Assembles All Cooperative Relationships*. Carlsbad, CA: Hay House, 2009.

Homes, Peter. *The Energetics of Western Herbs, Volumes One and Two*. Boulder, CO: Artemis Press, 1989.

Iyengar, B.K.S. *Light on Pranayama: The Yogic Art of Breathing*. New York: Crossroad Publishing Company, 2006.

Jarrett, Lonny S. *Nourishing Destiny: The Inner Tradition of Chinese Medicine*. Stockbridge, MA: Spirit Path Press, 1998.

Joy, W. Brugh, MD. *Joy's Way, A Map for the Transformational Journey: An Introduction to the Potentials for Healing with Body Energies.* Los Angeles: J. P. Tarcher, 1979.

Kabat-Zinn, John, PhD. *Full Catastrophe Living: Using the Wisdom of Your Body and Mind to Face Stress, Pain, and Illness.* New York: Bantam-Dell, 2005.

Kaminski, Patricia, and Richard Katz. *Flower Essence Repertory.* Nevada City, CA: Flower Essence Society, 1994.

Karpa, Kelly Dowhower, PhD, RPh. *Bacteria for Breakfast: Probiotics for Good Health.* Victoria, BC: Trafford Publishing, 2003.

Katz, Sandor Ellis. *Wild Fermentation: The Flavor, Nutrition and Craft of Live-Culture Foods.* White River Junction, VT: Chelsea Green, 2003.

Keith, Lierre. *The Vegetarian Myth: Food Justice and Sustainability.* Oakland, CA: PM Press, 2009.

Kendall, Philip C., PhD, editor. *Child and Adolescent Therapy: Cognitive-Behavioral Procedures,* third edition. New York: The Guilford Press, 2005.

Kurtz, Ron. *Body-Centered Psychotherapy: The Hakomi Method.* Mendocino, CA: LifeRhythm Books, 2007.

Lappé, Frances Moore. *Diet for a Small Planet* (20th Anniversary Edition). New York: Ballantine Books, 1991.

Lawless, Julia. *The Encyclopedia of Essential Oils.* Rockport, MA: Element Inc., 1992.

Lazarus, Arnold A. *Behavior Therapy & Beyond.* New York: McGraw-Hill, 1971.

Lazarus, Paul. *Healing the Mind the Natural Way: Nutritional Solutions to Psychological Problems.* New York: Tarcher-Putnam, 1995.

Lebeau, Jill. *Feng Shui Your Mind: Four Easy Steps to Rapidly Transform Your Life.* Indianapolis, IN: Dog Ear Publishing 2010.

Lee, Martin A. *Smoke Signals: A Social History of Marijuana.* New York: Scribner, 2012.

Levine, Peter A. *Waking the Tiger.* Berkeley, CA: North Atlantic Books, 1997.

Levine, Peter A. *Healing Trauma. A Pioneering Program for Restoring the Wisdom of Your Body,* includes a CD. Boulder, CO: Sounds True, Inc., 2005.

Leyel, C. F. *Elixirs of Life.* New York: Sam Weiser, 1970.

———. *Heart's-Ease: Herbs for the Heart.* London: Faber and Faber, 1941.

———. *Compassionate Herbs.* London: Faber and Faber, 1946.

Lipton, Bruce. *The Biology of Belief: Unleashing the Power of Consciousness, Matter and Miracles.* Santa Rosa, CA: Mountain of Love/Elite Books, 2005.

Lyubomirsky, Sonja. *The How of Happiness: A Scientific Approach to Getting the Life You Want.* New York: Penguin Press, 2008.

Mapel, Daniel, M. A. *Into the Heart of the Wild: Healing and Transformation with the Wild Earth Animal Essences.* Charlottesville, VA: Wild Earth, 2002.

Mees, L. F. C., MD. *Blessed By Illness.* Great Barrington, MA: Anthroposophic Press, 1990.

Miller, Jill Wright. *Exploring Body-Mind Centering: An Anthology of Experience and Method.* Berkeley, CA: North Atlantic Books, 2011.

Monroe, Robert. *Journeys Out of Body,* updated edition. New York: Doubleday, 1992.

———. *Far Journeys.* New York: Doubleday, 1985.

———. *Ultimate Journey.* New York: Three Rivers Press, 1996.

Moore, Michael. *Medicinal Plants of the Pacific West.* Santa Fe, NM: Red Crane Books, 1993.

Moorjani, Anita. *Dying to Be Me: My Journey from Cancer, to Near Death, to True Healing.* Carlsbad, CA: Hay House, 2012.

Morrison, Roger, MD. *Desktop Guide to Keynotes and Confirmatory Symptoms.* Grass Valley, CA: Hahnemann Clinic Publishing, 1993.

Myss, Caroline, PhD, and C. Norman Shealy, MD, PhD. *The Creation of Health: The Emotional, Psychological, and Spiritual Responses that Promote Health and Healing.* New York: Three Rivers Press, 1988, 1993.

Narby, Jeremy. *Intelligence in Nature: An Inquiry into Knowledge.* New York: Jeremy P. Tarcher/Penguin, 2006.

Nhat Hanh, Thich, *The Heart of the Buddha's Teaching: Transforming Suffering into Peace, Joy, and Liberation.* New York: Broadway Books, 1999.

———. *Peace is in Every Step: The Path of Mindfulness in Everyday Life.* New York: Bantam Books, 1991.

Oschman, James. *Energy Medicine: The Scientific Basis.* Philadelphia: Churchill Livingstone, 2000.

Overmyer, Luann. *Ortho-Bionomy: A Path to Self-Care.* Berkeley, CA: North Atlantic Books, 2009.

Peace Pilgrim. *Peace Pilgrim: Her Life and Work in Her Own Words.* Santa Fe, NM: Ocean Tree Books, 1982; www.peacepilgrim.org/.

Pert, Candace, PhD. *Molecules of Emotion.* New York: Scribner, 1997.

Pollan, Michael. *The Omnivore's Dilemma: A Natural History of Four Meals.* New

York: Penguin, 2007.

———. *In Defense of Food: An Eater's Manifesto.* New York: Penguin, 2009.

Prentice, Jessica. *Full Moon Feast: Food and the Hunger for Connection.* White River Junction, VT: Chelsea Green, 2006.

Price, Shirley. *Practical Aromatherapy: How to Use Essential Oils to Restore Vitality.* London: Thorsens, 1997.

Price, Weston A., DDS. *Nutrition and Physical Degeneration,* eighth edition. La Mesa, CA: Price Pottenger Nutrition, 2008.

Provine, Robert R., PhD. *Laughter: A Scientific Investigation.* New York: Penguin Books, 2001.

Ravnskov, Uffe, MD, PhD. *Fat and Cholesterol Are Good for You.* Sweden: GB Publishing, 2009.

———. *Ignore the Awkward: How the Cholesterol Myths Are Kept Alive.* Create Space Independent Publishing [digital], 2010.

———. *The Cholesterol Myths: Exposing the Fallacy that Saturated Fat and Cholesterol Cause Heart Disease.* Washington, DC: New Trends Publishing, 2000.

Reinecke, Mark A., Frank M. Dattilio, and A. Freeman, editors. *Cognitive Therapy with Children and Adolescents: A Casebook for Clinical Practice,* second edition. New York: The Guilford Press, 2006.

Roads, Michael. *Journey into Nature: A Spiritual Adventure.* Tiburon, CA: HJ Kramer, 1990.

———. *Talking with Nature: Sharing the Energies and Spirit of Trees, Plants, Birds, and Earth.* Tiburon, CA: HJ Kramer, 1997.

Ruiz, don Miguel. *The Four Agreements: A Practical Guide to Personal Freedom, A Toltec Wisdom Book.* San Rafael, CA: Amber-Allen, 2001.

Sands, Helen Raphael. *The Healing Labyrinth: Finding Your Path to Inner Peace.* Hauppage, NY: Barron Educational Series, 2001.

Scaer, Robert C. *The Body Bears the Burden: Trauma, Dissociation, and Disease.* Binghamton, NY: The Haworth Press, Inc., 2001.

Schaper, Donna, and Carole Ann Camp. *Labyrinths from the Outside: Walking to Spiritual Insight, A Beginner's Guide.* Woodstock, VT: Skylight Paths Publishing, 2000.

Schnaubelt, Kurt, PhD. *Advanced Aromatherapy: The Science of Essential Oil Therapy.* Rochester, VT: Healing Arts Press, 1995.

Seem, Mark, PhD (with Joan Kaplan). *Bodymind Energetics: Toward a Dynamic Model of Health*. Rochester, VT: Healing Arts Press, 1989.

Segerstrom, Suzanne, PhD. *Breaking Murphy's Law: How Optimists Get What They Want from Life—and Pessimists Can Too*. New York: The Guilford Press, 2007.

Seligman, Martin, PhD. *Authentic Happiness: Using the New Positive Psychology to Realize Your Potential for Lasting Fulfillment*. New York: The Free Press, Simon and Schuster, 2002.

————. *Flourish: A Visionary New Understanding of Happiness and Well-Being*. New York: Free Press, Simon and Schuster, 2011.

————. *Learned Optimism: How to Change Your Mind and Your Life*. New York: Pocket Books, 1998.

Shapiro, Francine, PhD. *Getting Past Your Past: Take Control of Your Life with Self-Help Techniques from EMDR*. New York: Rodale, Inc., 2012.

Shealy, C. Norman. *90 Days to Stress-Free Living: A Day-by-Day Health Plan Including Exercises, Diet and Relaxation Techniques*. Boston: Element, 1999.

Sheehan, Molly. *A Guide to Green Hope Farm Flower Essences*. Meriden, NH: Green Hope Farm, 2009.

Singer, Michael. *The Untethered Soul: The Journey Beyond Yourself*. Oakland, CA: New Harbinger Publications, 2007.

Sutherland, W. G., DO. *Contributions of Thought*. Yakima, WA: Sutherland Cranial Teaching Foundation, 1998.

————. *Teachings in the Science of Osteopathy*. Yakima, WA: Sutherland Cranial Teaching Foundation, 1990.

Talbot, Michael. *The Holographic Universe*. New York: Harper Collins, 1991.

Tang, W., and Eisenbrand, G. *Chinese Drugs of Plant Origin*. Heidelberg, Germany: Springer-Verlag, 1992.

Time Magazine, "The Science of Happiness" Issue, January 17, 2005.

Tisserand, Robert, and Tony Balacs. *Essential Oil Safety: A Guide for Health Professionals*. London: Churchill Livingstone, 1998.

Tiwari, Maya. *Ayurveda Secrets of Healing*. Twin Lakes, WI: Lotus Press, 1995.

Ullman, Dana, MPH. *Homeopathy A-Z*. Carlsbad, CA: Hay House, 1999.

Ullman, Robert, and Reichenberg-Ullman, Judith. *Homeopathic Self Care: The Quick and Easy Guide for the Whole Family*. New York: Three Rivers Press, 1997.

Voisin, Andre. *Soil, Grass and Cancer: The Link Between Human and Animal Health and the Mineral Balance of the Soil.* Austin, TX: Acres USA, 2000.

Watts, Alan. *The Book: On the Taboo Against Knowing Who You Are.* New York: Vintage Books, 1989.

———. *Behold the Spirit: A Study in the Necessity of Mystical Religion.* New York: Vintage, 1972.

West, Melissa Gayle: *Exploring the Labyrinth: A Guide for Healing and Spiritual Growth.* New York: Broadway Books, 2000.

White, Ian. *Australian Bush Flower Healing.* Sydney, Australia: Bantam Books, 1999.

———. *Australian Bush Flower Essences.* Sydney, Australia: Bantam Books, 2001.

Wildwood, Christine. *The Encyclopedia of Aromatherapy.* Rochester, VT: Healing Arts Press, 1996.

Williamson, Marianne. *A Return to Love: Reflections on the Principles of "A Course in Miracles."* New York: Harper Paperbacks, 1990.

Wood, Matthew. *The Book of Herbal Wisdom: Using Plants as Medicines.* Berkeley, CA: North Atlantic Books, 1997.

———. *Vitalism: The History of Herbalism, Homeopathy, and Flower Essences.* Berkeley, CA: North Atlantic Books, 2005.

Wormwood, Valerie Ann. *The Fragrant Mind: Aromatherapy for Personality, Mind, Mood, and Emotion.* Novato, CA: New Work Library, 1996.

About the Author

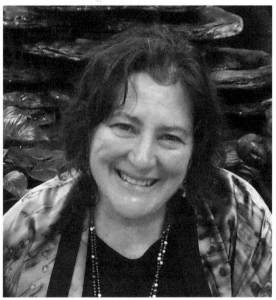

PHOTO: STAR WOODWARD

MARCEY SHAPIRO, MD, is a family physician with extensive training and experience in many areas of natural medicine including Western and Chinese herbal medicine, acupuncture, aromatherapy, flower essences, homeopathy, breathing techniques, nutritional therapies, Scenar®, and hands-on modalities such as Ortho-Bionomy® and the Biodynamics of Osteopathy. She works with patients to address the many facets of illness/imbalance—biophysical, psychological, and spiritual—and creates realistic treatment plans that incorporate a variety of modalities.

Marcey states: "There is a connection between emotional well being and physical health. Body, mind, and spirit form a cohesive whole. I believe my job as a physician, and a writer, is to help people come into balance and positive relationship with all parts of themselves, in order to lead full, joyous, and meaningful lives enriched by the best possible health."

Follow her on twitter: @MarceyShapiro
Facebook: Marcey Shapiro, MD Transforming the Nature of Health
View her personal and professional website: http://marceyshapiromd.com

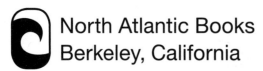 North Atlantic Books
Berkeley, California

Personal, spiritual, and planetary transformation

North Atlantic Books, a nonprofit publisher established in 1974, is dedicated to fostering community, education, and constructive dialogue. NABCommunities.com is a meeting place for an ever-growing membership of readers and authors to engage in the discussion of books and topics from North Atlantic's core publishing categories.

NAB Communities offer interactive social networks in these genres:

NOURISH: Raw Foods, Healthy Eating and Nutrition, All-Natural Recipes

WELLNESS: Holistic Health, Bodywork, Healing Therapies

WISDOM: New Consciousness, Spirituality, Self-Improvement

CULTURE: Literary Arts, Social Sciences, Lifestyle

BLUE SNAKE: Martial Arts History, Fighting Philosophy, Technique

Your free membership gives you access to:

Advance notice about new titles and exclusive giveaways

Podcasts, webinars, and events

Discussion forums

Polls, quizzes, and more!

Go to www.NABCommunities.com and join today.